CHILDHOOD PSYCHOSIS:
INITIAL STUDIES AND
NEW INSIGHTS

LEO KANNER

THE JOHNS HOPKINS UNIVERSITY SCHOOL OF MEDICINE

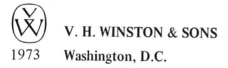 V. H. WINSTON & SONS

1973   Washington, D.C.

DISTRIBUTED BY THE HALSTED PRESS DIVISION OF

JOHN WILEY & SONS
New York   Toronto   London   Sydney

RJ499
.K322

V. H. Winston & Sons, Inc., Publishers
1511 K St. N.W., Washington, D.C. 20005

Distributed solely by Halsted Press Division, John Wiley & Sons, Inc. New York.

Library of Congress Cataloging in Publication Data

Kanner, Leo, 1894–
    Childhood psychosis: initial studies and new insights.

    1. Child psychiatry.   I. Title.
RJ499.K322   618.9'28'9   73–2855
ISBN 0-470-45610-8

TO JEFFREY ALAN KANNER

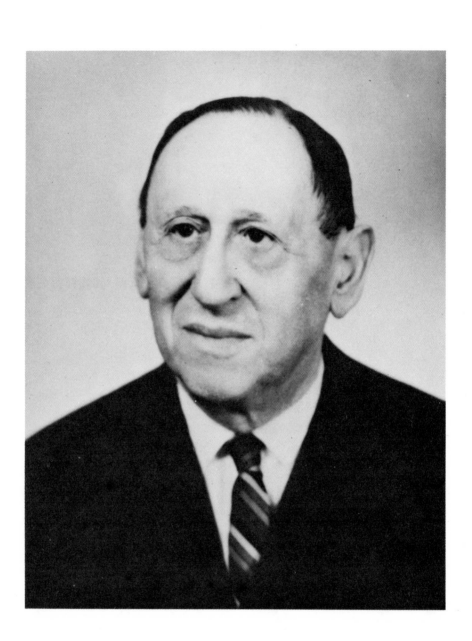

CONTENTS

The 1960's . . .

The 1970's . . .

FOREWORD

The field of childhood psychoses is strewn with descriptions of this or that syndrome which purport to represent some distinct entity. Most of these have passed into the sands of time but one—a careful clinical description of eleven children—remains as important today as when it first appeared some thirty years ago. During the early years of this century there had been a growing awareness of the existence of psychoses in childhood and by 1940 many workers appreciated the need to take into account developmental considerations when extending diagnostic criteria determined from adult psychotic patients to children. But before Kanner's description of "early infantile autism," only very limited progress had been made in this direction. His paper was a landmark in providing the first clear account of a disorder of psychotic intensity which had been present from the beginning without a previous period of normal development. It was important in tying psychosis to the process of development and the paper was a model of clarity in its combination of systematic, thorough and objective observations with deep clinical understanding and appreciation of the personal problems faced by each child and his family. Since 1943 Kanner has continued to develop and extend his concept of the autistic syndrome as shown in this volume of collected papers. Nearly all the basic points made in the original paper have been amply confirmed by other workers but in addition Kanner has himself done much to increase knowledge on the characteristics and course of the disorder and to determine its relationship to other conditions in childhood.

The initial description of infantile autism stressed the ways in which the syndrome differed from schizophrenia. This differentiation was rejected by other writers for many years but recent evidence has confirmed Kanner's view that autism and schizophrenia are separate conditions. He argued that there was an inborn defect in autism—a strange notion in an era of epidemic environmentalism. Again, research has pointed to the correctness of Kanner's suggestion, although the defect may be cognitive rather than affective. The children's excellent rote memory and visuo-spatial skills served to conceal the specific cognitive deficiencies which have now been shown to be present in autistic children.

Infantile autism is a syndrome fascinating in its own right and well worthy of study for this reason alone. But its investigation has reaped a richer harvest in throwing light on aspects of child development which extend well beyond the psychoses. The appreciation of the effect of an autistic child on the rest of the family and on parental attitudes and behavior has paralleled a revival of interest in the ways in which a child's characteristics may influence and modify parent-child interaction. Conversely, the benefits of educational methods in the treatment of autistic children emphasize that the presence of a biological handicap does not mean that behavior is fixed or resistant to environmental influences.

Collections of papers are usually the mark of respect to a great man on his retirement and frequently they serve as a reminder of past glories for a new generation of students who know the man only as a remnant of the past. The collections usually begin with scientific contributions of merit but all too often end with scholarly but dull historical reviews or papers giving mere light-hearted recollections. This collection of papers is quite different. A mark of respect, certainly, but there is no need to remind modern students of Kanner's existence. They are already reading his latest papers giving new findings on infantile autism (e.g., chapters 13 and 14) or providing new insights into old topics (e.g., chapters 12 and 15).

Childhood Psychosis: Initial Studies and New Insights comprises 16 papers presented in chronological sequence and covering three decades of study, from 1943 to 1973. Chapter 16, just recently completed for incorporation in this volume, represents the fascinating diagnostic evaluations and follow-up notes on 34 psychotic children; this material has not been published up to this time. The concern that new evidence be placed in an historical setting has been a feature of Kanner's writings from his early days (an example is his 1935 textbook) but his history has never been dull. Rather it has given a lively thoughtful perspective on the growth of knowledge. Over the years his papers have had a distinctive style which still persists—appreciative of others' achievements but irreverent of authority, scholarly but with a vital and compassionate concern for the individual, full of information but always interesting and readable. Edward Park's preface to the first (1935) edition of Kanner's textbook of "Child Psychiatry" stated "The book is full of wisdom and common sense. No other book is quite like it." That description could well be applied to the whole of Kanner's writings.

Kanner's contributions to child psychiatry, of course, range widely far beyond infantile autism. In a very real sense he can be regarded as the founder-father of child psychiatry in the English-speaking world. Visitors from all over the world went to Johns Hopkins while he headed the Department of Child Psychiatry there. His influence on child psychiatry in Europe has been very considerable and for this reason he has been the obvious first choice to deliver several key memorial or commemorative lectures this side of the Atlantic. His papers on many clinical topics have helped to shape psychiatric thinking. But none have been more formative than those on infantile autism included in this volume which serve both to add to our knowledge and to give a flavor of Kanner's rich contribution to child psychiatry.

Michael L. Rutter, M.D., MRCP, DPM
Honorary Consultant Psychiatrist
Maudsley Hospital, London

PREFACE

It is a very considerable honor to be invited to contribute prefatory remarks to a collection of papers that have become classics in child psychiatry. For a grateful pupil, it is an additional source of pleasure to be able to record my enormous debt of gratitude to a great teacher. Michael Rutter has indicated the seminal significance of Dr. Kanner's delineation of the syndrome of early infantile autism. What I should like to add is a personal memoir.

Dr. Kanner was a physician in the Yankton, South Dakota State Hospital when he applied to Professor Adolf Meyer for a special fellowship at the Phipps Clinic. Meyer recognized the young psychiatrist's aptitude for clinical investigation but responded with an ambiguous letter. On the one hand were the opportunities for academic training at Hopkins; on the other, contributions a bright young man could make at the state hospital. The letter seemed to say both yes and no to a recent migrant from Germany who did not trust his mastery of English. His hospital superintendent was no more able than he to decipher the language. With the bold ingenuity that was his hallmark, the young Kanner cut the Gordian knot by wiring Professor Meyer his projected date of arrival in Baltimore with a query as to its acceptability. It was and he came.

Upon completion of the fellowship, Professor Meyer and Edwards A. Park, the distinguished Professor of Pediatrics, had the vision to choose Dr. Kanner to start the first psychiatric service within a pediatric department in this country (1930). Beginning in a modest examining room with washbasin and table in the outpatient clinic, he went to work to teach himself with the aid of his patients and their families. Not more than five years later he had published the first American textbook of child psychiatry, a book that was to become the standard reference in its field! The ability to observe, to note similarities, to keep formulations tentative, and the distaste for metaphysics that enabled Dr. Kanner to see children as children and not miniature adults (as they had been viewed in previous psychiatric formulations) were the very same talents that enabled him to recognize in a group of eleven children a disorder sufficiently unique to warrant delineation as a new syndrome. The genius of the discovery was to detect the cardinal traits (aloneness and preoccupation with sameness) in the midst of phenomenology as diverse as muteness in one child and verbal precocity in another. Perhaps most remarkable of all, as Dr. Rutter points out, is the fact that the original report has been verified by subsequent investigations; from the first, Dr. Kanner had recognized the essential core of the disorder.

All of this was history by the time I arrived at the Children's Psychiatric Clinic of the Harriet Lane Home to seek training with Dr. Kanner. He listened graciously to the pretentions of a young resident who dilated on his intellectual reasons for choosing child psychiatry. Not until I declared my interest in people and my wish to understand in order to help did he smile warmly and agree to have me. Concern for human welfare was and is his ultimate criterion.

Dr. Kanner was then engaged in the sequential follow-up of his growing series of autistic patients and I was fortunate enough to participate in the study. It afforded me the rare privilege of observing a master clinician at work in return for the small chore of preparing the records.

His interview with parents is remarkable for its capacity to elicit a sequential account of the vicissitudes of development. A sensitive listener, he rarely interrupts. His questions are disarmingly gentle but shrewdly penetrating. Apparently looking at the ceiling or past the patient, he is alert to changes in physiognomy and shifts in posture that reveal underlying emotions, observations I all too frequently missed until the review of the case when what had been obscure to me was suddenly made crystal clear in his succinct summary.

Most astonishing of all is his capacity for entering the world of a child. Puffing away at his omnipresent cigar, he is a veritable pied piper whom no child can resist. He cares for them; they trust him and tell him what they choose to reveal to no other. Just as he would recall the minute details of an interview years earlier, they would affirm their recollection of what clearly had been a meaningful interchange with a man they regarded as friend as well as physician. To an observer, these were moving human encounters which still remain with me.

There can be no explaining the final alchemy of clinical greatness. Its ingredients are clarity of observation, freedom from theoretical preconceptions, personal humility, and human empathy. To Dr. Kanner, now as then, each patient remains a person; it is his individuality that is to be understood against the background of biological warp and cultural woof. His ability to look with a fresh eye—and to resort and reshape traditional categories in response to empirical data—has identified for us the one psychosis unique to childhood. Any hope of unraveling its mysteries begins with the study of the classic papers included in this volume. It is a major service to students of psychiatry, psychology, and pediatrics to have this material in a single collection.

Leon Eisenberg, M.D.
Professor of Psychiatry
Harvard Medical School

1

AUTISTIC DISTURBANCES OF AFFECTIVE CONTACT

Since 1938, there have come to our attention a number of children whose condition differs so markedly and uniquely from anything reported so far, that each case merits—and, I hope, will eventually receive—a detailed consideration of its fascinating peculiarities. In this place, the limitations necessarily imposed by space call for a condensed presentation of the case material. For the same reason, photographs have also been omitted. Since none of the children of this group has as yet attained an age beyond 11 years, this must be considered a preliminary report, to be enlarged upon as the patients grow older and further observation of their development is made.

Case 1

Donald T. was first seen in October, 1938, at the age of 5 years, 1 month. Before the family's arrival from their home town, the father sent a thirty-three-page typewritten history that, though filled with much obsessive detail, gave an excellent account of Donald's background. Donald was born at full term on September 8, 1933. He weighed nearly 7 pounds at birth. He was breast fed, with supplementary feeding, until the end of the eighth month; there were frequent changes of formulas. "Eating," the report said, "has always been a problem with him. He has never shown a normal appetite. Seeing children eating candy and ice cream has never been a temptation to him." Dentition proceeded satisfactorily. He walked at 13 months.

At the age of 1 year "he could hum and sing many tunes accurately." Before he was 2 years old, he had "an unusual memory for faces and names, knew the names of a great number of houses" in his home town. "He was encouraged by the family in learning and reciting short poems, and even learned the Twenty-third Psalm and twenty-five questions and answers of the Presbyterian Catechism." The parents observed that "he was not learning to ask questions or to answer questions unless they pertained to rhymes or things of this nature, and often then he would ask no question except in single words." His enunciation was clear. He became interested in pictures "and very soon knew an inordinate number of the pictures in a set of *Compton's Encyclopedia.*" He knew the pictures of the presidents "and knew most of the pictures of his ancestors and kinfolks on both sides of the house." He quickly learned the whole alphabet "backward as well as forward" and to count to 100.

It was observed at an early time that he was happiest when left alone, almost never cried to go with his mother, did not seem to notice his father's homecomings, and was indifferent to visiting relatives. The father made a special point of mentioning that Donald even failed to pay the slightest attention to Santa Claus in full regalia.

> He seems to be self-satisfied. He has no apparent affection when petted. He does not observe the fact that anyone comes or goes, and never seems glad to see father or mother or any playmate. He seems almost to draw into his shell and live within himself. We once secured a most attractive little boy of the same age from an orphanage and brought him home to spend the summer with Donald, but Donald has never asked him a question nor answered a question and has never romped with him in play. He seldom comes to anyone when called but has to be picked up and carried or led wherever he ought to go.

In his second year, he "developed a mania for spinning blocks and pans and other round objects." At the same time, he had

> A dislike for self-propelling vehicles, such as Taylor-tots, tricycles, and swings. He is still fearful of tricycles and seems to have almost a horror of

them when he is forced to ride, at which time he will try to hold onto the person assisting him. This summer [1937] we bought him a playground slide and on the first afternoon when other children were sliding on it he would not get about it, and when we put him up to slide down it he seemed horror-struck. The next morning when nobody was present, however, he walked out, climbed the ladder, and slid down, and he has slid on it frequently since, but slides only when no other child is present to join him in sliding. . . . He was always constantly happy and busy entertaining himself, but resented being urged to play with certain things.

When interfered with, he had temper tantrums, during which he was destructive. He was "dreadfully fearful of being spanked or switched" but "could not associate his misconduct with his punishment."

In August, 1937, Donald was placed in a tuberculosis preventorium in order to provide for him "a change of environment." While there, he had a "disinclination to play with children and do things children his age usually take an interest in." He gained weight but developed the habit of shaking his head from side to side. He continued spinning objects and jumped up and down in ecstasy as he watched them spin. He displayed

An abstraction of mind which made him perfectly oblivious to everything about him. He appears to be always thinking and thinking, and to get his attention almost requires one to break down a mental barrier between his inner consciousness and the outside world.

The father, whom Donald resembles physically, is a successful, meticulous, hard-working lawyer who has had two "breakdowns" under strain of work. He always took every ailment seriously, taking to his bed and following doctors' orders punctiliously even for the slightest cold. "When he walks down the street, he is so absorbed in thinking that he sees nothing and nobody and cannot remember anything about the walk." The mother, a college graduate, is a calm, capable woman, to whom her husband feels vastly superior. A second child, a boy, was born to them on May 22, 1938.

Donald, when examined at the Harriet Lane Home in October, 1938, was found to be in good physical condition. During the initial observation and in a two-week study by Drs. Eugenia S. Cameron and George Frankl at the Child Study Home of Maryland, the following picture was obtained:

There was a marked limitation of spontaneous activity. He wandered about smiling, making stereotyped movements with his fingers, crossing them about in the air. He shook his head from side to side, whispering or humming the same three-note tune. He spun with great pleasure anything he could seize upon to spin. He kept throwing things on the floor, seeming to delight in the sounds they made. He arranged beads, sticks, or blocks in groups of different series of colors. Whenever he finished one of these performances, he squealed and jumped up and down. Beyond this he showed no initiative, requiring constant instruction (from his mother) in any form of activity other than the limited ones in which he was absorbed.

Most of his actions were repetitions carried out in exactly the same way in which they had been performed originally. If he spun a block, he must always start with the same face uppermost. When he threaded buttons, he arranged them in a certain sequence that had no pattern to it but happened to be the order used by the father when he first had shown them to Donald.

There were also innumerable verbal rituals recurring all day long. When he desired to get down after his nap, he said, "Boo [his word for his mother], say 'Don, do you want to get down?' "

His mother would comply, and Don would say: "Now say 'All right.' "

The mother did, and Don got down. At mealtime, repeating something that had obviously been said to him often, he said to his mother, "Say 'Eat it or I won't give you tomatoes, but if you don't eat it I will give you tomatoes,' " or "Say 'If you drink to there, I'll laugh and I'll smile.' "

And his mother had to conform or else he squealed, cried, and strained every muscle in his neck in tension. This happened all day long about one thing or another. He seemed to have much pleasure in ejaculating words or phrases, such as "Chrysanthemum"; "Dahlia, dahlia, dahlia"; "Business"; "Trumpet vine"; "The right one is on, the left one off"; "Through the dark clouds shining." Irrelevant utterances such as these were his ordinary mode of speech. He always seemed to be parroting what he had heard said to him at one time or another. He used the personal pronouns for the persons he was quoting, even imitating the intonation. When he wanted his mother to pull his shoe off, he said: "Pull off your shoe." When he wanted a bath, he said: "Do you want a bath?"

Words to him had a specifically literal, inflexible meaning. He seemed unable to generalize, to transfer an expression to another similar object or situation. If he did so occasionally, it was a substitution, which then "stood" definitely for the original meaning. Thus he christened each of his water color bottles by the name of one of the Dionne quintuplets—Annette for blue, Cécile for red, etc. Then, going through a series of color mixtures, he proceeded in this manner: "Annette and Cécile make purple."

The colloquial request to "put that *down*" meant to him that he was to put the thing on the floor. He had a "milk glass" and a "water glass." When he spit some milk into the "water glass," the milk thereby became "white water."

The word "yes" for a long time meant that he wanted his father to put him up on his shoulder. This had a definite origin. His father, trying to teach him to say "yes" and "no," once asked him, "Do you want me to put you on my shoulder?"

Don expressed his agreement by repeating the question literally, echolalia-like. His father said, "If you want me to, say 'Yes'; if you don't want me to, say 'No.' "

Don said "yes" when asked. But thereafter "yes" came to mean that he desired to be put up on his father's shoulder.

He paid no attention to persons around him. When taken into a room, he completely disregarded the people and instantly went for objects, preferably those that could be spun. Commands or actions that could not possibly be disregarded were resented as unwelcome intrusions. But he was never angry at the interfering *person*. He angrily shoved away the *hand* that was in his way or the *foot* that stepped on one of his blocks, at one time referring to the foot on the block as "umbrella." Once the obstacle was removed, he forgot the whole affair. He gave no heed to the presence of other children but went about his favorite pastimes, walking off from the children if they were so bold as to join him. If a child took a toy from him, he passively permitted it. He scrawled lines on the picture books the other children were coloring, retreating or putting his hands over his ears if they threatened him in anger. His mother was the only person with whom he had any contact at all, and even she spent all of her time developing ways of keeping him at play with her.

After his return home, the mother sent periodic reports about his development. He quickly learned to read fluently and to play simple tunes on the piano. He began, whenever his attention could be obtained, to respond to questions "which require yes or no for an answer." Though he occasionally began to speak of himself as "I" and of the person addressed as "you," he continued for quite some time the pattern of pronominal reversals. When, for instance, in February, 1939, he stumbled and nearly fell, he said of himself, "*You* did not fall down."

He expressed puzzlement about the inconsistencies of spelling: "bite" should be spelled "bight" to correspond to the spelling of "light." He could spend hours writing on the blackboard. His play became more imaginative and varied, though still quite ritualistic.

He was brought back for a check-up in May, 1939. His attention and concentration were improved. He was in better contact with his environment, and there were some direct reactions to people and situations. He showed disappointment when thwarted, demanded bribes promised him, gave evidence of pleasure when praised. It was possible, at the Child Study Home, to obtain with constant insistence some conformity to daily routine and some degree of proper handling of objects. But he still went on writing letters with his fingers in the air, ejaculating words—"Semicolon"; "Capital"; "Twelve, twelve"; "Slain, slain"; "I could put a little comma or semicolon"—chewing on paper, putting food on his hair, throwing books into the toilet, putting a key down the water drain, climbing onto the table and bureau, having temper tantrums, giggling and whispering autistically. He got hold of an encyclopedia and learned about fifteen words in the index and kept repeating them over and over again. His mother was helped in trying to develop his interest and participation in ordinary life situations.

The following are abstracts from letters sent subsequently by Donald's mother:

September, 1939. He continues to eat and to wash and dress himself only at my insistence and with my help. He is becoming resourceful, builds things with his blocks, dramatizes stories, attempts to wash the car, waters the flowers with the hose, plays store with the grocery supply, tries to cut out pictures with the scissors. Numbers still have a great attraction for him. While his play is definitely improving, he has never asked questions about people and shows no interest in our conversation. . . .

October, 1939 [a school principal friend of the mother's had agreed to try Donald in the first grade of her school]. The first day was very trying for them but each succeeding day he has improved very much. Don is much more independent, wants to do many things for himself. He marches in line nicely, answers when called upon, and is more biddable and obedient. He never voluntarily relates any of his experiences at school and never objects to going. . . .

November, 1939. I visited his room this morning and was amazed to see how nicely he cooperated and responded. He was very quiet and calm and listened to what the teacher was saying about half the time. He does not squeal or run around but takes his place like the other children. The teacher began writing on the board. That immediately attracted his attention. She wrote:

> Betty may feed a fish.
> Don may feed a fish.
> Jerry may feed a fish.

In his turn he walked up and drew a circle around his name. Then he fed a goldfish. Next, each child was given his weekly reader, and he turned to the proper page as the teacher directed and read when called upon. He also answered a question about one of the pictures. Several times, when pleased, he jumped up and down and shook his head once while answering. . . .

March, 1940. The greatest improvement I notice is his awareness of things about him. He talks very much more and asks a good many questions. Not often does he voluntarily tell me of happenings at school, but if I ask leading questions, he answers them correctly. He really enters into the games with other children. One day he enlisted the family in one game he had just learned, telling each of us just exactly what to do. He feeds himself some better and is better able to do things for himself.

March, 1941. He has improved greatly, but the basic difficulties are still evident. . . .

Donald was brought for another check-up in April, 1941. An invitation to enter the office was disregarded, but he had himself led willingly. Once inside, he did not even glance at the three physicians present (two of whom he well remembered from his previous visits) but immediately made for the desk and handled papers and books. Questions at first were met with the stereotyped reply, "I don't know." He then helped himself to pencil and paper and wrote and drew pages and pages full of letters of the alphabet and a few simple designs. He arranged the letters in two or three lines, reading them in vertical rather than horizontal succession, and was very much pleased with the result. Occasionally he volunteered a statement or question: "I am going to stay for two days at the Child Study Home." Later he said, "Where is my mother?"

"Why do you want her?" he was asked.

"I want to hug her around the neck."

He used pronouns adequately and his sentences were grammatically correct.

The major part of his "conversation" consisted of questions of an obsessive nature. He was inexhaustible in bringing up variations: "How many days in a week, years in a century, hours in a day, hours in half a day, weeks in a century, centuries in half a millennium," etc., etc.; "How many pints in a gallon, how many gallons to fill four gallons?" Sometimes he asked, "How many hours in a minute, how many days in an hour?" etc. He looked thoughtful and always wanted an answer. At times he temporarily compromised by responding quickly to some other question or request but promptly returned to the same type of behavior. Many of his replies were metaphorical or otherwise peculiar. When asked to subtract 4 from 10, he answered: "I'll draw a hexagon."

He was still extremely autistic. His relation to people had developed only insofar as he addressed them when he needed or wanted to know something. He never looked at the person while talking and did not use communicative gestures. Even this type of contact ceased the moment he was told or given what he had asked for.

A letter from the mother stated in October, 1942:

> Don is still indifferent to much that is around him. His interests change often, but always he is absorbed in some kind of silly, unrelated subject. His literal-mindedness is still very marked, he wants to spell words as they sound and to pronounce letters consistently. Recently I have been able to have Don do a few chores around the place to earn picture show money. He really enjoys the movies now but not with any idea of a connected story. He remembers them in the order in which he sees them. Another of his recent hobbies is with old issues of *Time* magazine. He found a copy of the first issue of March 3, 1923, and has attempted to make a list of the dates of publication of each issue since that time. So far he has gotten to April, 1934. He has figured the number of issues in a volume and similar nonsense.

Case 2

Frederick W. was referred on May 27, 1942, at the age of 6 years, with the physician's complaint that his "adaptive behavior in a social setting is characterized by attacking as well as withdrawing behavior." His mother stated:

> The child has always been self-sufficient. I could leave him alone and he'd entertain himself very happily, walking around, singing. I have never known him to cry in demanding attention. He was never interested in hide-and-seek, but he'd roll a ball back and forth, watch his father shave, hold the razor box and put the razor back in, put the lid on the soap box. He never was very good with cooperative play. He doesn't care to play with the ordinary things that other children play with, anything with wheels on. He is afraid of mechanical things; he runs from them. He used to be afraid of my egg beater, is perfectly petrified of my vacuum cleaner. Elevators are simply a terrifying experience to him. He is afraid of spinning tops.
>
> Until the last year, he mostly ignored other people. When we had guests, he just wouldn't pay any attention. He looked curiously at small children and then would go off all alone. He acted as if people weren't there at all, even with his grandparents. About a year ago, he began showing more interest in observing them, would even go up to them.

But usually people are an interference. He'll push people away from him. If people come too close to him, he'll push them away. He doesn't want me to touch him or put my arm around him, but he'll come and touch *me*.

To a certain extent, he likes to stick to the same thing. On one of the bookshelves we had three pieces in a certain arrangement. Whenever this was changed, he always rearranged it in the old pattern. He won't try new things, apparently. After watching for a long time, he does it all of a sudden. He wants to be sure he does it right.

He had said at least two words ["Daddy" and "Dora," the mother's first name] before he was 2 years old. From then on, between 2 and 3 years, he would say words that seemed to come as a surprise to himself. He'd say them once and never repeat them. One of the first words he said was "overalls." [The parents never expected him to answer any of their questions, were *once* surprised when he did give an answer—"Yes"]. At about 2½ years, he began to sing. He sang about twenty or thirty songs, including a little French lullaby. In his fourth year, I tried to make him ask for things before he'd get them. He was stronger-willed than I was and held out longer, and he would not get it but he never gave in about it. Now he can count up to into the hundreds and can read numbers, but he is not interested in numbers as they apply to objects. He has great difficulty in learning the proper use of personal pronouns. When receiving a gift, he would say of himself: "You say 'Thank you.' "

He bowls, and when he sees the pins go down, he'll jump up and down in great glee.

Frederick was born May 23, 1936, in breech presentation. The mother had "some kidney trouble" and an elective cesarean section was performed about two weeks before term. He was well after birth; feeding presented no problem. The mother recalled that he was never observed to assume an anticipatory posture when she prepared to pick him up. He sat up at 7 months, walked at about 18 months. He had occasional colds but no other illness. Attempts to have him attend nursery school were unsuccessful: "he would either be retiring and hide in a corner or would push himself into the middle of a group and be very aggressive."

The boy is an only child. The father, aged 44, a university graduate and a plant pathologist, has traveled a great deal in connection with his work. He is a patient, even-tempered man, mildly obsessive; as a child he did not talk "until late" and was delicate, supposedly "from lack of vitamin in diet allowed in Africa." The mother, aged 40, a college graduate, successively a secretary to physicians, a purchasing agent, director of secretarial studies in a girls' school, and at one time a teacher of history, is described as healthy and even-tempered.

The paternal grandfather organized medical missions in Africa, studied tropical medicine in England, became an authority on manganese mining in Brazil, was at the same time dean of a medical school and director of an art museum in an American city, and is listed in *Who's Who* under two different names. He disappeared in 1911, his whereabouts remaining obscure for twenty-five years. It was then learned that he had gone to Europe and married a novelist, without obtaining a divorce from his first wife. The family considers him "a very strong character of the genius type, who wanted to do as much good as he could."

The paternal grandmother is described as "a dyed-in-the-wool missionary if ever there was one, quite dominating and hard to get along with, at present pioneering in the South at a college for mountaineers."

The father is the second of five children. The oldest is a well known newspaper man and author of a best-seller. A married sister, "high-strung and quite precocious," is a singer. Next comes a brother who writes for adventure magazines. The youngest, a painter, writer, and radio commentator, "did not talk until he was about 6 years old," and the first words he is reported to have spoken were, "When a lion can't talk he can whistle."

The mother said of her own relatives, "Mine are very ordinary people." Her family is settled in a Wisconsin town, where her father is a banker; her mother is "mildly interested" in church work, and her three sisters, all younger than herself, are average middle-class matrons.

Frederick was admitted to the Harriet Lane Home on May 27, 1942. He appeared to be well nourished. The circumference of his head was 21 inches, of his chest 22 inches, of his abdomen 21 inches. His occiput and frontal region were markedly prominent. There was a supernumerary nipple in the left axilla. Reflexes were sluggish but present. All other findings, including laboratory examinations and X-ray of his skull, were normal, except for large and ragged tonsils.

He was led into the psychiatrist's office by a nurse, who left the room immediately afterward. His facial expression was tense, somewhat apprehensive, and gave the impression of intelligence. He wandered aimlessly about for a few moments, showing no sign of awareness of the three adults present. He then sat down on the couch, ejaculating unintelligible sounds, and then abruptly lay down, wearing throughout a dreamy-like smile. When he responded to questions or commands at all, he did so by repeating them echolalia fashion. The most striking feature in his behavior was the difference in his reactions to objects and to people. Objects absorbed him easily and he showed good attention and perseverance in playing with them. He seemed to regard people as unwelcome intruders to whom he paid as little attention as they would permit. When forced to respond, he did so briefly and returned to his absorption in things. When a hand was held out before him so that he could not possibly ignore it, he played with it briefly as if it were a detached object. He blew out a match with an expression of satisfaction with the achievement, but did not look up to the person who had lit the match. When a fourth person entered the room, he retreated for a minute or two behind the bookcase, saying, "I don't want you," and waving him away, then resumed his play, paying no further attention to him or anyone else.

Test results (Grace Arthur performance scale) were difficult to evaluate because of his lack of cooperation. He did best with the Seguin form board (shortest time, 58 seconds). In the mare and foal completion test he seemed to be guided by form entirely, to the extent that it made no difference whether the pieces were right side up or not. He completed the triangle but not the rectangle. With all the form boards he showed good perseverance and concentration, working at them spontaneously and interestedly. Between tests, he wandered about the room examining various objects or fishing in the wastebasket without regard for the persons present. He made frequent sucking noises and occasionally kissed the dorsal surface of his hand. He became fascinated with the circle from the form board, rolling it on the desk and attempting, with occasional success, to catch it just before it rolled off.

Frederick was enrolled at the Devereux Schools on September 26, 1942.

Case 3

Richard M. was referred to the Johns Hopkins Hospital on February 5, 1941, at 3 years, 3 months of age, with the complaint of deafness because he did not talk and did not respond to questions. Following his admission, the interne made this observation:

> The child seems quite intelligent, playing with the toys in his bed and being adequately curious about instruments used in the examination. He seems quite self-sufficient in his play. It is difficult to tell definitely whether he hears, but it seems that he does. He will obey commands, such as "Sit up" or "Lie down," even when he does not see the speaker. He does not pay attention to conversation going on around him, and although he does make noises, he says no recognizable words.

His mother brought with her copious notes that indicated obsessive preoccupation with details and a tendency to read all sorts of peculiar interpretations into the child's performances. She watched (and recorded) every gesture and every "look," trying to find their specific significance and finally deciding on a particular, sometimes very farfetched explanation. She thus accumulated an account that, though very elaborate and richly illustrated, on the whole revealed more of her own version of what had happened in each instance than it told of what had actually occurred.

Richard's father is a professor of forestry in a southern university. He is very much immersed in his work, almost entirely to the exclusion of social contacts. The mother is a college graduate. The maternal grandfather is a physician, and the rest of the family, in both branches, consists of intelligent professional people. Richard's brother, thirty-one months his junior, is described as a normal, well developed child.

Richard was born on November 17, 1937. Pregnancy and birth were normal. He sat up at 8 months and walked at 1 year. His mother began to "train" him at the age of 3 weeks, giving him a suppository every morning "so his bowels would move by the clock." The mother, in comparing her two children, recalled that while her younger child showed an active anticipatory reaction to being picked up, Richard had not shown any physiognomic or postural sign of preparedness and had failed to adjust his body to being held by her or the nurse. Nutrition and physical growth proceeded satisfactorily. Following smallpox vaccination at 12 months, he had an attack of diarrhea and fever, from which he recovered in somewhat less than a week.

In September, 1940, the mother, in commenting on Richard's failure to talk, remarked in her notes:

> I can't be sure just when he stopped the imitation of word sounds. It seems that he has gone backward mentally gradually for the last two years. We have thought it was because he did not disclose what was in his head, that it was there all right. Now that he is making so many sounds, it is disconcerting because it is now evident that he can't talk. Before, I thought he could if he only would. *He gave the impression of silent wisdom to me.* . . . . One puzzling and discouraging thing is the great difficulty one has in getting his attention.

On physical examination, Richard was found to be healthy except for large tonsils and adenoids, which were removed on February 8, 1941. His head circumference was 54½ cm. His electroencephalogram was normal.

He had himself led willingly to the psychiatrist's office and engaged at once in active play with the toys, paying no attention to the persons in the room. Occasionally, he looked up at the walls, smiled and uttered short staccato forceful sounds—"Ee! Ee! Ee!" He complied with a spoken and gestural command of his mother to take off his slippers. When the command was changed to another, this time without gestures, he repeated the original request and again took off his slippers (which had been put on again). He performed well with the unrotated form board but not with the rotated form board.

Richard was again seen at the age of 4 years, 4 months. He had grown considerably and gained weight. When started for the examination room, he screamed and made a great fuss, but once he yielded he went along willingly. He immediately proceeded to turn the lights on and off. He showed no interest in the examiner or any other person but was attracted to a small box that he threw as if it were a ball.

At 4 years, 11 months, his first move in entering the office (or any other room) was to turn the lights on and off. He climbed on a chair, and from the chair to the desk in order to reach the switch of the wall lamp. He did not communicate his wishes but went into a rage until his mother guessed and procured what he wanted. He had no contact with people, whom he definitely regarded as an interference when they talked to him or otherwise tried to gain his attention.

The mother felt that she was no longer capable of handling him, and he was placed in a foster home near Annapolis with a woman who had shown a remarkable talent for dealing with difficult children. Recently, this woman heard him say clearly his first intelligible words. They were, "Good night."

Case 4

Paul G. was referred in March, 1941, at the age of 5 years, for psychometric assessment of what was thought to be a severe intellectual defect. He had attended a private nursery school, where his incoherent speech, inability to conform, and reaction with temper outbursts to any interference created the impression of feeblemindedness.

Paul, an only child, had come to this country from England with his mother at nearly 2 years of age. The father, a mining engineer, believed to be in Australia now, had left his wife shortly before that time after several years of an unhappy marriage. The mother, supposedly a college graduate, a restless, unstable, excitable woman, gave a vague and blatantly conflicting history of the family background and the child's development. She spent much time emphasizing and illustrating her efforts to make Paul clever by teaching him to memorize poems and songs. At 3 years, he knew the words of not less than thirty-seven songs and various and sundry nursery rhymes.

He was born normally. He vomited a great deal during his first year, and feeding formulas were changed frequently with little success. He ceased vomiting when he was started on solid food. He cut his teeth, held up his head, sat up, walked, and established bowel and bladder control at the usual age. He had measles, chickenpox, and pertussis without complications. His tonsils were removed when he was 3 years old. On physical examination, phimosis was found to be the only deviation from otherwise good health.

The following features emerged from observation on his visits to the clinic, during five weeks' residence in a boarding home, and during a few days stay in the hospital.

Paul was a slender, well built, attractive child, whose face looked intelligent and animated. He had good manual dexterity. He rarely responded to any form of address, even to the calling of his name. At one time he picked up a block from the floor on request. Once he copied a circle immediately after it had been drawn before him. Sometimes an energetic "Don't!" caused him to interrupt his activity of the moment. But usually, when spoken to, he went on with whatever he was doing as if nothing had been said. Yet one never had the feeling that he was willingly disobedient or contrary. He was obviously so remote that the remarks did not reach him. He was always vivaciously occupied with something and seemed to be highly satisfied, unless someone made a persistent attempt to interfere with his self-chosen actions. Then he first tried impatiently to get out of the way and, when this met with no success, screamed and kicked in a full-fledged tantrum.

There was a marked contrast between his relations to people and to objects. Upon entering the room, he instantly went after objects and used them correctly. He was not destructive and treated the objects with care and even affection. He picked up a pencil and scribbled on paper that he found on the table. He opened a box, took out a toy telephone, singing again and again: "He wants the telephone," and went around the room with the mouthpiece and receiver in proper position. He got hold of a pair of scissors and patiently and skillfully cut a sheet of paper into small bits, singing the phrase "Cutting paper," many times. He helped himself to a toy engine, ran around the room holding it up high and singing over and over again, "The engine is flying." While these utterances, made always with the same inflection, were clearly connected with his actions, he ejaculated others that could not be linked up with immediate situations. These are a few examples: "The people in the hotel"; "Did you hurt your leg?" "Candy is all gone, candy is empty"; "You'll fall off the bicycle and bump your head." However, some of those exclamations could be definitely traced to previous experiences. He was in the habit of saying almost every day, "Don't throw the dog off the balcony." His mother recalled that she had said those words to him about a toy dog while they were still in England. At the sight of a saucepan he would invariably exclaim, "Peter-eater." The mother remembered that this particular association had begun when he was 2 years old and she happened to drop a saucepan while reciting to him the nursery rhyme about "Peter, Peter, pumpkin eater." Reproductions of warnings of bodily injury constituted a major portion of his utterances.

None of these remarks was meant to have communicative value. There was, on his side, no affective tie to people. He behaved as if people as such did not matter or even exist. It made no difference whether one spoke to him in a friendly or a harsh way. He never looked up at people's faces. When he had any dealings with persons at all, he treated them, or rather parts of them, as if they were objects. He would use a hand to lead him. He would, in playing, butt his head against his mother as at other times he did against a pillow. He allowed his boarding mother's hands to dress him, paying not the slightest attention to *her*. When with other children, he ignored them and went after their toys.

His enunciation was clear and he had a good vocabulary. His sentence construction was satisfactory, with one significant exception. He never used the pronoun of the first person, nor did he refer to himself as Paul. All statements pertaining to himself were made in the second person, as literal repetitions of things that had been said to him before. He would express his desire for candy by saying, "*You* want candy." He would pull his hand away from a hot radiator and say "*You* get hurt." Occasionally there were parrot-like repetitions of things said to him.

Formal testing could not be carried out, but he certainly could not be regarded as feebleminded in the ordinary sense. After hearing his boarding mother say grace three times, he repeated it without a flaw and has retained it since then. He could count and name colors. He learned quickly to identify his favorite victrola records from a large stack and knew how to mount and play them.

His boarding mother reported a number of observations that indicated compulsive behavior. He often masturbated with complete abandon. He ran around in circles emitting phrases in an ecstatic-like fashion. He took a small blanket and kept shaking it, delightedly shouting, "Ee! Ee!" He could continue in this manner for a long time and showed great irritation when he was interfered with. All these and many other things were not only repetitions but recurred day after day with almost photographic sameness.

Case 5

Barbara K. was referred in February, 1942, at 8 years, 3 months of age. Her father's written note stated:

> First child, born normally October 30, 1933. She nursed very poorly and was put on bottle after about a week. She quit taking any kind of nourishment at 3 months. She was tube-fed five times daily up to 1 year of age. She began to eat then, though there was much difficulty until she was about 18 months old. Since then she has been a good eater, likes to experiment with food, tasting, and now fond of cooking.
>
> Ordinary vocabulary at 2 years, but always slow at putting words into sentences. Phenomenal ability to spell, read, and a good writer, but still has difficulty with verbal expression. Written language has helped the verbal. Can't get arithmetic except as a memory feat.
>
> Repetitious as a baby, and obsessive now: holds things in hands, takes things to bed with her, repeats phrases, gets stuck on an idea, game, etc., and rides it hard, then goes to something else. She used to talk using "you" for herself and "I" for her mother or me, as if she were saying things as we would in talking to her.
>
> Very timid, fearful of various and changing things, wind, large animals, etc. Mostly passive, but passively stubborn at times. Inattentive to the point where one wonders if she hears. (She does!) No competitive spirit, no desire to please her teacher. If she knew more than any other member in the class about something, she would give no hint of it, just keep quiet, maybe not even listen.
>
> In camp last summer she was well liked, learned to swim, is graceful in water (had always appeared awkward in her motility before), overcame fear of ponies, played best with children of 5 years of age. At camp she slid into avitaminosis and malnutrition but offered almost no verbal complaints.

Barbara's father is a prominent psychiatrist. Her mother is a well educated, kindly woman. A younger brother, born in 1937, is healthy, alert, and well developed.

Barbara "shook hands" upon request (offering the left upon coming, the right upon leaving) by merely raising a limp hand in the approximate direction of the examiner's proffered hand; the motion definitely lacked the implication of greeting. During the entire interview there was no indication of any kind of affective contact. A pin prick resulted in withdrawal of her arm, a fearful glance at the pin (not the examiner), and utterance of the word "Hurt!" not addressed to anyone in particular.

She showed no interest in test performances. The concept of test, of sharing an experience or situation, seemed foreign to her. She protruded her tongue and played with her hand as one would with a toy. Attracted by a pen on the desk stand, she said: "Pen like yours at home." Then, seeing a pencil, she inquired: "May I take this home?"

When told that she might, she made no move to take it. The pencil was given to her, but she shoved it away, saying, "It's not my pencil."

She did the same thing repeatedly in regard to other objects. Several times she said, "Let's see Mother" (who was in the waiting room).

She read excellently, finishing the 10-year Binet fire story in thirty-three seconds and with no errors, but was unable to reproduce from memory anything she had read. In the Binet pictures, she saw (or at least reported) no action or relatedness between the single items, which she had no difficulty enumerating. Her handwriting was legible. Her drawing (man, house, cat sitting on six legs, pumpkin, engine) was unimaginative and stereotyped. She used her right hand for writing, her left for everything else; she was left-footed and right-eyed.

She knew the days of the week. She began to name them: "Saturday, Sunday, Monday," then said, "You go to school" (meaning, "on Monday"), then stopped as if the performance were completed.

Throughout all these procedures, in which—often after several repetitions of the question or command—she complied almost automatically, she scribbled words spontaneously: "oranges"; "lemons"; "bananas"; "grapes"; "cherries"; "apples"; "apricots"; "tangerine"; "grapefruits"; "watermelon juice"; the words sometimes ran into each other and were obviously not meant for others to read.

She frequently interrupted whatever "conversation" there was with references to "motor transports" and "piggy-back," both of which—according to her father—had preoccupied her for quite some time. She said, for instance, "I saw motor transports"; "I saw piggy-back when I went to school."

Her mother remarked, "Appendages fascinate her, like a smoke stack or a pendulum." Her father had previously stated: "Recent interest in sexual matters, hanging about when we take a bath, and obsessive interest in toilets."

Barbara was placed at the Devereux Schools, where she is making some progress in learning to relate herself to people.

Case 6

Virginia S., born September 13, 1931, has resided at a state training school for the feebleminded since 1936, with the exception of one month in 1938, when she was paroled to a school for the deaf "for educational opportunity." Dr. Esther L. Richards, who saw her several times, clearly recognized that she was neither deaf nor feebleminded and wrote in May, 1941:

> Virginia stands out from other children [at the training school] because she is absolutely different from any of the others. She is neat and tidy, does not play with other children, and does not seem to be deaf from gross tests, but does not talk. The child will amuse herself by the hour putting picture puzzles together, sticking to them until they are done. I have seen her with a box filled with the parts of two puzzles gradually work out the pieces for each. All findings seem to be in the nature of a congenital abnormality which looks as if it were more of a personality abnormality than an organic defect.

Virginia, the younger of two siblings, was the daughter of a psychiatrist, who said of himself (in December, 1941): "I have never liked children, probably a reaction on my part to the restraint from movement (travel), the minor interruptions and commotions."

Of Virginia's mother, her husband said: "She is not by any means the mother type. Her attitude [toward a child] is more like toward a doll or pet than anything else."

Virginia's brother, Philip, five years her senior, when referred to us because of severe stuttering at 15 years of age, burst out in tears when asked how things were at home and he sobbed: "The only time my father has ever had anything to do with me was when he scolded me for doing something wrong."

His mother did not contribute even that much. He felt that all his life he had lived in "a frosty atmosphere" with two inapproachable strangers.

In August, 1938, the psychologist at the training school observed that Virginia could respond to sounds, the calling of her name, and the command, "Look!"

> She pays no attention to what is said to her but quickly comprehends whatever is expected. Her performance reflects discrimination, care, and precision.

With the nonlanguage items of the Binet and Merrill-Palmer tests, she achieved an IQ of 94. "Without a doubt," commented the psychologist,

> Her intelligence is superior to this.... She is quiet, solemn, composed. Not once have I seen her smile. She retires within herself, segregating herself from others. She seems to be in a world of her own, oblivious to all but the center of interest in the presiding situation. She is mostly self-sufficient and independent. When others encroach upon

her integrity, she tolerates them with indifference. There was no manifestation of friendliness or interest in persons. On the other hand, she finds pleasure in dealing with things, about which she shows imagination and initiative. Typically, there is no display of affection. . . .

Psychologist's note, October, 1939. Today Virginia was much more at home in the office. She remembered (after more than a year) where the toys were kept and helped herself. She could not be persuaded to participate in test procedures, would not wait for demonstrations when they were required. Quick, skilled moves. Trial and error plus insight. Very few futile moves. Immediate retesting reduced the time and error by more than half. There are times, more often than not, in which she is completely oblivious to all but her immediate focus of attention. . . .

January, 1940. Mostly she is quiet, as she has always worked and played alone. She has not resisted authority or caused any special trouble. During group activities, she soon becomes restless, squirms, and wants to leave to satisfy her curiosity about something elsewhere. She does make some vocal sounds, crying out if repressed or opposed too much by another child. She hums to herself, and in December I heard her hum the perfect tune of a Christmas hymn while she was pasting paper chains.

June, 1940. The school girls have said that Virginia says some words when at the cottage. They remember that she loves candy so much and says "Chocolate," "Marshmallow," also "Mama" and "Baby."

When seen on October 11, 1942, Virginia was a tall, slender, very neatly dressed 11-year-old girl. She responded when called by getting up and coming nearer, without ever looking up to the person who called her. She just stood listlessly, looking into space. Occasionally, in answer to questions, she muttered, "Mamma, baby." When a group was formed around the piano, one child playing and the others singing, Virginia sat among the children, seemingly not even noticing what went on, and gave the impression of being self-absorbed. She did not seem to notice when the children stopped singing. When the group dispersed she did not change her position and appeared not to be aware of the change of scene. She had an intelligent physiognomy, though her eyes had a blank expression.

Case 7

Herbert B. was referred on February 5, 1941, at 3 years, 2 months of age. He was thought to be seriously retarded in intellectual development. There were no physical abnormalities except for undescended testicles. His electroencephalogram was normal.

Herbert was born November 16, 1937, two weeks before term by elective cesarean section; his birth weight was 6¼ pounds. He vomited all food from birth through the third month. Then vomiting ceased almost abruptly and, except for occasional regurgitation, feeding proceeded satisfactorily. According to his mother, he was "always slow and quiet." For a time he was believed to be deaf because "he did not register any change of expression when spoken to or when in the presence of other people; also, he made no attempt to speak or to form words." He held up his head at 4 months and sat at 8 months, but did not try to walk until 2 years old, when suddenly "he began to walk without any preliminary crawling or assistance by chairs." He persistently refused to take fluid in any but an all-glass container. Once, while at a hospital, he went three days without fluid because it was offered in tin cups. He was "tremendously frightened by running water, gas burners, and many other things." He became upset by any change of an accustomed pattern: "if he notices change, he is very fussy and cries." But he himself liked to pull blinds up and down, to tear cardboard boxes into small pieces and play with them for hours, and to close and open the wings of doors.

Herbert's parents separated shortly after his birth. The father, a psychiatrist, is described as "a man of unusual intelligence, sensitive, restless, introspective, taking himself very seriously, not interested in people, mostly living within himself, at times alcoholic." The mother, a physician, speaks of herself as "energetic and outgoing, fond of people and children but having little insight into their problems, finding it a great deal easier to accept people rather than try to understand them." Herbert is the youngest of three children. The second is a normal, healthy boy. The oldest, Dorothy, born in June, 1934, after thirty-six hours of hard labor, seemed alert and responsive as an infant and said many words at 18 months, but toward the end of the second year she "did not show much progression in her play relationships or in contacts with other people." She wanted to be left alone, danced about in circles, made queer noises with her mouth, and *ignored persons completely* except for her mother, to whom she clung "in panic and general agitation." (Her father hated her ostensibly.) "Her speech was very meager and expression of ideas completely lacking. She had *difficulties with her pronouns* and would repeat 'you' and 'I' instead of using them for the proper persons." She was first declared to be feebleminded, then schizophrenic, but after the parents separated (the children remaining with their mother), she "blossomed out." She now attends school, where she makes good progress; she talks well, has an IQ of 108, and—though sensitive and moderately apprehensive—is interested in people and gets along reasonably well with them.

Herbert, when examined on his first visit, showed a remarkably intelligent physiognomy and good motor coordination. Within certain limits, he displayed astounding purposefulness in the pursuit of self-selected goals. Among a group of blocks, he instantly recognized those that were glued to a board and those that were detachable. He could build a tower of blocks as skillfully and as high as any child of his age or even older. He could not be diverted from his self-chosen occupations. He was annoyed by any interference, shoving intruders away (without ever looking at them), or screaming when the shoving had no effect.

He was again seen at 4 years, 7 months, and again at 5 years, 2 months of age. He still did not speak. Both times he entered the office without paying the slightest attention to the people present. He went after the Seguin form board and instantly busied himself putting the figures into their proper spaces and taking them out again adroitly and quickly. When interfered with he whined impatiently. When one figure was stealthily removed, he immediately noticed its absence, became disturbed, but promptly forgot all about it when it was put back. At times, after he had finally quieted down following the upset caused by the removal of the form board, he jumped up and down on the couch with an ecstatic expression on his face. He did not respond to being called or to any other words addressed to him. He was completely absorbed in whatever he did. He never smiled. He sometimes uttered inarticulate sounds in a monotonous singsong manner. At one time he gently stroked his mother's leg and touched it with his lips. He very frequently brought blocks and other objects to his lips. There was an almost photographic likeness of his behavior during the two visits, with the main exception that at 4 years he showed apprehension and shrank back when a match was lighted, while at 5 years he reacted by jumping up and down ecstatically.

Case 8

Alfred L. was brought by his mother in November, 1935, at 3½ years of age with this complaint:

> He has gradually shown a marked tendency toward developing one special interest which will completely dominate his day's activities. He talks of little else while the interest exists, he frets when he is not able to indulge in it (by seeing it, coming in contact with it, drawing pictures of it), and it is difficult to get his attention because of his preoccupation. . . . There has also been the problem of an overattachment to the world of objects and failure to develop the usual amount of social awareness.

Alfred was born in May, 1932, three weeks before term. For the first two months, "the feeding formula caused considerable concern but then he gained rapidly and became an unusually large and vigorous baby." He sat up at 5 months and walked at 14.

Language developed slowly; he seemed to have no interest in it. He seldom tells experience. He still confuses pronouns. He never asks questions in the form of questions (with the appropriate inflection). Since he talked, there has been a tendency to repeat over and over one word or statement. He almost never says a sentence without repeating it. Yesterday, when looking at a picture, he said many times, "Some cows standing in the water." We counted fifty repetitions, then he stopped after several more and then began over and over.

He had a good deal of "worrying":

He frets when the bread is put in the oven to be made into toast, and is afraid it will get burned and be hurt. He is upset when the sun sets. He is upset because the moon does not always appear in the sky at night. He prefers to play alone; he will get down from a piece of apparatus as soon as another child approaches. He likes to work out some project with large boxes (make a trolley, for instance) and does not want anyone to get on it or interfere.

When infantile thumb sucking was prevented by mechanical devices, he gave it up and instead put various objects into his mouth. On several occasions pebbles were found in his stools. Shortly before his second birthday, he swallowed cotton from an Easter rabbit, aspirating some of the cotton, so that tracheotomy became necessary. A few months later, he swallowed some kerosene "with no ill effects."

Alfred was an only child. His father, 30 years old at the time of his birth, "does not get along well with people, is suspicious, easily hurt, easily roused to anger, has to be dragged out to visit friends, spends his spare time reading, gardening, and fishing." He is a chemist and a law school graduate. The mother, of the same age, is a "clinical psychologist," very obsessive and excitable. The paternal grandparents died early; the father was adopted by a minister. The maternal grandfather, a psychologist, was severely obsessive, had numerous tics, was given to "repeated hand washing, protracted thinking along one line, fear of being alone, cardiac fears." The grandmother, "an excitable, explosive person, has done public speaking, published several books, is an incessant solitaire player, greatly worried over money matters." A maternal uncle frequently ran away from home and school, joined the marines, and later "made a splendid adjustment in commercial life."

The mother left her husband two months after Alfred's birth. The child has lived with his mother and maternal grandparents. "In the home is a nursery school and kindergarten (run by the mother), which creates some confusion for the child." Alfred did not see his father until he was 3 years, 4 months old, when the mother decided that "he should know his father" and "took steps to have the father come to the home to see the child."

Alfred, upon entering the office, paid no attention to the examiner. He immediately spotted a train in the toy cabinet, took it out, and connected and disconnected the cars in a slow, monotonous manner. He kept saying many times, "More train—more train—more train." He repeatedly "counted" the car windows: "One, two windows—one, two windows—one, two windows—four window, eight window, eight windows." He could not in any way be distracted from the trains. A Binet test was attempted in a room in which there were no trains. It was possible with much difficulty to pierce from time to time through his preoccupations. He finally complied in most instances in a manner that clearly indicated that he wanted to get through with the particular intrusion; this was repeated with each individual item of the task. In the end he achieved an IQ of 140.

The mother did not bring him back after this first visit because of "his continued distress when confronted with a member of the medical profession." In August, 1938, she sent upon request a written report of his development. From this report, the following passages are quoted:

> He is called a lone wolf. He prefers to play alone and avoids groups of children at play. He does not pay much attention to adults except when demanding stories. He avoids competition. He reads simple stories to himself. He is very fearful of being hurt, talks a great deal about the use of the electric chair. He is thrown into a panic when anyone accidentally covers his face.

Alfred was again referred in June, 1941. His parents had decided to live together. Prior to that the boy had been in eleven different schools. He had been kept in bed often because of colds, bronchitis, chickenpox, streptococcus infection, impetigo, and a vaguely described condition which the mother—the assurances of various pediatricians to the contrary notwithstanding—insisted was "rheumatic fever." While in the hospital, he is said to have behaved "like a manic patient." The mother liked to call herself a psychiatrist and to make "psychiatric" diagnoses of the child. From the mother's report, which combined obsessive enumeration of detailed instances with "explanations" trying to prove Alfred's "normalcy," the following information was gathered.

He had begun to play with children younger than himself, "using them as puppets—that's all." He had been stuffed with music, dramatics, and recitals, and had an excellent rote memory. He still was "terribly engrossed" in his play, didn't want people around, just couldn't relax:

> He had many fears, almost always connected with mechanical noise (meat grinders, vacuum cleaners, streetcars, trains, etc.). Usually he winds up with an obsessed interest in the things he was afraid of. Now he is afraid of the shrillness of a dog's barking.

Alfred was extremely tense during the entire interview, and very serious-minded, to such an extent that had it not been for his juvenile voice, he might have given the impression of a worried and preoccupied little old man. At the same time, he was very restless and showed considerable pressure of talk, which had nothing personal in it but consisted of obsessive questions about windows, shades, dark rooms, especially the X-ray room. He never smiled. No change of topic could get him away from the topic of light and darkness. But in between he answered the examiner's questions, which often had to be repeated several times, and to which he sometimes responded as the result of a bargain—"You answer my question, and I'll answer yours." He was painstakingly specific in his definitions. A balloon "is made out of lined rubber and has air in it and some have gas and sometimes they go up in the air and sometimes they can hold up and when they got a hole in it they'll bust up; if people squeeze they'll bust. Isn't it right?" A tiger "is a thing, animal, striped, like a cat, can scratch, eats people up, wild, lives in the jungle sometimes and in the forests, mostly in the jungle. Isn't it right?" This question "Isn't it right?" was definitely meant to be answered; there was a serious desire to be assured that the definition was sufficiently complete.

He was often confused about the meaning of words. When shown a picture and asked, "What is this picture about?" he replied, "People are moving *about*."

He once stopped and asked, very much perplexed, why there was "The Johns Hopkins Hospital" printed on the history sheets: "Why do they have to say it?" This, to him, was a real problem of major importance, calling for a great deal of thought and discussion. Since the histories were taken at the hospital, why should it be necessary to have the name on every sheet, though the person writing on it knew where he was writing? The examiner, whom he remembered very well from his visit six years previously, was to him nothing more nor less than a person who was expected to answer his obsessive questions about darkness and light.

Case 9

Charles N. was brought by his mother on February 2, 1943, at 4½ years of age, with the chief complaint, "The thing that upsets me most is that I can't reach my baby." She introduced her report by saying: "I am trying hard not to govern my remarks by professional knowledge which has intruded in my own way of thinking by now."

As a baby, the boy was inactive, "slow and phlegmatic." He would lie in the crib, just staring. He would act almost as if hypnotized. He seemed to concentrate on doing one thing at a time. Hypothyroidism was suspected, and he was given thyroid extract, without any change of the general condition.

> His enjoyment and appreciation of music encouraged me to play records. When he was 1½ years old, he could discriminate between eighteen symphonies. He recognized the composer as soon as the first movement started. He would say "Beethoven." At about the same age, he began to spin toys and lids of bottles and jars by the hour. He had a lot of manual dexterity in ability to spin cylinders. He would watch it and get severely excited and jump up and down in ecstasy. Now he is interested in reflecting light from mirrors and catching reflections. When he is interested in a thing, you cannot change it. He would pay no attention to me and show no recognition of me if I enter the room. . . .
>
> The most impressive thing is his detachment and his inaccessibility. He walks as if he is in a shadow, lives in a world of his own where he cannot be reached. No sense of relationship to persons. He went through a period of quoting another person; never offers anything himself. His entire conversation is a replica of whatever has been said to him. He used to speak of himself in the second person, now he uses the third person at times; he would say, "He wants"—never "I want.". . .
>
> He is destructive; the furniture in his room looks like it has hunks out of it. He will break a purple crayon into two parts and say, "*You* had a beautiful purple crayon and now it's two pieces. Look what *you* did."
>
> He developed an obsession about feces, would hide it anywhere (for instance, in drawers), would tease me if I walked into the room: "You soiled your pants, now you can't have your crayons!"
>
> As a result, he is still not toilet trained. He never soils himself in the nursery school, always does it when he comes home. The same is true of wetting. He is proud of wetting, jumps up and down with ecstasy, says, "Look at the big puddle *he* made."

When he is with other people, he doesn't look up at them. Last July, we had a group of people. When Charles came in, it was just like a foal who'd been let out of an enclosure. He did not pay attention to them but their presence was felt. He will mimic a voice and he sings and some people would not notice any abnormality in the child. At school, he never envelops himself in a group, he is detached from the rest of the children, except when he is in the assembly; if there is music, he will go to the front row and sing.

He has a wonderful memory for words. Vocabulary is good, except for pronouns. He never initiates conversation, and conversation is limited, extensive only as far as objects go.

Charles was born normally, a planned and wanted child. He sat up at 6 months and walked at less than 15 months—"just stood up and walked one day—no preliminary creeping." He has had none of the usual children's diseases.

Charles is the oldest of three children. The father, a high-school graduate and a clothing merchant, is described as a "self-made, gentle, calm, and placid person." The mother has "a successful business record, theatrical booking office in New York, of remarkable equanimity." The other two children were 28 and 14 months old at the time of Charles' visit to the Clinic. The maternal grandmother, "very dynamic, forceful, hyperactive, almost hypomanic," has done some writing and composing. A maternal aunt, "psychoneurotic, very brilliant, given to hysterics," has written poems and songs. Another aunt was referred to as "the amazon of the family." A maternal uncle, a psychiatrist, has considerable musical talent. The paternal relatives are described as "ordinary simple people."

Charles was a well developed, intelligent-looking boy, who was in good physical health. He wore glasses. When he entered the office, he paid not the slightest attention to the people present (three physicians, his mother, and his uncle). Without looking at anyone, he said, "Give me a pencil!" and took a piece of paper from the desk and wrote something resembling a figure 2 (a large desk calendar prominently displayed a figure 2; the day was February 2). He had brought with him a copy of *Readers Digest* and was fascinated by a picture of a baby. He said, "Look at the funny baby," innumerable times, occasionally adding, "Is he not funny? Is he not sweet?"

When the book was taken away from him, he struggled with the hand that held it, without looking at the *person* who had taken the book. When he was pricked with a pin, he said, "What's this?" and answered his own question: "It is a needle."

He looked timidly at the pin, shrank from further pricks, but at no time did he seem to connect the pricking with the *person* who held the pin. When the *Readers Digest* was taken from him and thrown on the floor and a foot placed over it, he tried to remove the foot as if it were another detached and interfering object, again with no concern for the *person* to whom the foot belonged. He once turned to his mother and excitedly said, "Give it to you!"

When confronted with the Seguin form board, he was mainly interested in the names of the forms, before putting them into their appropriate holes. He often spun the forms around, jumping up and down excitedly while they were in motion. The whole performance was very repetitious. He never used language as a means of communicating with people. He remembered names, such as "octagon," "diamond," "oblong block," but nevertheless kept asking, "What is this?"

He did not respond to being called and did not look at his mother when she spoke to him. When the blocks were removed, he screamed, stamped his feet, and cried, "I'll give it to you!" (meaning "You give it to me"). He was very skillful in his movements.

Charles was placed at the Devereux Schools.

Case 10

John F. was first seen on February 13, 1940, at 2 years, 4 months of age.

The father said: "The main thing that worries me is the difficulty in feeding. That is the essential thing, and secondly his slowness in development. During the first days of life he did not take the breast satisfactorily. After fifteen days he was changed from breast to bottle but did not take the bottle satisfactorily. There is a long story of trying to get food down. We have tried everything under the sun. He has been immature all along. At 20 months he first started to walk. He sucks his thumb and grinds his teeth quite frequently and rolls from side to side before sleeping. It we don't do what he wants, he will scream and yell."

John was born September 19, 1937; his birth weight was 7½ pounds. There were frequent hospitalizations because of the feeding problem. No physical disorder was ever found, except that the anterior fontanelle did not close until he was 2½ years of age. He suffered from repeated colds and otitis media, which necessitated bilateral myringotomy.

John was an only child until February, 1943. The father, a psychiatrist, is "a very calm, placid, emotionally stable person, who is the soothing element in the family." The mother, a high school graduate, worked as secretary in a pathology laboratory before marriage—"a hypomanic type of person; sees everything as a pathological specimen rather than well; throughout the pregnancy she was very apprehensive, afraid she would not live through the labor." The paternal grandmother is "obsessive about religion and washes her hands every few minutes." The maternal grandfather was an accountant.

John was brought to the office by both parents. He wandered about the room constantly and aimlessly. Except for spontaneous scribbling, he never brought two objects into relation to each other. He did not respond to the simplest commands, except that his parents with much difficulty elicited bye-bye, pat-a-cake, and peek-a-boo gestures, performed clumsily. His typical attitude toward objects was to throw them on the floor.

Three months later, his vocabulary showed remarkable improvement, though his articulation was defective. Mild obsessive trends were reported, such as pushing aside the first spoonful of every dish. His excursions about the office were slightly more purposeful.

At the end of his fourth year, he was able to form a very limited kind of affective contact, and even that only with a very limited number of people. Once such a relationship had been established, it had to continue in exactly the same channels. He was capable of forming elaborate and grammatically correct sentences, but he used the pronoun of the second person when referring to himself. He used language not as a means of communication but mainly as a repetition of things he had heard, without alteration of the personal pronoun. There was very marked obsessiveness. Daily routine must be adhered to rigidly; any slightest change of the pattern called forth outbursts of panic. There was endless repetition of sentences. He had an excellent rote memory and could recite many prayers, nursery rhymes, and songs "in different languages"; the mother did a great deal of stuffing in this respect and was very proud of these "achievements": "He can tell victrola records by their color and if one side of the record is identified, he remembers what is on the other side."

At 4½ years, he began gradually to use pronouns adequately. Even though his direct interest was in objects only, he took great pains in attracting the attention of the examiner (Dr. Hilde Bruch) and in gaining her praise. However, he never addressed her directly and spontaneously. He wanted to make sure of the sameness of the environment literally by keeping doors and windows closed. When his mother opened the door "to pierce through his obsession," he became violent in closing it again and finally, when again interfered with, burst helplessly into tears, utterly frustrated.

He was extremely upset upon seeing anything broken or incomplete. He noticed two dolls to which he had paid no attention before. He saw that one of them had no hat and became very much agitated, wandering about the room to look for the hat. When the hat was retrieved from another room, he instantly lost all interest in the dolls.

At 5½ years, he had good mastery of the use of pronouns. He had begun to feed himself satisfactorily. He saw a group photograph in the office and asked his father, "When are they coming out of the picture and coming in here?"

He was very serious about this. His father said something about the pictures they have at home on the wall. This disturbed John somewhat. He corrected his father: "We have them *near* the wall" ("on" apparently meaning to him "above" or "on top").

When he saw a penny, he said, "Penny. That's where you play tenpins." He had been given pennies when he knocked over tenpins while playing with his father at home.

He saw a dictionary and said to his father, "That's where you left the money?"

Once his father had left some money in a dictionary and asked John to tell his mother about it.

His father whistled a tune and John instantly and correctly identified it as "Mendelssohn's violin concerto." Though he could speak of things as big or pretty, he was utterly incapable of making comparisons ("Which is the bigger line? Prettier face?" etc.).

In December, 1942, and January, 1943, he had two series of predominantly right-sided *convulsions*, with conjugate deviation of the eyes to the right and transient paresis of the right arm. Neurologic examination showed no abnormalities. His eyegrounds were normal. An electroencephalogram indicated "focal disturbance in the left occipital region," but "a good part of the record could not be read because of the continuous marked artefacts due to the child's lack of cooperation."

Case 11

Elaine C. was brought by her parents on April 12, 1939, at the age of 7 years, 2 months, because of "unusual development": "She doesn't adjust. She stops at all abstractions. She doesn't understand other children's games, doesn't retain interest in stories read to her, wanders off and walks by herself, is especially fond of animals of all kinds, occasionally mimics them by walking on all fours and making strange noises."

Elaine was born on February 3, 1932, at term. She appeared healthy, took feedings well, stood up at 7 months and walked at less than a year. She could say four words at the end of her first year but made no progress in linguistic development for the following four years. Deafness was suspected but ruled out. Because of a febrile illness at 13 months, her increasing difficulties were interpreted as possible postencephalitic behavior disorder. Others blamed the mother, who was accused of inadequate handling of the child. Feeblemindedness was another diagnosis. For eighteen months, she was given anterior pituitary and thyroid preparations. "Some doctors," struck by Elaine's intelligent physiognomy, "thought she was a normal child and said that she would outgrow this."

At 2 years, she was sent to a nursery school, where "she independently went her way, not doing what the others did. She, for instance, drank the water and ate the plant when they were being taught to handle flowers." She developed an early interest in pictures of animals. Though generally restless, she could for hours concentrate on looking at such pictures, "especially engravings."

When she began to speak at about 5 years, she started out with complete though simple sentences that were "mechanical phrases" not related to the situation of the moment or related to it in a peculiar metaphorical way. She had an excellent vocabulary, knew especially the names and "classifications" of animals. She did not use pronouns correctly, but used plurals and tenses well. She "could not use negatives but recognized their meaning when others used them."

There were many peculiarities in her relation to situations:

> She can count by rote. She can set the table for numbers of people if the names are given her or enumerated in any way, but she cannot set the table "for three." If sent for a specific object in a certain place, she cannot bring it if it is somewhere else but still visible.

She was "frightened" by noises and anything moving toward her. She was so afraid of the vacuum cleaner that she would not even go near the closet where it was kept, and when it was used, ran out into the garage, covering her ears with her hands.

Elaine was the older of two children. Her father, aged 36, studied law and the liberal arts in three universities (including the Sorbonne), was an advertising copy writer, "one of those chronically thin persons, nervous energy readily expended." He was at one time editor of a magazine. The mother, aged 32, a "self-controlled, placid, logical person," had done editorial work for a magazine before marriage. The maternal grandfather was a newspaper editor, the grandmother was "emotionally unstable."

Elaine had been examined by a Boston psychologist at nearly 7 years of age. The report stated among other things:

> Her attitude toward the examiner remained vague and detached. Even when annoyed by restraint, she might vigorously push aside a

table or restraining hand with a scream, but she made no personal appeal for help or sympathy. At favorable moments she was competent in handling her crayons or assembling pieces to form pictures of animals. She could name a wide variety of pictures, including elephants, alligators, and dinosaurs. She used language in simple sentence structure, but rarely answered a direct question. As she plays, she repeats over and over phrases which are irrelevant to the immediate situation.

Physically the child was in good health. Her electroencephalogram was normal.

When examined in April, 1939, she shook hands with the physician upon request, without looking at him, then ran to the window and looked out. She automatically heeded the invitation to sit down. Her reaction to questions—after several repetitions—was an echolalia type reproduction of the whole question or, if it was too lengthy, of the end portion. She had no real contact with the persons in the office. Her expression was blank, though not unintelligent, and there were no communicative gestures. At one time, without changing her physiognomy, she said suddenly: "Fishes don't cry." After a time, she got up and left the room without asking or showing fear.

She was placed at the Child Study Home of Maryland, where she remained for three weeks and was studied by Drs. Eugenia S. Cameron and George Frankl. While there, she soon learned the names of all the children, knew the color of their eyes, the bed in which each slept, and many other details about them, but never entered into any relationship with them. When taken to the playgrounds, she was extremely upset and ran back to her room. She was very restless but when allowed to look at pictures, play alone with blocks, draw, or string beads, she could entertain herself contentedly for hours. Any noise, any interruption disturbed her. Once, when on the toilet seat, she heard a knocking in the pipes; for several days thereafter, even when put on a chamber pot in her own room, she did not move her bowels, anxiously listening for the noise. She frequently ejaculated stereotyped phrases, such as, "Dinosaurs don't cry"; "Crayfish, sharks, fish, and rocks"; "Crayfish and forks live in children's tummies"; "Butterflies live in children's stomachs, and in their panties, too"; "Fish have sharp teeth and bite little children"; "There is war in the sky"; "Rocks and crags, I will kill" (grabbing her blanket and kicking it about the bed); "Gargoyles bite children and drink oil"; "I will crush old angle worm, he bites children" (gritting her teeth and spinning around in a circle, very excited); "Gargoyles have milk bags"; "Needle head. Pink wee-wee. Has a yellow leg. Cutting the dead deer. Poison deer. Poor Elaine. No tadpoles in the house. Men broke deer's leg" (while cutting the picture of a deer from a book); "Tigers and cats"; "Seals and salamanders"; "Bears and foxes."

A few excerpts from the observations follow:

> Her language always has the same quality. Her speech is never accompanied by facial expression or gestures. She does not look into one's face. Her voice is peculiarly unmodulated, somewhat hoarse; she utters her words in an abrupt manner.
>
> Her utterances are impersonal. She never uses the personal pronouns of the first and second persons correctly. She does not seem able to conceive the real meaning of these words.
>
> Her grammar is inflexible. She uses sentences just as she has heard them, without adapting them grammatically to the situation of the moment. When she says, "Want me to draw a spider," she means, "I want you to draw a spider."
>
> She affirms by repeating a question literally, and she negates by not complying.
>
> Her speech is rarely communicative. She has no relation to children, has never talked to them, to be friendly with them, or to play with them. She moves among them like a strange being, as one moves between the pieces of furniture of a room.
>
> She insists on the repetition of the same routine always. Interruption of the routine is one of the most frequent occasions for her outbursts. Her own activities are simple and repetitious. She is able to spend hours in some form of daydreaming and seems to be very happy with it. She is inclined to rhythmical movements which always are masturbatory. She masturbates more in periods of excitement than during calm happiness. . . . Her movements are quick and skillful.

Elaine was placed in a private school in Pennsylvania. In a recent letter, the father reported "rather amazing changes":

> She is a tall, husky girl with clear eyes that have long since lost any trace of that animal wildness they periodically showed in the time you knew her. She speaks well on almost any subject, though with something of an odd intonation. Her conversation is still rambling talk, frequently with an amusing point, and it is only occasional, deliberate, and announced. She reads very well, but she reads fast, jumbling words, not pronouncing clearly, and not making proper emphases. Her range of information is really quite wide, and her memory almost infallible. It is obvious that Elaine is not "normal." Failure in anything leads to a feeling of defeat, of despair, and to a momentary fit of depression.

Discussion

The eleven children (eight boys and three girls) whose histories have been briefly presented offer, as is to be expected, individual differences in the degree of their disturbance, the manifestation of specific features, the family constellation, and the step-by-step development in the course of years. But even a quick review of the material makes the emergence of a number of essential common characteristics appear inevitable. These characteristics form a unique "syndrome," not heretofore reported, which seems to be rare enough, yet is probably more frequent than is indicated by the paucity of observed cases. It is quite possible that some such children have been viewed as feebleminded or schizophrenic. In fact, several children of our group were introduced to us as idiots or imbeciles, one still resides in a state school for the feebleminded, and two had been previously considered as schizophrenic.

The outstanding, "pathognomonic," fundamental disorder is the children's *inability to relate themselves* in the ordinary way to people and situations from the beginning of life. Their parents referred to them as having always been "self-sufficient"; "like in a shell"; "happiest when left alone"; "acting as if people weren't there"; "perfectly oblivious to everything about him"; "giving the impression of silent wisdom"; "failing to develop the usual amount of social awareness"; "acting almost as if hypnotized." This is not, as in schizophrenic children or adults, a departure from an initially present relationship; it is not a "withdrawal" from formerly existing participation. There is from the start an *extreme autistic aloneness* that, whenever possible, disregards, ignores, shuts out anything that comes to the child from the outside. Direct physical contact or such motion or noise as threatens to disrupt the aloneness is either treated "as if it weren't there" or, if this is no longer sufficient, resented painfully as distressing interference.

According to Gesell, the average child at 4 months of age makes an anticipatory motor adjustment by facial tension and shrugging attitude of the shoulders when lifted from a table or placed on a table. Gesell commented:

> It is possible that a less definite evidence of such adjustment may be found as low down as the neonatal period. Although a habit must be conditioned by experience, the opportunity for experience is almost universal and the response is sufficiently objective to merit further observation and record.

This universal experience is supplied by the frequency with which an infant is picked up by his mother and other persons. It is therefore highly significant that almost all mothers of our patients recalled their astonishment at the children's *failure to assume at any time an anticipatory posture* preparatory to being picked up. One father recalled that his daughter (Barbara) did not for years change her physiognomy or position in the least when the parents, upon coming home after a few hours' absence, approached her crib talking to her and making ready to pick her up.

The average infant learns during the first few months to adjust his body to the posture of the person who holds him. Our children were not able to do so for two or three years. We had an opportunity to observe 38-month-old Herbert in such a situation. His mother informed him in appropriate terms that she was going to lift him up, extending her arms in his direction. There was no response. She proceeded to take him up, and he allowed her to do so, remaining completely passive as if he were a sack of flour. It was the mother who had to do all the adjusting. Herbert was at that time capable of sitting, standing, and walking.

Eight of the eleven children acquired the *ability to speak* either at the usual age or after some delay. Three (Richard, Herbert, Virginia) have so far remained "mute." In none of the eight "speaking" children has language over a period of years served to convey meaning to others. They were, with the exception of John F., capable of clear articulation and phonation. Naming of objects presented no difficulty; even long and unusual words were learned and retained with remarkable facility. Almost all the parents reported, usually with much pride, that the children had learned at an early age to repeat an inordinate number of nursery rhymes, prayers, lists of animals, the roster of presidents, the alphabet forward and backward, even foreign-language (French) lullabies. Aside from the recital of sentences contained in the ready-made poems or other remembered pieces, it took a long time before they began to put words together. Other than that, "language" consisted mainly of "naming," of nouns identifying objects, adjectives indicating colors, and numbers indicating nothing specific.

Their *excellent rote memory,* coupled with the inability to use language in any other way, often led the parents to stuff them with more and more verses, zoologic and botanic names, titles and composers of victrola record pieces, and the like. Thus, from the start, language—which the children did not use for the purpose of communication—was deflected in a considerable measure to a self-sufficient, semantically and conversationally valueless or grossly distorted memory exercise. To a child 2 or 3 years old, all these words, numbers, and poems ("questions and answers of the Presbyterian Catechism"; "Mendelssohn's violin concerto"; the "Twenty-third Psalm"; a French lullaby; an encyclopedia index page) could hardly have more meaning than sets of nonsense syllables to adults. It is difficult to know for certain whether the stuffing as such has contributed essentially to the course of the psychopathologic condition. But it is also difficult to imagine that it did not cut deeply into the development of language as a tool for receiving and imparting meaningful messages.

As far as the communicative functions of speech are concerned, there is no fundamental difference between the eight speaking and the three mute children. Richard was once overheard by his boarding mother to say distinctly, "Good night." Justified skepticism about this observation was later dispelled when this "mute" child was seen in the office shaping his mouth in silent repetition of words when asked to say certain things. "Mute" Virginia—so her cottage mates insisted—was heard repeatedly to say, "Chocolate"; "Marshmallow"; "Mama"; "Baby."

When sentences are finally formed, they are for a long time mostly parrot-like repetitions of heard word combinations. They are sometimes echoed immediately, but they are just as often "stored" by the child and uttered at a later date. One may, if one wishes, speak of *delayed echolalia.* Affirmation is indicated by literal repetition of a question. "Yes" is a concept that it takes the children many years to acquire. They are incapable of using it as a general symbol of assent. Donald learned to say "Yes" when his father told him that he would put him on his shoulders if he said "Yes." This word then came to "mean" only the desire to be put on his father's shoulders. It took many months before he could detach the word "yes" from this specific situation, and it took much longer before he was able to use it as a general term of affirmation.

The same type of *literalness* exists also with regard to prepositions. Alfred, when asked, "What is this picture about?" replied: "People are moving *about*."

John F. corrected his father's statement about pictures on the wall; the pictures were "*near* the wall." Donald T., requested to put something *down*, promptly put it on the floor. Apparently the meaning of a word becomes inflexible and cannot be used with any but the originally acquired connotation.

There is no difficulty with plurals and tenses. But the absence of spontaneous sentence formation and the echolalia type reproduction has, in every one of the eight speaking children, given rise to a peculiar grammatical phenomenon. *Personal pronouns are repeated just as heard,* with no change to suit the altered situation. The child, once told by his mother, "Now I will give you your milk," expresses the desire for milk in exactly the same words. Consequently, he comes to speak of himself always as "you," and of the person addressed as "I." Not only the words, but even the intonation is retained. If the mother's original remark has been made in form of a question, it is reproduced with the grammatical form and the inflection of a question. The repetition "Are you ready for your dessert?" means that the child is ready for his dessert. There is a set, not-to-be-changed phrase for every specific occasion. The pronominal fixation remains until about the sixth year of life, when the child gradually learns to speak of himself in the first person, and of the individual addressed in the second person. In the transitional period, he sometimes still reverts to the earlier form or at times refers to himself in the third person.

The fact that the children echo things heard does not signify that they "attend" when spoken to. It often takes numerous reiterations of a question or command before there is even so much as an echoed response. Not less than seven of the children were therefore considered as deaf or hard of hearing. There is an all-powerful need for being left undisturbed. Everything that is brought to the child from the outside, everything that changes his external or even internal environment, represents a dreaded intrusion.

Food is the earliest intrusion that is brought to the child from the outside. David Levy observed that affect-hungry children, when placed in foster homes where they are well treated, at first demand excessive quantities of food. Hilde Bruch, in her studies of obese children, found that overeating often resulted when affectionate offerings from the parents were lacking or considered unsatisfactory. Our patients, reversely, anxious to keep the outside world away, indicated this by the refusal of food. Donald, Paul ("vomited a great deal during the first year"), Barbara ("had to be tube-fed until 1 year of age"), Herbert, Alfred, and John presented severe feeding difficulty from the beginning of life. Most of them, after an unsuccessful struggle, constantly interfered with, finally gave up the struggle and all of a sudden began eating satisfactorily.

Another intrusion comes from *loud noises and moving objects*, which are therefore reacted to with horror. Tricycles, swings, elevators, vacuum cleaners, running water, gas burners, mechanical toys, egg beaters, even the wind could on occasions bring about a major panic. One of the children was even afraid to go near the closet in which the vacuum cleaner was kept. Injections and examinations with stethoscope or otoscope created a grave emotional crisis. Yet it is not the noise or motion itself that is dreaded. The disturbance comes from the noise or motion that intrudes itself, or threatens to intrude itself, upon the child's aloneness. The child himself can happily make as great a noise as any that he dreads and move objects about to his heart's desire.

But the child's noises and motions and all of his performances are as *monotonously repetitive* as are his verbal utterances. There is a marked limitation in the variety of his spontaneous activities. The child's behavior is governed by an *anxiously obsessive desire for the maintenance of sameness* that nobody but the child himself may disrupt on rare occasions. Changes of routine, of furniture arrangement, of a pattern, of the order in which everyday acts are carried out, can drive him to despair. When John's parents got ready to move to a new home, the child was frantic when he saw the moving men roll up the rug in his room. He was acutely upset until the moment when, in the new home, he saw his furniture arranged in the same manner as before. He looked pleased, all anxiety was suddenly gone, and he went around affectionately patting each piece. Once blocks, beads, sticks have been put together in a certain way, they are always regrouped in exactly the same way, even though there was no definite design. The children's memory was phenomenal in this respect. After the lapse of several days, a multitude of blocks could be rearranged in precisely the same unorganized pattern, with the same color of each block turned up, with each picture or letter on the upper surface of each block facing in the same direction as before. The absence of a block or the presence of a supernumerary block was noticed immediately, and there was an imperative demand for the restoration of the missing piece. If someone removed a block, the child struggled to get it back, going into a panic tantrum until he regained it, and then promptly and with sudden calm after the storm returned to the design and replaced the block.

This insistence on sameness led several of the children to become greatly disturbed upon the sight of anything broken or incomplete. A great part of the day was spent in demanding not only the sameness of the wording of a request but also the sameness of the sequence of events. Donald would not leave his bed after his nap until after he had said, "Boo, say 'Don, do you want to get down?'" and the mother had complied. But this was not all. The act was still not considered completed. Donald would continue, "Now say 'All right.'" Again the mother had to comply, or there was screaming until the performance was completed. All of this ritual was an indispensable part of the act of getting up after a nap. Every other activity had to be completed from beginning to end in the manner in which it had been started originally. It was impossible to return from a walk without having covered the same ground as had been covered before. The sight of a broken crossbar on a garage door on his regular daily tour so upset Charles that he kept talking and asking about it for weeks on end, even while spending a few days in a distant city. One of the children noticed a crack in the office ceiling and kept asking anxiously and repeatedly who had cracked the ceiling, not calmed by any answer given her. Another child, seeing one doll with a hat and another without a hat, could not be placated until the other hat was found and put on the doll's head. He then immediately lost interest in the two dolls; sameness and completeness had been restored, and all was well again.

The dread of change and incompleteness seems to be a major factor in the explanation of the monotonous repetitiousness and the resulting *limitation in the variety of spontaneous activity*. A situation, a performance, a sentence is not regarded as complete if it is not made up of exactly the same elements that were present at the time the child was first confronted with it. If the slightest ingredient is altered or removed, the total situation is no longer the same and therefore is not accepted as such, or it is resented with impatience or even with a reaction of profound frustration. The inability to experience wholes without full attention to the constituent parts is somewhat reminiscent of the plight of children with specific reading disability who do not respond to the modern system of configurational reading instruction but must be taught to build up words from their alphabetic elements. This is perhaps one of the reasons why those children of our group who were old enough to be instructed in reading immediately became excessively preoccupied with the "spelling" of words, or why Donald, for example, was so disturbed over the fact that "light" and "bite," having the same phonetic quality, should be spelled differently.

Objects that do not change their appearance and position, that retain their sameness and never threaten to interfere with the child's aloneness, are readily accepted by the autistic child. He has a good *relation to objects*; he is interested in them, can play with them happily for hours. He can be very fond of them, or get angry at them if, for instance, he cannot fit them into a certain space. When with them, he has a gratifying sense of undisputed power and control. Donald and Charles began in the second year of life to exercise this power by spinning everything that could be possibly spun and jumping up and down in ecstasy when they watched the objects whirl about. Frederick "jumped up and down in great glee" when he bowled and saw the pins go down. The children sensed and exercised the same power over their own bodies by rolling and other rhythmic movements. These actions and the accompanying ecstatic fervor strongly indicate the presence of *masturbatory orgastic gratification*.

The children's *relation to people* is altogether different. Every one of the children, upon entering the office, immediately went after blocks, toys, or other objects, without paying the least attention to the persons present. It would be wrong to say that they were not aware of the presence of persons. But the people, so long as they left the child alone, figured in about the same manner as did the desk, the bookshelf, or the filing cabinet. When the child was addressed, he was not bothered. He had the choice between not responding at all or, if a question was repeated too insistently, "getting it over with" and continuing with whatever he had been doing. Comings and goings, even of the mother, did not seem to register. Conversation going on in the room elicited no interest. If the adults did not try to enter the child's domain, he would at times, while moving between them, gently touch a hand or a knee as on other occasions he patted the desk or the couch. But he never looked into anyone's face. If an adult forcibly intruded himself by taking a block away or stepping on an object that the child needed, the child struggled and became angry with the hand or the foot, which was dealt with per se and not as a part of a person. He never addressed a word or a look to the owner of the hand or foot. When the object was retrieved, the child's mood changed abruptly to one of placidity. When pricked, he showed fear of the *pin* but not of the person who pricked him.

The relation to the members of the household or to other children did not differ from that to the people at the office. Profound aloneness dominates all behavior. The father or mother or both may have been away for an hour or a month; at their homecoming, there is no indication that the child has been even aware of their absence. After many outbursts of frustration, he gradually and reluctantly learns to compromise when he finds no way out, obeys certain orders, complies in matters of daily routine, but always strictly insists on the observance of his rituals. When there is company, he moves among the people "like a stranger" or, as one mother put it, "like a foal who had been let out of an enclosure." When with other children, he does not play with them. He plays alone while they are around, maintaining no bodily, physiognomic, or verbal contact with them. He does not take part in competitive games. He just is there, and if sometimes he happens to stroll as far as the periphery of a group, he soon removes himself and remains alone. At the same time, he quickly becomes familiar with the names of all the children of the group, may know the color of each child's hair, and other details about each child.

There is a far better relationship with pictures of people than with people themselves. Pictures, after all, cannot interfere. Charles was affectionately interested in the picture of a child in a magazine advertisement. He remarked repeatedly about the child's sweetness and beauty. Elaine was fascinated by pictures of animals but would not go near a live animal. John made no distinction between real and depicted people. When he saw a group photograph, he asked seriously when the people would step out of the picture and come into the room.

Even though most of these children were at one time or another looked upon as feebleminded, they are all unquestionably endowed with good *cognitive potentialities.* They all have strikingly intelligent physiognomies. Their faces at the same time give the impression of *serious-mindedness* and, in the presence of others, an anxious *tenseness*, probably because of the uneasy anticipation of possible interference. When alone with objects, there is often a placid smile and an expression of beatitude, sometimes accompanied by happy though monotonous humming and singing. The astounding vocabulary of the speaking children, the excellent memory for events of several years before, the phenomenal rote memory for poems and names, and the precise recollection of complex patterns and sequences, bespeak good intelligence in the sense in which this word is commonly used. Binet or similar testing could not be carried out because of limited accessibility. But all the children did well with the Seguin form board.

Physically, the children were essentially normal. Five had relatively large heads. Several of the children were somewhat clumsy in gait and gross motor performances, but all were very skillful in terms of finer muscle coordination. Electroencephalograms were normal in the case of all but John, whose anterior fontanelle did not close until he was 2½ years old, and who at 5¼ years had two series of predominantly right-sided convulsions. Frederick had a supernumerary nipple in the left axilla; there were no other instances of congenital anomalies.

There is one other very interesting common denominator in the backgrounds of these children. *They all come of highly intelligent families.* Four fathers are psychiatrists, one is a brilliant lawyer, one a chemist and law school graduate employed in the government Patent Office, one a plant pathologist, one a professor of forestry, one an advertising copy writer who has a degree in law and has studied in three universities, one is a mining engineer, and one a successful business man. Nine of the eleven mothers are college graduates. Of the two who have only high school education, one was secretary in a pathology laboratory, and the other ran a theatrical booking office in New York City before marriage. Among the others, there was a free-lance writer, a physician, a psychologist, a graduate nurse, and Frederick's mother was successively a purchasing agent, the director of secretarial studies in a girls' school, and a teacher of history. Among the grandparents and collaterals there are many physicians, scientists, writers, journalists, and students of art. All but three of the families are represented either in *Who's Who in America* or in *American Men of Science*, or in both.

Two of the children are Jewish, the others are all of Anglo-Saxon descent. Three are "only" children, five are the first-born of two children in their respective families, one is the oldest of three children, one is the younger of two, and one the youngest of three.

COMMENT

The combination of extreme autism, obsessiveness, stereotypy, and echolalia brings the total picture into relationship with some of the basic schizophrenic phenomena. Some of the children have indeed been diagnosed as of this type at one time or another. But in spite of the remarkable similarities, the condition differs in many respects from all other known instances of childhood schizophrenia.

First of all, even in cases with the earliest recorded onset of schizophrenia, including those of De Sanctis' dementia praecocissima and of Heller's dementia infantilis, the first observable manifestations were preceded by at least two years of essentially average development; the histories specifically emphasize a more or less gradual *change* in the patients' behavior. The children of our group have all shown their extreme aloneness from the very beginning of life, not responding to anything that comes to them from the outside world. This is most characteristically expressed in the recurrent report of failure of the child to assume an anticipatory posture upon being picked up, and of failure to adjust the body to that of the person holding him.

Second, our children are able to establish and maintain an excellent, purposeful, and "intelligent" relation to objects that do not threaten to interfere with their aloneness, but are from the start anxiously and tensely impervious to people, with whom for a long time they do not have any kind of direct affective contact. If dealing with another person becomes inevitable, then a temporary relationship is formed with the person's hand or foot as a definitely detached object, but not with the person himself.

All of the children's activities and utterances are governed rigidly and consistently by the powerful desire for aloneness and sameness. Their world must seem to them to be made up of elements that, once they have been experienced in a certain setting or sequence, cannot be tolerated in any other setting or sequence; nor can the setting or sequence be tolerated without all the original ingredients in the identical spatial or chronologic order. Hence the obsessive repetitiousness. Hence the reproduction of sentences without altering the pronouns to suit the occasion. Hence, perhaps, also the development of a truly phenomenal memory that enables the child to recall and reproduce complex "nonsense" patterns, no matter how unorganized they are, in exactly the same form as originally construed.

Five of our children have by now reached ages between 9 and 11 years. Except for Vivian S., who has been dumped in a school for the feebleminded, they show a very interesting course. The basic desire for aloneness and sameness has remained essentially unchanged, but there has been a varying degree of emergence from solitude, an acceptance of at least some people as being within the child's sphere of consideration, and a sufficient increase in the number of experienced patterns to refute the earlier impression of extreme limitation of the child's ideational content. One might perhaps put it this way: While the schizophrenic tries to solve his problem by stepping out of a world of which he has been a part and with which he has been in touch, our children gradually *compromise* by extending cautious feelers into a world in which they have been total strangers from the beginning. Between the ages of 5 and 6 years, they gradually abandon the echolalia and learn spontaneously to use personal pronouns with adequate reference. Language becomes more communicative, at first in the sense of a question-and-answer exercise, and then in the sense of greater spontaneity of sentence formation. Food is accepted without difficulty. Noises and motions are tolerated more than previously. The panic tantrums subside. The repetitiousness assumes the form of obsessive preoccupations. Contact with a limited number of people is established in a twofold way: people are included in the child's world to the extent to which they satisfy his needs, answer his obsessive questions, teach him how to read and to do things. Second, though people are still regarded as nuisances, their questions are answered and their commands are obeyed reluctantly, with the implication that it would be best to get these interferences over with, the sooner to be able to return to the still much desired aloneness. Between the ages of 6 and 8 years, the children begin to play in a group, still never *with* the other members of the play group, but at least on the periphery *alongside* the group. Reading skill is acquired quickly, but the children read monotonously, and a story or a moving picture is experienced in unrelated portions rather than in its coherent totality. All of this makes the family feel that, in spite of recognized "difference" from other children, there is progress and improvement.

It is not easy to evaluate the fact that all of our patients have come of highly intelligent parents. This much is certain, that there is a great deal of obsessiveness in the family background. The very detailed diaries and reports and the frequent remembrance, after several years, that the children had learned to recite twenty-five questions and answers of the Presbyterian Catechism, to sing thirty-seven nursery songs, or to discriminate between eighteen symphonies, furnish a telling illustration of parental obsessiveness.

One other fact stands out prominently. In the whole group, there are very few really warmhearted fathers and mothers. For the most part, the parents, grandparents, and collaterals are persons strongly preoccupied with abstractions of a scientific, literary, or artistic nature, and limited in genuine interest in people. Even some of the happiest marriages are rather cold and formal affairs. Three of the marriages were dismal failures. The question arises whether or to what extent this fact has contributed to the condition of the children. The children's aloneness from the beginning of life makes it difficult to attribute the whole picture exclusively to the type of the early parental relations with our patients.

We must, then, assume that these children have come into the world with innate inability to form the usual, biologically provided affective contact with people, just as other children come into the world with innate physical or intellectual handicaps. If this assumption is correct, a further study of our children may help to furnish concrete criteria regarding the still diffuse notions about the constitutional components of emotional reactivity. For here we seem to have pure-culture examples of *inborn autistic disturbances of affective contact.*†

†Reset from the original published in *Nervous Child*, Volume 2, pp. 217–250, 1943.

IRRELEVANT AND METAPHORICAL LANGUAGE IN EARLY INFANTILE AUTISM

During the past few years, I have had occasion to observe 23 children whose extreme withdrawal and disability to form the usual relations to people were noticed from the beginning of life. I have designated this condition as "early infantile autism." Phenomenologically, excessive aloneness and an anxiously obsessive desire for the preservation of sameness are the outstanding characteristics. Memory is often astounding. Cognitive endowment, masked frequently by limited responsiveness, is at least average. Most patients stem from psychometrically superior, though literal-minded and obsessive, families.

This condition offers fascinating problems and opportunities for study from the points of view of genetics, of the psychodynamics of earliest parent-infant relationship, and of its resemblances to the schizophrenias. Among numerous other features, the peculiarities of language present an important and promising basis for investigation. I should like to mention briefly the "mutism" of 8 of the 23 children, which is on rare occasions interrupted by the utterance of a whole

45

sentence in emergency situations; the use of simple verbal negation as magic protection against unpleasant occurrences; the literalness which cannot accept synonyms or different connotations of the same preposition; the self-absorbed inaccessibility which has caused most of the parents to suspect deafness; the echolalia-type repetition of whole phrases; and the typical, almost pathognomonic, pronominal reversals which consist of the child's reference to himself as "you" and to the person spoken to as "I."

Frequently these children say things which seem to have no meaningful connection with the situation in which they are voiced. The utterances impress the audience as "nonsensical," "silly," "incoherent," and "irrelevant." These are the terms used by the reporting parents, physicians and nursery school teachers.

We were fortunate in having opportunities to trace some of these "irrelevant" phrases to earlier sources and to learn that, whenever such tracing was possible, the utterances, though still peculiar and out of place in ordinary conversation, assume definite meaning. I should like to illustrate this with a few characteristic examples:

Paul G., while observed at our clinic at 5 years of age, was heard saying: "Don't throw the dog off the balcony." There was neither a dog nor a balcony around. The remark therefore sounded irrelevant. It was learned that three years previously he had thrown a toy dog down from the balcony of a London hotel at which the family was staying. His mother, tired of retrieving the toy, had said to him, with some irritation: "Don't throw the dog off the balcony." Since that day, Paul, whenever tempted to throw anything, used these words to admonish and check himself.

"Peter eater" was another of Paul's "nonsensical," "irrelevant" expressions. It seemed to have no association with his experiences of the moment. His mother related that, when Paul was 2 years old, she once recited to him the nursery rhyme about "Peter, Peter, pumpkin eater," while she was busy in the kitchen; just then she dropped a saucepan. Ever since that day Paul chanted the words "Peter eater" whenever he saw anything resembling a saucepan. There was, indeed, in the playroom a toy stove on which sat a miniature pan. It was noted then that Paul, while saying these words, glanced in the direction of the stove and finally picked up the pan, running wildly around with it and chanting "Peter eater" over and over again.

John F., at 5 years of age, saw Webster's Unabridged Dictionary in the office. He turned to his father and said: "That's where you left the money." In this instance the connection was established by the fact that John's father was in the habit of leaving money for his wife in the dictionary which they had at home. Upon being shown a penny, John said: "That's where play ten pins," as a sort of definition of penny. His father was able to supply the clue. He and John played ten pins at home with a children's set. Every time that John knocked over one of the ten pins, his father gave him a penny.

Elaine C. had been surrounded in her infancy with toy animals of which she was very fond. When she cried, her mother used to point out to her that the toy dog or toy rabbit did not cry. When Elaine was seen at 7 years of age, she still kept saying when she was fearful and on the verge of tears: "Rabbits don't cry." "Dogs don't cry." She added a large number of other animals. She went about, when in distress, reiterating the seemingly irrelevant words: "Seals don't cry." "Dinosaurs don't cry." "Crayfishes don't cry." She came to use the names of these and other animals in a great variety of connections.

Jay S., not quite 4 years old, referred to himself as "Blum" whenever his veracity was questioned by his parents. The mystery of this "irrelevance" was explained when Jay, who could read fluently, once pointed to the advertisement of a furniture firm in the newspapers, which said in large letters: "Blum tells the truth." Since Jay had told the truth, he *was* Blum. This analogy between himself as a teller of the truth and Blum does not differ essentially from the designation of a liar as Ananias, a lover as Romeo, or an attractive lad as Adonis. But while these designations are used with the expectation that the listener is familiar with the analogy, the autistic child has his own private, original, individualized references, the semantics of which are transferable only to the extent to which any listener can, through his own efforts, trace the source of the analogy.

The cited examples represent in the main metaphorical expressions which, instead of relying on accepted or acceptable substitutions as encountered in poetry and conversational phraseology, are rooted in *concrete, specific, personal* experiences of the child who uses them. So long as the listener has no access to the original source, the meaning of the metaphor must remain obscure to him, and the child's remark is not "relevant" to any sort of verbal or other situational interchange. Lack of access to the source shuts out any comprehension, and the baffled listener, to whom the remark means nothing, may too readily assume that it has no meaning at all. If the metaphorical reference to Ananias, Romeo or Adonis is not understood, dictionaries, encyclopedias or informed persons can supply the understanding. But the personal metaphors of the autistic children can convey "sense" only through acquaintance with the singular, unduplicated meaning which they have to the children themselves. The only clue can be supplied by the direct observation and recall of the episode which started off the use of each particular metaphorical expression.

Occasionally, though not very often, a chance gesture or remark of the child himself may lead to the understanding of a metaphor. This was the case when

Jay S. happened to point to the Blum advertisement. This was also the case when 5-year-old Anthony F. solved the puzzle of his frequently expressed fondness of "55." On one occasion, he spoke of his two grandmothers. We knew that one of them had shown little interest in him, while the other had reared him with much patience and affection. Anthony said: "One is 64 [years old], and one is 55. I like 55 best." The seemingly irrelevant preoccupation with a seemingly arbitrary number can now be recognized as being heavily endowed with meaning. It is Anthony's private way of expressing affection for his grandmother.

This phenomenon of metaphorical substitution is very common among our autistic children. Donald T., at 7 years of age, was asked the Binet question: "If I were to buy 4 cents worth of candy and give the storekeeper 10 cents, how much money would I get back?" He obviously knew the answer. His reply, however, was not "6 cents" but: "I'll draw a hexagon." Two years previously, at 5 years of age, Donald had been scribbling with crayons; all the while he kept saying seriously and with conviction: "Annette and Cecile make purple." It was learned that Donald had at home five bottles of paint. He named each after one of the Dionne quintuplets. Blue became "Annette," and red became "Cecile." After that, Annette became his word for blue, and Cecile for red. Purple, not being one of the five colors, remained "purple."

It is mainly the private, original frame of reference which makes these substitutions seem peculiar. We witness similar processes in the introduction of trade names for perfumes, wines, cigarettes, cigars, paints and many other items. Etymology abounds with similar derivations. Common usage makes it unnecessary to know the original source in order to get the meaning. An ulster is a certain type of top coat whether or not you connect it with the county in Ireland from which it has its name. You need not know that a serpent is a "creeper" or that a dromedary is a "runner." It does not matter whether or not you know that filibuster is a corrupted form of "freebooter."

The autistic child does not depend upon such prearranged semantic transfers. He makes up his own as he goes along. In fact, he can keep transferring and retransferring to his heart's desire, Gary T., at 5 years, designated a bread basket as "home bakery." He did not stop there. After this, *every* basket to him became a "home bakery." This was his term for coal basket, waste basket or sewing basket. This procedure, too, has its etymological counterparts. The original meaning of "caput" is transferred from anatomy to anything which, literally or figuratively, is at the top or at the "head," whether this be "captain," the head of a group of people, "capitol," at the top of a pillar, or "chapter," the inscription over a section of a book. The transfer does not even stop there, for a "chapter" then becomes not only the "heading" of the section but the whole section itself.

From these observations we may safely draw a number of significant conclusions:

1. The seemingly irrelevant and nonsensical utterances of our autistic children are metaphorical expressions in the sense that they represent "figures of speech by means of which one thing is put for another which it only resembles." The Greek work metapherein means "to transfer."

2. The transfer of meaning is accomplished in a variety of ways:

a. Through substitutive analogy: Bread basket becomes "home bakery"; Annette and Cecile become "red" and "blue"; penny becomes "that's where play ten pin."

b. Through generalization: *Totum pro parte.* "Home bakery" becomes the term for *every* basket; "Don't throw the dog off the balcony" assumes the meaning of self-admonition in *every* instance when the child feels the need for admonishing himself.

c. Through restriction: *Pars pro toto.* The 55-year-old grandmother becomes "55"; a teller of truth becomes "Blum"; the number 6 is referred to as "hexagon."

3. The linguistic processes through which the transfers are achieved do not as such differ essentially from poetical and ordinary phraseological metaphors. Etymologically, much of our language is made up of similar transfers of meaning through substitutions, generalizations and restrictions.

4. The basic difference consists of the autistic privacy and original uniqueness of the transfers, derived from the children's situational and emotional experiences. Once the connection between experience and metaphorical utterance is established, and only then, does the child's language become meaningful. The goal of the transfer is intelligible only in terms of its source.

5. In contrast to poetry and etymology, the metaphorical language in early infantile autism is not directly communicable. It is not primarily intended as a means of inviting other people to understand and to share the child's symbols. Though it is undoubtedly creative, the creation is in the main self-sufficient and self-contained.

"The abnormality of the autistic person," say Whitehorn and Zipf, "lies only in ignoring the other fellow: that is, it lies in his disregard of the social obligation to make only those changes which are socially acceptable in the sense that they are both understandable and serviceable in the group. Naturally, once the autistic person pursues his own linguistic and semantic paths of least effort, the result may well appear to his perplexed auditor as a disorder of meanings, or even as a disorder of association. Yet the autistic speaker, in making his own language, without the nuisance of satisfying the auditor's needs, may employ the same principles of linguistic and semantic change as does the normal person, though not with the same care to insure community acceptance."

The above observations and conclusions gain additional importance because they give concrete evidence to the long-felt assumption that similar mechanisms prevail in the "irrelevant," "incoherent," and metaphorical language of adult schizophrenics. In the case of the latter, the earlier and earliest connections and pertinences have often been lost irretrievably, as they have been even for some of the expressions of our children at so early an age. But the examples cited (and the study by Whitehorn and Zipf) justify the conviction that schizophrenic "irrelevance" is not irrelevant to the patient himself and could become relevant to the audience to the extent to which it were possible to find the clues to his private and self-contained metaphorical transfers.†

REFERENCES

Kanner, L. Autistic disturbances of affective contact. *The Nervous Child,* 1943, 2, 217–250.
Kanner, L. Early infantile autism. *Journal of Pediatrics,* 1944, 25, 211–217.
Whitehorn, J. C., & Zipf, G. K. Schizophrenic language. *Archives of Neurology and Psychiatry,* 1943, 49, 831–851.

†Reset from the original published in *American Journal of Psychiatry,* Volume 103, pp. 242–246, 1946. Copyright 1946, American Psychiatric Association.

3

1950's

PROBLEMS OF NOSOLOGY AND PSYCHODYNAMICS IN EARLY INFANTILE AUTISM

In 1943, under the title *Autistic Disturbances of Affective Contact*, I published 11 cases of infantile psychosis noticed as early as in the first two years of life. Since then, I have seen more than 50 such children, and knowledge of many others has come to me from psychiatrists and pediatricians in this country and abroad. To satisfy the need for some terminological identification of the condition, I have come to refer to it as "early infantile autism."

Briefly, the characteristic features consist of a profound withdrawal from contact with people, an obsessive desire for the preservation of sameness, a skillful and even affectionate relation to objects, the retention of an intelligent and pensive physiognomy, and either mutism or the kind of language which does not seem intended to serve the purpose of interpersonal communication. An analysis of this language has revealed a peculiar reversal of pronouns, neologisms, metaphors, and apparently irrelevant utterances which become meaningful to

51

the extent to which they can be traced to the patient's experiences and their emotional implications.

The syndrome of early infantile autism is by now reasonably well established and commonly accepted as a psychopathologic pattern. The symptom combination in most instances warrants an unequivocal diagnostic formulation. Once I became impressed by the syndrome, my first interests went in the direction of observation and description.

In the early days of scientific psychiatry, the singling out of a pathologic behavior syndrome was deemed fully sufficient. A certain type of symptom mosaic was lifted out of the diagnostic diffuseness and given a distinctive name, which was viewed as the designation of a disease entity. This happened, for instance, to Hecker's hebephrenia and Kahlbaum's catatonia.

Nowadays, the study of a psychotic pattern imposes two major obligations. Kraepelin introduced one of these by emphasizing similarities and dissimilarities of clinical pictures. He was able to find a common denominator for hebephrenia, catatonia, and other apparently heterogeneous phenomena.

Now that early infantile autism has a well-defined symptomatology and the syndrome as such can be recognized with relative ease, it is ready to apply for a place in the existing psychiatric nosology. In accepting this application, I am less interested in terminological allocation than in the intrinsic nature of the condition as related or unrelated to the intrinsic nature of other conditions.

Recent experiences with Heller's disease have pointed out the importance of this necessity. Heller's disease, or dementia infantilis, was first described in 1908. A child develops normally for a period of about two years, then loses the ability to speak, has no interest in his toys, and deteriorates rapidly to the point of idiocy. It has been customary to assign to Heller's disease a place among the forms of childhood schizophrenia. Corberi in Italy did a biopsy of cortical tissue in two cases and found wide areas of ganglion cell degeneration and shrinkage of the cell processes. This was fully verified in two cases of my own observation. It is therefore appropriate to separate Heller's disease from the schizophrenias and to align it with the organic degenerative disorders akin to the Tay-Sachs disease group.

Early infantile autism bears no resemblance to Heller's disease or to any other organic condition. Heller's disease has a definite onset; the child impresses people as feeling and being sick. In fact, Zappert counted this initial malaise, or *Krankheitsgefühl*, among the essential features of Heller's disease; it was reported in the few cases which I had an opportunity to study and was one of the guides to diagnosis. Our autistic children did not go through such a prodromal stage. It is true that I have not considered a brain tissue biopsy in any of the autistic patients. Neither the clinical neurological findings nor the electroencephalograms nor the subsequent developments seemed to me to justify such a procedure. Even those patients who have withdrawn to the point of functional idiocy or imbecility show, especially in their behavior with puzzles and form boards, residual oases of planned mental activity which should deter one from thinking in terms of a degenerative organic process.

It has been suggested by some that early infantile autism is basically an aphasic phenomenon related to so-called congenital word deafness. This assumption can be understood in view of the mutism of many of the children and in view of all the patients' lack of response to verbal address. But here the resemblance stops. It can, of course, be imagined that aphasic children, cut off from linguistic contact with the environment, may find it difficult to connect in other respects as well. I have seen word-deaf children who were shy, apprehensive, lacking in spontaneity, pathetically bewildered, and insecure. But they all responded promptly to gestures, were keenly sensitive to physiognomies, and had a definite relation to their mothers, mostly one of clinging dependence. None showed the isolation, obsessiveness, and fragmentation of interests typical of early infantile autism. Certainly, there are enough autistic children who have amazingly large vocabularies; one patient who was brought to me from South Africa could speak English, French, and Afrikaans. Even some of the mute children have astounded their parents by uttering well-formed sentences in emergency situations. One 5-year-old boy, who had never been heard to pronounce one articulate word in his life, became distressed when the skin of a prune stuck to his palate. He exclaimed distinctly, "Take it out of there!" and then resumed his muteness. Another mute boy, 4 years old, was examined in a pediatrician's office and was annoyed by the physical contact. He cried out, "Want to go home!" About a year later, when left in a hospital because of bronchitis, he was heard saying, "Want to go back!" These—and other—examples are convincing proof that even the mute autistic children do not suffer from either sensory or motor aphasia. Those who eventually begin to talk give evidence that during the silent period they have accumulated a considerable store of readily available linguistic material.

The extreme emotional isolation from other people, which is the foremost characteristic of early infantile autism, bears so close a resemblance to schizophrenic withdrawal that the relationship between the two conditions deserves serious consideration. My first observations impressed me with the difference from the current experiences with, and concept of, childhood schizophrenia. The second of nine criteria presented by Bradley, as a result of his review of the literature, postulated: "His (the patient's) mental disorder must have appeared without known or obvious cause after a period in earlier life when he was comparatively free from mental disorder." This criterion does not apply to early infantile autism. The disturbance, though commonly misjudged at first, is apparent as early as in the second half-year of life. The infants seem unusually apathetic, do not react to the approach of people, fail to assume an anticipatory posture preparatory to being picked up and, when they are picked up, do not adjust their posture to the person who holds them. They shrink from anything that encroaches on their isolation: persons, noises, moving objects, and often even food. They seem happiest when left alone. Persistent lack of responsiveness raises doubts about the child's hearing acuity. When it becomes obvious that hearing as such is not impaired, poor test performances lead to the assumption of innate feeblemindedness. This succession of a first diagnosis of deafness and a second diagnosis of mental deficiency is almost invariably a part of the case histories of autistic children. It indicates that a disturbance of relationships has been recognized by the parents from an early date. There is no period in the child's development in which there has been a comparatively normal adjustment.

In view of this beginning, the question arises: Must we assume that early infantile autism represents a syndrome which is not in any way related to the known psychopathologic patterns, or are we justified in correlating the essential features of the syndrome with the essential features of a condition which it most closely resembles, namely, schizophrenia?

After the publication of my first report, I received a very thoughtful letter from Dr. Louise Despert. I should like to quote from it. She wrote: "If, leaving aside the nature of etiology, we agree on the descriptive definition of schizophrenia as a withdrawal of affect from reality, then where are we going to draw the line? At adolescence? During pre-adolescent years? During childhood? In early childhood years? Obviously the symptoms which are an expression of the withdrawal of affect must vary according to the developmental level and the structure of personality at various age levels. It cannot be accidentally that the symptoms described by you have an almost word-for-word similarity with the symptoms which I, for instance, have described regarding the language-sign and language function, the fear of noise, the compulsive acts, the need for things to be the same, etc." In a later, equally thoughtful letter, Dr. Despert stated: "You certainly have clearly and concisely defined a clinical entity which had baffled many observers. It (the report) will do much to bring order and clarity in the confused mass of mental illnesses of the earliest years. Whether or not the similarities with the previously described schizophrenia in childhood should be later established, is an issue to be resolved after further study."

Further study has prompted the following considerations:

1. Early infantile autism is a well-defined syndrome which an experienced observer has little difficulty in recognizing in the course of the first two years of the life of the patient.

2. The basic nature of its manifestations is so intimately related to the basic nature of childhood schizophrenia as to be indistinguishable from it, especially from the cases with insidious onset discussed by Ssucharewa, Grebelskaya-Albatz, and Despert.

3. Nevertheless, one can hardly speak of an insidious onset of early infantile autism, except perhaps with reference to the first semester of life. By that time, or slightly later, the withdrawal, the detachment, the disability to relate to people are accomplished phenomena. There may be a slow onset of the ability to recognize the child's behavior for what it represents but the condition as such is unquestionably there.

4. Early infantile autism may therefore be looked upon as the earliest possible manifestation of childhood schizophrenia. As such, because of the age at the time of the withdrawal, it presents a clinical picture which has certain characteristics of its own, both at the start and in the course of later development. I have tried to do justice to this by including the discussion of early infantile autism in the schizophrenia chapter of the rewritten edition of my textbook of *Child Psychiatry* (published in 1948), at the same time acknowledging its special features by dealing with it under a special subheading.

5. I do not believe that there is any likelihood that early infantile autism will at any future time have to be separated from the schizophrenias, as was the case with Heller's disease or with many instances of so-called dementia praecocissima of De Sanctis.

6. Nosologically, therefore, the great importance of the group which I have described as early infantile autism lies in the correction of the impression that a comparatively normal period of adjustment must precede the development of schizophrenia. Furthermore, this group shows that schizophrenic withdrawal can and does begin as early as in the diaper stage. It also confirms the observation, made of late by many authors, that childhood schizophrenia is not so rare as was believed as recently as twenty years ago.

These points should take care of the first of two postulates regarding a psychopathologic syndrome, to wit, its nosological allocation. The second postulate calls for etiological orientation.

Not one of the 55 patients studied has had in his infancy any disease or physical injury to which his behavior could be possibly ascribed by any stretch of the imagination. Only one began having convulsions at the age of 4 years and had a correspondingly abnormal electroencephalogram. All others remained physically healthy, except for mild colds, children's diseases, and minor ailments. There was nothing which could be interpreted as encephalitis or other cerebal illness. Endocrine functioning was unimpaired. There were no cogenital abnormalities of the body. On the whole, the children were well formed, well developed, rather slender, and attractive. The absence of allergies, asthma, urticarial and eczematous skin eruptions may be incidental but is certainly worth mentioning.

It is customary to evaluate the hereditary element in the schizophrenias. Such an inquiry into the ancestral background of the autistic children is entirely fruitless if one limits the investigation to overtly psychotic or hospitalized relatives. It is indeed remarkable that, with the exception of the paternal aunt of one of the children, there is no history of psychosis, at least of committable mental disorder, in any of the antecedents. There is no instance of schizophrenia, manic-depressive psychosis, or even senile psychosis among the parents, grandparents, uncles, and aunts of the autistic children.

It is even more remarkable that almost all adult relatives have been rather successful in their chosen careers. The fathers are scientists, college professors, artists, clergymen, business executives; there are a few psychologists and psychiatrists among them. Many of the fathers, grandfathers, and uncles are listed in some of the *Who's Who* compilations or in *American Men of Science*. All but five of the mothers of the 55 children have attended college. All but one have been active vocationally before, and some also after, marriage as scientists, laboratory technicians, nurses, physicians, librarians, or artists. One mother who was not a college graduate was a busy and well-known theatrical agent in New York City. One, who has a Ph.D. degree, collaborated in the publication of a Middle English dictionary. One stated: "I majored in zoology and could have majored in music. I play the organ, piano, and cello. I wanted to be a doctor but my family didn't have the stamina. I have often regretted it. I taught school for two years, then worked in an endocrinology laboratory."

My search for autistic children of unsophisticated parents has remained unsuccessful to date. This astounding fact has created a curiosity about the personalities of the parents, their attitudes and resulting behavior toward the patients, and the possible relationship between these factors and the presence and structure of the children's psychopathologic manifestations.

It is admittedly a hazardous undertaking to try to present a composite characterization of any group of individuals. There will always be variations and fluctuations within the group, and one person or another will stand out in sharp contrast to such an extent that the uniform application of any general statement will be jeopardized. This has always been the bane of many a statistical approach to the evaluation of personality traits.

Nevertheless, aside from the indisputably high level of intelligence, the vast majority of the parents of the autistic children have features in common which it would be impossible to disregard. The oustanding attributes may be summed up as follows:

One is struck again and again by what I should like to call a mechanization of human relationships. Most of the parents declare outright that they are not comfortable in the company of people; they prefer reading, writing, painting, making music, or just "thinking." Those who speak of themselves as sociable tend to qualify this by explaining that they have no use for ordinary chatter. They are, on the whole, polite and dignified people who are impressed by seriousness and disdainful of anything that smacks of frivolity.

They describe themselves and their marital partners as undemonstrative. This adjective and all that it implies is not offered apologetically by the parent as it refers to himself or herself, nor in any way critically as it refers to the spouse. Often parents of other children brought because of emotional problems complain with some bitterness about the husband's or wife's lack of outward show of affection. The parents of autistic children do not seem to mind. Matrimonial life is a rather cold and formal affair. There is no glamor of romance in premarital courtship, no impetuousness in postnuptial mating. On the other hand, there are no major animosities. There has been only one separation or divorce of any of the 55 couples. The parents treat each other with faultless respect, talk things over calmly and earnestly, and give to outsiders the impression of mutual loyalty. So far as can be ascertained, there are no extramarital sex relations. One father, ready after much persuasion to yield to the temptations of an amateur actress, suddenly found himself sexually impotent; he went home, told his wife about it, and it was she who, without rancor, asked me for suggestions in a long-distance telephone call.

The parents' behavior toward the children must be seen to be fully appreciated. Maternal lack of genuine warmth is often conspicuous in the first visit to the clinic. As they come up the stairs, the child trails forlornly behind the mother, who does not bother to look back. The mother accepts the invitation to sit down in the waiting room, while the child sits, stands, or wanders about at a distance. Neither makes a move toward the other. Later, in the office, when the mother is asked under some pretext to take the child on her lap, she usually does so in a dutiful, stilted manner, holding the child upright and using her arms solely for the mechanical purpose of maintaining him in his position. I saw only one mother of an autistic child who proceeded to embrace him warmly and bring her face close to his. Some time ago, I went to see an autistic child, the son of a brilliant lawyer. I spent an evening with the family.

Donald, the patient, sat down next to his mother on the sofa. She kept moving away from him as though she could not bear the physical proximity. When Donald moved along with her, she finally told him coldly to go and sit on a chair.

Many of the fathers hardly know their autistic children. They are outwardly friendly, admonish, teach, observe "objectively," but rarely step down from the pedestal of somber adulthood to indulge in childish play. One father, a busy and competent surgeon, had three children. The first, a girl, was docile, submissive, and gave no cause for concern to the parents. The second, a boy, was very insecure and stuttered badly. The third, George, was an extremely withdrawn, typically autistic child. The father, who once told me proudly that he never wasted his time talking to his patients' relatives, did not see anything wrong with George, who was merely "a little slow" and would "catch up" eventually. When nothing could shake this man's smiling impassiveness, I tried to arouse his anger by asking him if he would recognize any of his children if they passed him on a busy street. Far from being irked, he deliberated for a while and replied, just as impassively, that he was not sure that he would. This seemingly unemotional objectivity, applied to oneself and to others, is a frequent expression of the mechanization of human relationships.

The void created by the absence of wholehearted interest in people is occupied by a devotion to duty. Most of the fathers are, in a sense, bigamists. They are wedded to their jobs at least as much as they are married to their wives. The job, in fact, has priority. Many of the fathers remind one of the popular conception of the absent-minded professor who is so engrossed in lofty abstractions that little room is left for the trifling details of everyday living. Many of the fathers and most of the mothers are perfectionists. Obsessive adherence to set rules serves as a substitute for the enjoyment of life. These people, who themselves had been reared sternly in emotional refrigerators, have found at an early age that they could gain approval only through unconditional surrender to standards of perfection. It is interesting that, despite their high intellectual level, not one of the parents has displayed any really creative abilities. They make good teachers in the sense that they can transmit that which they have learned. They are essentially conservative repeaters of that which they have been taught. This is not quite true of many of the grandfathers, some of whom have established flourishing businesses, expounded original theories, or produced fairly successful pieces of fiction and art. One grandfather, whose recently published autobiography tells of a life of uncanny versatility, was at various times a medical missionary, professor of tropical medicine, dean of a large medical school, curator of an art museum, manganese mining engineer, novelist, painter who exhibited in Paris, the representative of a sewing machine firm and, if this also is an achievement, pretty much of a Don Juan. One of his sons is a much-read novelist, another the author of adventure and horror stories, and a third a radio news commentator. His daughter is a singer. Our patient's father, who is the second of the five children, is a plant pathologist, a very conscientious and reliable scientist.

The obsessiveness of the parents of the autistic children was a veritable boon to me with regard to the case histories. Few children have ever been observed by their parents with such minute precision. Every smallest detail of the child's development, utterances, and activities had either been recorded in voluminous diaries or were remembered by heart. The parents recalled the exact number of words which the child knew at a certain time, the exact number of nursery rhymes the children could recite, the exact body weights at specified intervals. Even the surgeon who was not certain that he would recognize his children if he met them on the street knew promptly and correctly all about the patient's developmental data.

But the same obsessiveness was a major contribution to the impersonal, mechanized relation with the children. The parents, apparently unable to derive enjoyment from the children as they are, work for the attainment of goodness, obedience, quiet, good eating, earliest possible control of elimination, large vocabularies, memory feats. One father had the ambition to see his son walk alone at the age of 3 months; he held the baby up and moved his legs forward. Another procured Compton's *Encyclopedia* for his 2-year-old son and noted with pride that, while the child was progressively withdrawing from contact with people, he could identify all the pictures by name.

The child is essentially the object of an interesting experiment and can be put aside when he is not needed for this purpose. While in most instances this is justified by the parent on the basis of some form of rationalization, one couple made this their conscious and deliberate endeavor. The father was a business manager of whom his wife said: "He is the best-natured person you'll ever find; he is only interested in business." The mother was a graduate nurse. When they had two children, a boy and a girl, they felt that they had done their duty by society and posterity. An "accidental" third pregnancy came as a great inconvenience. The mother's fleeting thought of an induced abortion was counteracted by the firm determination to rear "a perfect baby." She decided that, to achieve this goal, she should leave Patricia alone and give her no more attention than was deemed necessary for obsessively regulated feeding and change of diapers. The baby seemed to reward her fully. She cried very little after the first few weeks of intensive yammering, gave no further trouble, took her bottle mechanically, and submitted passively to manipuation. She showed no anticipatory reaction to being picked up (something that happened very rarely). The first intimation that all was not well came to the parents when the child was 13 months old and they returned from a trip which had taken them away from home for several days. Patricia did not even look up when they came close to her and, when touched, seemed "stiff and indifferent." When seen at our clinic at 5½ years, she was extremely withdrawn, obsessive, had a phenomenal memory for names, was "marvelous with blocks," and could, as the mother reported, identify by name ten of the fifty victrola records which the parents had. They would turn on a record and the child would say: "Scheherazade—Rimsky-Korsakoff." She did not use speech for the purpose of communication. There was typical reversal of pronouns. The parents concluded reluctantly that their experiment had not worked.

It can be said only of several of the children that they were rejected in the sense in which this term is commonly understood. The majority of the children were not unwanted; the pregnancy as such was not unwelcome. Childbearing was an accepted part of the parents' conception of matrimony. No contraceptive precautions were taken, and there was not even a fleeting thought of abortion. The children were, as modern phraseology usually has it, "planned and wanted." Yet the parents did not seem to know what to do with the children when they had them. They lacked the warmth which the babies needed. The children did not seem to fit into their established scheme of living. The mothers felt duty-bound to carry out to the letter the rules and regulations which they were given by their obstetricians and pediatricians. They were anxious to do a good job, and this meant mechanized service of the kind which is rendered by an overconscientious gasoline station attendant.

One New England mother, a Methodist minister's only child, who had studied child psychology and majored in English and music, taught school before marriage but was unhappy because it was a progressive school and she was a strong believer in discipline. She shared with the late George Apley an interest in "birds." She never held a bird in her hand. She "roamed around" and made notes, referring to her excursions as "observation trips," which she identified both by dates and ordinal numbers. She married a Harvard graduate chemist whose description of himself as an introvert was offered with a bland smile. They decided that it was the proper thing to have a child. Said the mother at the clinic: "I felt it was my duty to have a child, and we planned to have him. I am not very attached to children, it upsets me when he cries; maybe I should have a sympathetic nerve cut. I am more interested in my birds than I am in people."

The arrival of the child reduced the number of her ornithologic excursions and because of this she "felt resentment" against him; though she added: "Of course, I am always glad to see him when I come back from my trips." She ministered painstakingly to the baby's material needs and took care of the rest by reading to him from books on bird lore. When he was seen at the clinic at slightly more than 2½ years of age, he was oblivious to people but performed skillfully with blocks, was amazingly adroit in spinning objects, was repetitious in his activities, and seemed happy and pensive when left alone but became very much upset when the slightest attempt was made to interfere with his privacy.

I have dwelt at some length on the personalities, attitudes, and behavior of the parents because they seem to throw considerable light on the dynamics of the children's psychopathologic condition. Most of the patients were exposed from the beginning to parental coldness, obsessiveness, and a mechanical type of attention to material needs only. They were the objects of observation and experiment conducted with an eye on fractional performance rather than with genuine warmth and enjoyment. They were kept neatly in refrigerators which did not defrost. Their withdrawal seems to be an act of turning away from such a situation to seek comfort in solitude.

I believe that the children's memory feats, their obsessive preoccupation with names, watches, maps or calendar dates represent a plea for parental approval. The children, who have good cognitive endowment, find that their parents encourage such performances. How else would a 3-year-old be able to name all the Presidents and Vice-Presidents, to recite 37 nursery rhymes (counted by the parents), or to rattle off 25 questions and answers of the Presbyterian catechism, at an age when these things have no semantic value to him? The obsessiveness at the same time seems to serve another function. While an obsessive adult tries to fight his ruminative needs out with himself, the autistic children, who otherwise have little dealing with the parents, force them with the tyranny of temper outbursts to participate in their sometimes very elaborate obsessive-compulsive schemes. This seems to me to serve as an opportunity—the only available opportunity—for retaliation.

I wish to repeat, in conclusion, that I have presented a composite picture, got together from the case histories and observation of 55 autistic children and their parents. There were very few exceptions, but the existence of these exceptions is puzzling. One is also entitled to wonder why some of these parents have been able to rear other children who did not withdraw. Furthermore, I have seen parent couples who answered the above characterization to the fullest extent, yet whose offspring, far from withdrawing autistically, responded with restless aggressiveness. It is not easy to account for this difference of reaction. It is also very tempting to ponder about the psychodynamic relationship between early infantile autism, schizophrenia of later childhood, and the "hospitalism" studied by Goldfarb. Further, do not the personalities of the parents indicate that there are milder degrees of detachment and obsessiveness which enable a person to function and even gain a certain type of success in a nonpsychotic existence? These are highly important questions which await much further thought and study.†

REFERENCES

Corberi, G. Sindromi di regressione mentale infanto-giovanile. *Revista di patologia nervosa e mentale,* 1962, **31**, 6–45.

De Sanctis, S. *Neuropsichiatria infantile.* Rome: Stock, 1925.

Despert, J. L. Schizophrenia in children. *Psychiatric Quarterly,* 1938, **12**, 366–371.

Goldfarb, H. Effects of psychological deprivation in infancy and subsequent stimulation. *American Journal of Psychiatry,* 1945, **102**, 18–33.

Grebelskaya-Albatz, E. Zur klinik der schizophrenie des frühen kindesalters. *Schweizerisches Archiv für Neurologie und Psychiatrie,* 1934, **34**, 274–283.

Grebelskaya-Albatz, E. Zur klinik der schizophrenie des frühen kindesalters. *Schweizerisches Archiv für Neurologie und Psychiatrie,* 1935, **35**, 30–40.

Heller, T. Über dementia infantilis. *Archiv für Kinderheilkunde,* 1930, **37**, 661–667.

Kanner, L. Autistic disturbances of affective contact. *Nervous Child,* 1943, **2**, 217–250.

Kanner, L. Early infantile autism. *Journal of Pediatrics,* 1944, **25**, 211–217.

Kanner, L. Irrelevant and metaphorical language in early infantile autism. *American Journal of Psychiatry,* 1946, **103**, 242–245.

Ssucharewa, G. Über den verlauf der schizophrenien im kindesalter. *Zeitschrifte für die gesamte Neurologie und Psychiatrie,* 1932, **142**, 309–321.

Zappert, J. Dementia infantilis (Heller). *Zeitschrift für Kinderpsychiatrie,* 1938, **4**, 161–169.

†Reset from the original published in *American Journal of Orthopsychiatry,* Volume 19, pp. 416–426, 1949.

1950's

4

THE CONCEPTION OF WHOLES
AND PARTS IN EARLY
INFANTILE AUTISM

The peculiarities of early infantile autism and its close relation to the schizophrenias invite a detailed study of the various features of the illness. A previous investigation of apparently irrelevant speech and metaphoric utterances yielded highly instructive material. In this study, an attempt is made to learn how these patients view their world in terms of appraising and integrating their surroundings.

The autistic child desires to live in a static world, a world in which no change is tolerated. The status quo must be maintained at all cost. Only the child himself may sometimes take it upon himself to modify existing combinations. But no one else may do so without arousing unhappiness and anger. It is remarkable to what extent the children will go to assure the preservation of sameness. The totality of an experience that comes to the child from the outside must be reiterated, often with all its constituent details, in complete photographic and phonographic identity. No one part of this totality may be altered in terms of shape, sequence, or space. The slightest change of arrangement, sometimes so minute that it is hardly perceived by others, may evoke a violent outburst of rage.

This behavior differs from ordinary obsessive ritualism in one significant respect: The autistic child forces the people in his world to be even more obsessive than he is himself. While he may make occasional concessions, he does not grant this privilege to others. He is a stern and unrelenting judge and critic. When one watches such a child for any length of time, it becomes evident that, unless he is completely alone, most of his activities go into the job of serious, solemn, sacerdotal enforcement of the maintenance of sameness, of absolute identity.

It is, of course, impossible to live even in Kaspar Hauser fashion without the introduction of new situations. A child is weaned from the breast, then from the bottle; new food stuffs are introduced; he is taken out for his first walk; the family may move to a different location; he learns new songs and nursery rhymes, is given new toys.

The reports of the parents of our autistic children indicate, indeed, how exceedingly difficult it is to "teach" them these, or any, innovations. One may even say that these children learn while they resist being taught. Several children kept on crawling at a time when the parents felt that they could be walking. Much effort was expended in propping them up and encouraging them to make steps. There was no success. But one day, suddenly, when it was least expected, the children got up and walked. The parents of Frederick W. spent hours each day "teaching" him to talk. They begged him to repeat words after them. He remained "mute," except for two words ("Daddy" and "Dora") that he had never been taught to say. But one day, at about 2½ years of age, he spoke up and said: "Overalls," a word which was decidedly not a part of the teaching repertoire.

But once a new acquisition has been made or a new situation incorporated in the child's routine, he clings to it with exasperating tenacity and watches over its unaltered reproduction. This pertains to things said to him as well as to things done to him.

The mother of Joseph C. stated: "If I have read a story [to him] and used some pronunciation, his daddy has to do it the same way; else he is upset about it."

Since the whole must be preserved in its entirety, the children become greatly disturbed at the sight of anything broken or incomplete. The sight of a broken cross-bar on a garage door that he passed on his regular daily walk so upset Charles N. that he kept talking and asking about it for weeks on end, even while spending a few days in a distant city and even after the cross on the bar had been fixed.

Among the toys laid out for John F. were two dolls, one of which had a cap, while the other was bareheaded. Generally, John paid little or no attention to dolls. When he noticed that the cap of one of the dolls was missing, he immediately asked for "the hat," picked up the doll and ran up and down with it, shouting for the hat. He was not reassured until the cap was produced. He made sure that it fitted, then put the doll down and lost all interest in it.

Susan T. noticed some cracks in the office ceiling and walls. She kept asking anxiously and repeatedly who had cracked the ceiling and could not be calmed by any answer given her. She was obviously unhappy and every time she was in the office, she kept exclaiming: "Who cracked the ceiling?" "How did it crack itself?" Anthony F. became aware of the same cracks and asked almost literally the same questions as Susan. He touched some of the cracks within his reach and said, very seriously: "I don't know whether it's right or not—the wall."

People as well as objects must be "whole." A visible scar or wart evokes instant comment. There is no sympathy, no solicitude for the person as such. The attitude is rather one of annoyance—again not with the person but with the fact itself. Susan T., on the train, became upset and talked obsessively about "that one man sleeping with an open mouth." When a taxi driver cleared his throat, she kept asking him: "Did you have phlegm in your throat?" While she was fully absorbed and seemingly inaccessible in the office, I happened to clear my throat. Susan instantly looked up and asked: "What was that?"

Once blocks, beads, or sticks have been put together by the child in a certain way, they are often regrouped later in exactly the same way, even though there was no definite design. The children's memory is phenomenal in this respect. After the lapse of several days, a multitude of blocks could be rearranged, most astonishingly by Donald T. and Susan T., in precisely the same unorganized pattern, with the same color of each block turned up, with each picture or letter on the upper surface of each block facing in the same direction as before. The absence of a block or the presence of a supernumerary block was noticed immediately, and there was an imperative demand for the restoration of the missing piece. If someone removed a block, the child struggled to get it back, hitting the hand which held it and going into a crescendo panic tantrum until he regained it, and then promptly and with sudden calm after the storm returned to the design and replaced the block.

At home, the furniture arrangement, the location of bed and high chair, the position of the dishes on the table must not be changed. Frederick W.'s mother reported: "On one of the bookshelves we had three pieces in a certain arrangement. When this was changed, he always rearranged it in the old pattern." Herbert B. "wants the same arrangement at the dining table, the same dishes; if he notices changes, he is very fussy and cries." Jay S. "is very fussy about where things go, for instance, a certain tea set; he fusses till it is put right, cups, handles, etc.,–just so." Joseph C. even "sees to it that the coal bucket is always turned in the same certain position." Gary T.'s father related: "Everything must be put in its proper place. He insists on closet doors being closed, rugs being straightened. He is very upset if the table order is changed and makes an effort to bring it back to the pattern he knows. He has a plaque of a sandman over his bed, of which he is very fond; it was moved to another wall but he moved it right back. The furniture was rearranged lately and it bothers him. We bought him a new bed, and he was looking for the old one." Gary originally lived in Philadelphia; the family then moved to Greenbelt, to Chicago, and back to Greenbelt. At 5½ years, about 3 years since they had left Philadelphia, he still kept saying insistently: "Let's go back to the old house," meaning the home in Philadelphia, which he could describe in every detail. Richard F.'s high chair "always has to be in a certain place." Susan T.'s father said: "When we would sit down on a certain chair on which another member of the family usually sits, she would scream." Stephen N. "just can't stand things different from their usual appearance; for example, if my dress slips over my knee, he will pull it down."

Joseph C. had a definite notion about the arrangement of the parts of human bodies. While being observed, he at once became aware of an assistant's foot up on a chair. He became upset and rushed to the chair, saying: "Down, down," took her leg and put it down. When she put it up again, he repeated the procedure. He also became upset when a person had the legs crossed. He objected to hands being on the table or a person resting the chin on a hand. He demanded: "Down, down," and if his wish was not complied with, he became agitated and tried forcibly to bring the limbs into the position that seemed proper to him. Feet belonged on the floor, and arms alongside the trunk; no deviation was tolerated. He saw me smoke a cigar; he did not seem to notice it so long as the cigar was in my mouth. When I held it in my hand, he took my hand and pointed to my mouth, indicating that the cigar should be there. When he did not get his wish, he impatiently pulled the cigar out of my hand, pushed it between my lips, drew my hands down, and placidly turned to other pursuits.

Anthony F. was given the Seguin form board test, which he completed in 25 seconds. But he became disgusted with the star-shaped form. While quickly fitting it in the appropriate space, he said: "Star, you are bad." He took it out, hit it violently, and shouted: "Stay up in the sky!" He returned to the form board several times afterwards and each time again became angry at the wooden "star" which was not up in the sky. He was then presented with the Healy Picture Completion set. He picked out the clock, found the right place for it, put it there with considerable anger and vehemence and said to it: "Stay there, you." He then had some difficulty in fitting the other pieces. This disturbed him very much. At first he "revenged himself" by squeezing the pieces wherever they would go, laughing uneasily and uproariously. Then he no longer could stand it, suddenly got up, ran to the door and, slamming it, went out, saying: "I think I go."

Malcolm H. liked to sit for hours turning the pages of books and magazines. Once he saw a picture in an encyclopedia and asked his mother what it was. She said that it was the Taj Mahal in India. He then went through the whole library for days looking for another picture of "India" (the Taj Mahal), really found two (one in a book on India, the other in a volume on architecture), and recognized them even though one was much smaller and the other was presented from a different angle. But he was very unhappy because of these differences, growing steadily unhappier and more agitated when further search proved unproductive. He finally found solace in getting the encyclopedia and looking at the picture he had seen there first.

The retention of sequences is as important to the children as the maintenance of appearances and space relations. Malcolm H., when taken for a walk, "insists on covering the same ground that has been covered on previous walks, resisting strongly any change in the route." Stephen N.'s mother stated: "Daily walks, when changed, used to make him furious; now he can be persuaded with some difficulty to go in a different direction." Richard F.'s father gives him a bath every night: "They go through a ritual. When I [the mother] give him a bath, he pulls me to show me what to do next. If the things on his bed aren't just right he won't go to bed." When Elaine C. was sent to fetch a specific object, she always brought it if it was in the place where she knew it usually to be; if it was not there, she would not bring it even if it was very near and plainly visible. If Herbert B.'s bath time was changed in relation to supper, he became very upset; usually he got his bath after supper. Of John F., his father said: "The daily routine, the route taken on the daily walks with his mother, the succession of events must be repeated in the same manner. Any change, even the slightest, gives rise to unhappiness and temper on his part." Donald T. would not leave his bed after his nap until after he had said: "Boo, say: Don, do you want to get down?" and his mother (whom he called "Boo") had complied. Donald then climbed out of bed. But this was not all; the act was not considered completed. Donald continued: "Now say: 'All right.'" Again the mother had to comply, or there was screaming until the performance had run its prescribed course.

The same Donald T., at 9½ years of age, had been "going to school" since he was 6 years old; a school principal friend of the mother's had agreed to let him attend. On one afternoon, the session had been dispensed with; no one in the family knew about this. Donald went to school as usual. Though no other child was in the classroom, he sat down in his seat, took out his books, did some writing, and left when the bell rang. He evidently could not accept an "irregular" free afternoon contrary to established routine. The part had to be made to fit in with the accustomed whole, regardless of whether or not the teacher and the classmates chose to disrupt the ordinary sequence of events.

In summary, it can be said that autistic children show a peculiar type of obsessiveness that forces them to postulate imperiously a static, unchanged environment. Any modification meets with perplexity and major discomfort. The patients find security in sameness, a security that is very tenuous because changes do occur constantly and the children are therefore threatened perpetually and try tensely to ward off this threat to their security.†

References

Kanner, L. Autistic disturbances of affective contact. *Nervous Child,* 1943, **2**, 217–250.

Kanner, L. Early infantile autism. *Journal of Pediatrics,* 1944, **25**, 211–217.

Kanner, L. Irrelevant and metaphorical language in early infantile autism. *American Journal of Psychiatry,* 1946, **103**, 242–246.

Kanner, L. Problems of nosology and psychodynamics in early infantile autism. *American Journal of Orthopsychiatry,* 1949, **19**, 416–426.

5

TO WHAT EXTENT IS EARLY INFANTILE AUTISM DETERMINED BY CONSTITUTIONAL INADEQUACIES ?

Early infantile autism was singled out in 1938 as a psychotic illness presenting a set of characteristics worthy of special consideration. The first observations were reported in 1943. Since then, a sufficient number of patients has been studied in this country and abroad to substantiate the uniqueness of the syndrome. Our own case material (Kanner, 1944, 1946, 1949, 1951) now comprises exactly 100 children who can be so diagnosed with reasonable certainty. The common denominator consists of certain essential features in a combination not encountered in any other disease.

The first signs are noticed some time during the first two years of life. It would be difficult to pinpoint an exact time of onset. It is probably safe to say that the emergence from the neonatal stage of biological helplessness is not, as in the average infant, accompanied by a progressively differentiated contact with the human environment. Many mothers recall that they have never been able to "reach" their child, who lay "apathetically" in his crib and did not display an infant's usual anticipatory reaction when someone came to pick him up. Persistent absence of response to verbal address has almost invariably created the suspicion of deafness, which was later dispelled by otological examination and other evidences of normal hearing acuity. As the child grew older, the lack of response to attempted psychometry gave the impression of a markedly inadequate intellectual endowment; it must, indeed, be assumed that, prior to the delineation of the syndrome, autistic children were regarded as severe mental defectives.

This early self-isolation has been compared to schizophrenic withdrawal. The analogy is not incorrect insofar as the clinical appearance is one of a child out of contact with the people about him. It is true that the histories of three or, at most, four of our patients indicate some preliminary reaching out of affective tentacles which were pulled in more or less abruptly within a few months before the end of the second year. But in most instances there never has been any real relationship with the mother or anybody else. The isolation is not so much an event or a process as it is a status, an existence, which the child strives anxiously to maintain. It might be better to speak of it as *aloneness* rather than as withdrawal. The patient is an unrelenting guardian of his privacy. When he is left to himself, he can be happy, smile, hum a tune, play with his toys. When there is interference, he disregards it as long as he can. When the intrusion becomes too insistent, he fights it off with tantrums which appear to be the result of panic rather than anger.

The autistic child, ever ready to fend off other persons' encroachments on his capsulated inner world, is equally fearful of happenings in his surroundings which might necessitate a readaptation—that is, a modification—on his part. Changes of routine, of the furniture arrangement in his room, of the accustomed route when he is taken for a walk can precipitate a major burst of deep distress. The sight of a broken toy, a crack in the wall, or some other deviation from completeness as conceived by the child can become a disturbing experience, long remembered and brooded over. The patient is extremely cautious in enlarging the scope of his activities, which are limited in number and repeated again and again. Resisting innovations, he struggles to live in a static world, and much of his behavior is governed by a powerful *desire for the preservation of sameness.*

Aloneness and obsessive insistence on sameness are the two principal diagnostic criteria of early infantile autism. All other symptoms can be explained on that basis. There is no felt need for communication. Some of the children have remained mute, though the rare utterances of a whole sentence in emergency situations certainly prove the ability to store up and use language. It takes the speaking children a long time before they enter upon anything resembling ordinary conversation. Parroted phrases are retained and later, in a sort of delayed echolalia, employed exactly as heard, even with the same intonation; this accounts for the phenomenon of pronominal reversals which persists for several years. Thus, when the child wishes to retire, he may echo a sentence used often by his mother: "Now *I* am going to put *you* to bed." Spontaneous language consists for a long time of rote enumerations and seemingly irrelevant utterances not intended for communication.

The child's relation to obects is better than that to persons. He can manipulate them in his own obsessive way. He is skillful and nimble in his handling of them. He has a phenomenal memory for arrangements and can after days reconstruct a complex block design. He can become angry at objects if they do not conform to his preconceived pattern. One of the children scolded the star-shaped piece of the Seguin form board because it was not up in the sky where stars belong.

Many are the peculiarities of autistic children. There are differences in degree and in the number and nature of accessory symptoms. But the developmental history and the two pathognomonic features of aloneness and insistence on sameness are always present and indispensable for the inclusion of any child in the category of early infantile autism.

There has been justified puzzlement about the nosological position of the autistic illness. Van Krevelen (1952a, 1952b) saw in it an "oligophrenia with concomitant emotional defects." This assumption can be disproved by the observation that a few of the patients, who functioned at an idiot or imbecile level in preschool age, achieved intelligence quotients of well over 100 in their early teens. The possibility of prenatal organic damage has been considered but thorough physical and laboratory examinations have yielded no consistent clue of any kind. The relation to schizophrenia is more difficult to determine; it is possible to regard early infantile autism as the earliest form of this illness, the specific features of which are influenced by the age at which they develop. Mahler (1952) has distinguished convincingly between an autistic and symbiotic form of infantile psychosis, depending on the type of mother-child relationship. For the time being, it seems practical to follow the advice given by Stern and Schachter (1953) to study autism as a specific phenomenon. At any rate, the inclusion of these children in any broader diagnostic group would seem at present to shove such a study out of focus and to ignore the developmental and symptomatic peculiarities.

Of the 100 children of our series, 80 were boys and 20 were girls. The number of published cases other than our own is too small to allow any comparisons. But the ratio of 4:1 in the largest existing collection certainly indicates a male predominance.

The vast majority is made up of children of either Anglo-Saxon or Jewish descent. Not less than 27 were of Jewish origin. There was only a small sprinkling of patients who came of Italian, French, German, Scotch, or Irish stock. Clarification of this issue may come in the not too distant future from the fact that observations, as yet too sporadic, are beginning to be reported from European countries.

No generalizations can be made on the basis of the patients' physical condition or the circumstances surrounding birth. Difficult labor was reported in 11 cases, precipitous in 2, prolonged in 7, and placenta praevia in 2. Four were delivered by caesarean section, and one sustained a fracture of an arm at birth. Difficulties in breathing were stated to be present in 3 of those and in 3 others who were delivered without mishap. As for congenital anomalies, one had a clubfoot, one had strabismus. One boy began having grand mal seizures at 5 years of age. Twelve were reported to have been premature; of these, 8 weighed less than 6 pounds at birth.

The position in the order of birth was distributed as follows: At the time when last seen, 15 were only children, 43 were first-born, 23 were second, 13 were third, and 6 were fourth or fifth.

A statistical evaluation of the role of heredity is not easy if one thinks exclusively in terms of psychotic illness. To assure maximal accuracy, we have, for the purpose of this investigation, limited ourselves to parents, grandparents, uncles and aunts, and siblings.

Of the 200 parents, only one had a major mental illness, a postpartum psychosis following the birth of her autistic child's older sibling. One mother and one father were alcoholics, and one, who has a responsible secretarial position, is epileptic. One father, a prominent lawyer, had twice interrupted his college studies because of anxiety neurosis. Another father, a well-known scientist, had convulsions in infancy and has marked digital tremors.

Of the 400 grandparents, a paternal grandfather, a paternal grandmother, and maternal grandfather committed suicide. One maternal grandmother had an unidentified "nervous breakdown" at 50 years, and one had Friedreich's ataxia. One maternal grandfather, a noted psychologist, was an obsessive-compulsive person, another had a "nervous breakdown" at 30 years.

The number of the parents' siblings and entries about their histories of major illnesses are contained in 70 of our case records. Of the 373 uncles and aunts thus accounted for, a maternal aunt and a paternal uncle were schizophrenic, one paternal and one maternal aunt were depressed, two maternal aunts were feebleminded, two others (sisters) had a fear of leaving home, a paternal uncle had a psychotic episode while in college, and a maternal uncle and a paternal uncle were hospitalized for mental illness the nature of which could not be specified by the informants. One maternal aunt was epileptic.

Thus, among 973 parents, grandparents, uncles and aunts, there were a total of 13 psychotic individuals, 2 alcoholics, 2 epileptics, and 2 mental defectives.

Of the children's own 131 siblings, 117 were considered normal. Of the others, one each had epilepsy, sensory aphasia, mental retardation, specific reading disability, celiac disease, and Christian-Schüller's disease. One is said to have perished from "thymus death." One can be designated as a psychopathic personality, and 2 were severe stutterers. It is significant that 3 of our patients have siblings who, though not seen in our clinic, could be diagnosed as autistic children; one has, in addition, a brother who shows marked schizoid tendencies in his behavior.

These figures indicate that, from a genetic point of view, it would be difficult to see a meaningful positive correlation between early infantile autism and the occurrence of psychiatric and neurological diseases in the patients' ancestries. However, our attention has been drawn to certain items which seem to us to be of great significance.

The autistic children come from intelligent, sophisticated stock. Of the 100 fathers, 96 were high school graduates. Of these 87 had been to college, 74 were college graduates, and 38 had postgraduate training. Two of the 4 who did not finish high school were immigrants from countries in which their poor economic condition precluded secondary schooling; the father of one of them became municipal band leader in a large city. As regards occupations, there were 31 businessmen, 12 engineers, 11 physicians (including 5 psychiatrists), 10 lawyers, 8 tradesmen, 5 chemists, 5 army or navy officers, 4 writers, 3 Ph.D.'s in the sciences, 2 Ph.D.'s in the humanities, 2 teachers, 2 rabbis, and one each a psychologist, a dentist, a publisher, a forester, and a photographer.

Of the mothers, 92 were high school graduates. Of these, 70 had been to college, 49 were college graduates, and 11 had postgraduate training. Not less than 70 had been active in a variety of endeavors and some continued their occupations after marriage. There were 17 secretaries, 16 teachers, 6 business women, 6 librarians, 4 artists, 4 social workers, 3 writers, 3 nurses, 3 telephone operators, 2 psychologists, and one each a physician, a lawyer, a chemist, a Ph.D. in the humanities, a physiotherapist, and a laboratory technician.

To this day, we have not encountered any one autistic child who came of unintelligent parents. This fact gains added meaning if the personalities of the parents are subjected to careful scrutiny. Even though a study of this nature seems to elude the requirements for statistical deposition, it is safe to say that at least 85 per cent of the fathers and mothers present similar characterological features of a specific nature. Much caution has gone into the evaluation which resulted in the establishment of this percentage figure. It is, further, necessary to mention that in every one of the 100 cases at least one of the parents conforms to these characterological criteria.

As a rule, the parents of our autistic children are cold, humorless perfectionists; a general description of their personalities and interaction with children has been presented elsewhere (Kanner, 1949; see also this volume pp. 51 to 62). This picture of the parents' personalities was drawn and reported originally on the basis of the observation of the first 55 cases. Now that we have seen almost twice as many patients, it emerges with even greater consistency and clarity.

It has been said that the described parental behavior toward the autistic children could be merely an understandable reaction to the offspring's isolation and lack of response. It is, indeed, easy to see that it would be impossible for anyone to maintain a satisfactory relationship with an infant whose aloneness brushes off attempts at creating a feeling of togetherness. But the fact remains that these parents *are* the kind of detached people that they are, and that they would be known as such even if they had never had an autistic child. There is a resemblance between their make-up and that of their children, except that their aloofness has not reached the gross proportions of a psychotic illness. One is tempted to think of them as successfully autistic adults, in the sense that they do a creditable job in their chosen occupations and quite a few have attained sufficient recognition to be listed in some of the *Who's Who* compilations.

CONCLUSIONS

1. Physical and laboratory examinations have failed to furnish any consistent clues regarding the constitutional background of early infantile autism.

2. There is, in the families of autistic children, a remarkable paucity of psychoses and handicapping neuroses. Considerably fewer than 5% have progenitors or other kin who can be so designated.

3. The autistic children come from intelligent, sophisticated stock. Not less than 94 per cent of the parents, both fathers and mothers, are high school graduates; 74 per cent of the fathers and 49 per cent of the mothers have completed college.

4. The vast majority of the parents, though competent in their chosen vocations, are cold, detached, humorless perfectionists, more at home in the realm of abstractions than in the world of people. They deal with their fellow men on the basis of what one might call a mechanization of human relationships.

They treat their children about as meticulously and impersonally as they treat their automobiles.

5. The parents themselves have escaped the psychotic proportions of their offspring's aloneness and sterile obsessiveness. It is possible to speak of them as successfully autistic adults.

6. One is, therefore, led to think of a familial trend toward detached, obsessive, mechanical living. At the same time, it should not be forgotten that the emotional refrigeration which the children experience from such parents cannot but be a highly pathogenic element in the patients' early personality development, superimposed powerfully on whatever predisposition has come from inheritance.

7. These provocative findings warrant further research and classification.†

REFERENCES

Kanner, L. Autistic disturbances of affective contact. *Nervous Child,* 1943, **2**, 217–250.

Kanner, L. Early infantile autism. *Journal of Pediatrics,* 1944, **25**, 211–217.

Kanner, L. Irrelevant and metaphorical language in early infantile autism. *American Journal of Psychiatry,* 1946, **103**, 242–245.

Kanner, L. Problems of nosology and psychodynamics of early infantile autism. *American Journal of Orthopsychiatry,* 1949, **19**, 416–426.

Kanner, L. The conception of wholes and parts in early infantile autism. *American Journal of Psychiatry,* 1951, **108**, 23–26.

van Krevelen, D. A. Early infantile autism. *Zeitschrift fur Kinderpsychiatrie,* 1952, **19**, 91–97. (a)

van Krevelen, D. A. Een geval van early infantile autism. *Nederlands Tijdschrift voor Geneeskunde,* 1952, **96**, 202–205. (b)

Mahler, M. A. On child psychosis and schizophrenia. *The Psychoanalytic Study of the Child,* 1952, 7, 286–305.

Stern, E., & Schachter, M. Zum problem des frühkindlichen autismus. *Praxis der Kinderpsychologie und Kinderpsychiatrie,* 1953, 2, 113–118.

†Revised from the original published in *Genetics and the Inheritance of Integrated Neurological and Psychiatric Patterns,* edited by D. Hooker and C. C. Hare, pp. 378–385, 1954.

NOTES ON THE FOLLOW-UP STUDIES OF AUTISTIC CHILDREN

The syndrome of early infantile autism was first reported in 1943 under the heading, "autistic disturbances of affective contact." The eleven patients, who had been observed in the course of the preceding five years, showed characteristic peculiarities intrinsically similar to each other, yet different from any of the known psychopathologic patterns of infant and child behavior. The uniqueness of the symptom combination suggested as the first task an orienting study of the specific features and an attempt to view them not merely in enumerative juxtaposition but with an eye on their meaningful interconnection. The two principal *diagnostic criteria*, presenting themselves as extreme self-isolation and the obsessive insistence on sameness, could be recognized as the source from which the other clinical manifestations derived. One may, therefore, not unmindful of Bleuler's systematic grouping of schizophrenic

[1] Co-author: Leon Eisenberg, M.D.

phenomena, refer to the two consistent, pathognomonic matrices as "primary" and assign to the derivatives a position of "secondary" value. This is of major importance for purposes of the differentiation from other conditions in which a few corresponding behavior items may raise the question of nosologic allocation. In our experience, caution has been indicated, especially in some instances of congenital sensory aphasia, the incipient stages of Heller's disease, and—with increasing frequency—severe inherent intellectual deficiency with behavioral oddities bearing superficial resemblance to some of the "secondary" symptoms observed in the majority of our autistic patients.

A group of disturbed children was thus singled out whose distinctive design, not encountered in any other disease, called for some form of terminologic identification. The choice of the designation, "early infantile autism," was suggested by the unmistakable evidence of the typical symptoms in the first two years of life and the self-centered, at least in the beginning often impenetrable, aloneness. Since the initial publication, many more cases have come to our attention; at the time of this writing our material comprises 105 children. Additional observations were made and reported by Despert, Mahler, Rank, Weil, Murphy and others in this country, Cappon in Canada, Creak in England, Stern and Schachter in France, and van Krevelen in Holland.

We are justified in regarding the job of description and diagnostic formulation as reasonably accomplished. The details of the symptomatology—the detachment from people, the peculiarities of linguistic and motor performance, the type of relationship to objects, the conceptual fragmentation, the obsessive trends as shown through repetitiousness and ritualism—are well known and need not be reiterated. But once the matter of phenomenology had been settled, a number of significant issues arose which required further elucidation.

Paramount among them was the question of *etiology*. In this respect, no valid help came from the exploration of somatic factors; physical and laboratory examinations failed to furnish leading clues that might point to specific acquired or constitutional organic anomalies. A consideration of genetics, if confined to the incidence of psychoses and socially or vocationally handicapping neuroses, produced a figure of less than 5 per cent for progenitors and other kin, including collaterals. Our attention was directed to the undisputable fact that the patients came from intelligent, sophisticated stock: not less than 94 per cent of the parents, both fathers and mothers, were high school graduates and 74 per cent of the fathers and 49 per cent of the mothers had completed college. The majority of the parents, though competent in their chosen vocations, were cold, detached, humorless perfectionists, more at home in the world of abstractions than among people, dealing with their fellow men on the basis of what one might call a mechanization of human relationships; they themselves had escaped the psychotic proportions of their offsprings' aloneness and sterile obsessiveness. One is therefore led to think of a familial trend toward detached, obsessive, mechanical living. At the same time, it cannot be forgotten that the emotional refrigeration which the children experienced from such parents could not but be a highly pathogenic determinant of their early personality development, superimposed powerfully on whatever predisposition may have come through inheritance.

The *dynamic aspects* of the interplay between the patients and their parents have been made the focus of thoughtful investigation on the part of several authors. Three points of view have been put forth in the literature. One regards the parental behavior as a reaction to peculiarities which have existed *a priori*: the parent's personality has no etiologic significance and matters only insofar as it governs the nature of the response to the sick child's needs and demands. At the opposite pole, there is an insistence on considering the parents, and more especially the mother, as the basic source of pathogenicity; the assumption is that a healthier maternal attitude would have precluded the psychotic development of the child. A third group of investigators feels that the patient, endowed with an innate disability to relate himself to people, is further influenced adversely by the personality deviations of the parents and their resulting manner of handling him; this in no way discounts the possibility of a reciprocal relationship which, in turn, causes the parent to shrink from the child or to "overprotect" him in a more or less stilted fashion.

Similar divergencies exist also with regard to *nosology*. Van Krevelen argues that early infantile autism represents an "oligophrenia with affective defect." It is true that the solid barrier between mental deficiency and psychotic illness has been removed, or at least allowed to crumble, thanks to the efforts of Clemens Benda and others. It is also true that Weygandt, as far back as 1915, has described varieties of psychotic behavior in children thought to be idiotic or imbecile. Nevertheless, the observed fundamental differences between autistic and oligophrenic children cannot be simply dismissed as differently structured variants of essential feeblemindedness. Proceeding, therefore, on the conviction that early infantile autism is a true psychosis, the next issue was one of seeing whether it could be linked up with the category of childhood schizophrenia. Stern and Schachter suggest that, at least for the time being, it be kept apart as a syndrome *sui generis*. It certainly does present a picture of sufficient specificity to be sifted out and recognized as being unlike other psychotic behavior constellations, but there surely can be no objection to its inclusion in a broadly conceived framework of "schizophrenia." Differences in onset, content and course of schizophrenia in children have been discussed for some time. Ssucharewa and Grebelskaya-Albatz in Russia and Despert in this country have distinguished cases with acute onset and cases with insidious onset. After the publication of the first eleven cases of autism from our clinic, Despert and Mahler were among the first to study autistic children concurrently with our own work. It was Mahler who, on the basis of phenomenology and the nature of mother-child relationship, eventually worked out the helpful division between autistic and symbiotic infantile psychoses, presented in her excellent papers of 1949 and 1952.

Enough time has elapsed since the initial observation of many of our patients to enable us to follow their destinies over a period of years. It was felt that a follow-up study might throw some light on prognostic evaluations and, if subsequent events could be correlated with the absence or presence and mode of treatment, might give some indications of the most promising therapeutic approach to the problem. Letters were written to the parents or to the hospitals or residential schools in which the children were living. The age range at the time of this inquiry extended from 8 to 24 years (average of 14 years), the interval between the first acquaintance and the present from 4 to 19 years (average of 8½ years). The total number thus reached was 42. Wherever possible, a return visit was arranged and the patients examined again.

Before launching on a discussion of our data, we should like to mention a report by Darr and Worden about the condition of a woman 28 years after she had been seen (at 4 years of age) at the Henry Phipps Psychiatric Clinic by Drs. Meyer and Richards with what undoubtedly was an infantile autistic disorder. Even though no formal diagnosis was made, the child's behavior and the parents' personalities corresponded in every detail to the typical findings in early infantile autism. Dr. Richards wrote: "From the examination it seems probable that defectiveness and mental retardation are not responsible (or at least not wholly so) for the child's peculiar behavior. The mental picture seems to be more frankly that of a psychopathological condition characterized by preoccupation and impulsiveness." Dr. Meyer suggested "a natural, direct and affectionate handling without any pushing or undue demands." The mother carried this out by hiring people to take care of the child, who was placed in a home for special training; then spent three years in the care of a man interested in the treatment of the mentally ill; lived at home and was privately tutored for one year; from 10 to 17 she lived with a psychiatrist who looked after a number of problem children; then for about six years back home with her mother and—the father having died and the mother remarried—her stepfather. Following this, she was sent to live with a series of four companions during the next four years. She took piano and voice lessons, learned to speak Spanish fluently, and was able to take care of her personal needs. But at the same time, she lacked any intuitive social sense, had temper tantrums when thwarted, seemed most comfortable when she lived by precise routine, and showed marked hypochondriac tendencies which caused her to go into seclusion when contact with people became too upsetting. At the age of 27 years, she was sent to a school for disturbed children, but soon the authorities insisted that she be removed because of severe temper outbursts. She was transferred to another school, where she remained for two years. On a home visit for the Christmas holidays, there was an acutely psychotic exacerbation of her symptoms. Deep coma insulin and electroshock resulted in a brief period of remission. A second series, instituted because of a recurrence of her outbursts and occasional assaultive episodes, brought no improvement. After nine months of group and individual intensive psychotherapy, it was reported that she had established no particular relationship with either patients or personnel in the private sanitarium where she was being treated. There was an apparent lack of relatedness to other persons, real or imaginary, in the content of her psychosis. The authors state specifically that "none of her productions has indicated delusional content."

We have dwelt on the study by Darr and Worden at some length because it represents the first opportunity to follow an autistic child into adulthood. It is offered by the authors correctly as "one example" of how such a person has adjusted over a period of years. A more generalized prognostic statement was made by Mahler as a result of her rich experience. She wrote: "Establishment of contact and substitution therapy over a long period of time may sometimes give spurts of impressive and gratifying results. But they are usually followed by an insuperable plateau of arrested progress, which usually taxes the patience and frustrates the renewed hopes of the parents. Impatient reactions and pressures are then exercised and progress forced. But, if the autistic type is forced too rapidly into social contact, . . . he is often thrown into a catatonic state and then into a fulminant psychotic process. . . . If such catastrophic reactions cannot be avoided, it seems that such autistic infants are better off if allowed to remain in their autistic shell, even though in 'a daze of restricted orientation' they may drift into a very limited degree of reality adjustment only. Diagnosis of their 'original condition,' of course, then usually escapes recognition; they are thrown into the category of the feebleminded."

Every point of this statement was borne out by our follow-up studies: the spurts of gratifying results, the insuperable plateau, and the more or less permanent capsulation, occurring in different patients under different circumstances. Our findings suggest strongly that there are, from the beginning, differences in the intensity of autistic aloneness and fragmentation. We have as yet been unable to match them even approximately with somatic, genetic or dynamic factors which might possibly be held responsible. But they do exist and it would be a mistake to assume, as has been done sometimes, that autistic children are exactly alike in the manner in which, let us say, mongolian children are expected by some to be exactly alike. In this respect, a clear distinction between "primary" and "secondary" features proves of great value. Presence of the primary signs of aloneness and insistence on sameness is a sure diagnostic guide and holds the group together, regardless of the number and nature of the secondary manifestations.

When the children were first seen at our clinic, and on subsequent visits, we were impressed by differences in speech development. Some of the patients had completely renounced the use of speech; they either were mute throughout, or began to avail themselves sparingly of the linguistic tool only after five or more years of age, or—having said a few words—abandoned articulate language altogether. The utterance of whole sentences by some of these patients in emergency situations gave substance to the impression that a working vocabulary and at least a modicum of grammatic competence had been stored up but, except for those rare occasions, were kept locked up in storage. There were 19 of these children in our follow-up series. The other group comprised 23 patients who had begun to speak either at the usual age or after a slight delay. The mechanics of articulation presented no problem; phonation was either normal or manneristically altered to sing-song or a sort of Donald Duck quality. The children had learned at an early age to repeat an inordinate number of nursery rhymes, prayers, lists of animals, the roster of presidents, the alphabet forward and backward. Aside from the recital of sentences contained in the ready-made poems or other remembered pieces, it took a long time before they put words together for the purpose of oral communication with others. Even then, phrases heard were taken over in their totality, often with the same inflection, and reproduced in the form of what one might call delayed echolalia. This brought about the phenomenon of pronominal reversals, which continued into or beyond the sixth year of life, until eventually a give-and-take kind of conversation could be established with varying degrees of spontaneously communicating content.

Our follow-up survey indicates that the distinction between the mute and the speaking patients may have some useful prognostic implications. Of the 19 children who did not talk at around 4 years of age, 18 are still firmly enveloped in their autistic shell and would, as Mahler pointed out, impress a casual observer as essentially feebleminded. One brief case abstract may serve as an illustration:

John T. was first seen at 3 years and 2 months because of suspected mental deficiency. Undescended testicles were the only physical anomaly. Electroencephalogram was normal. He had been delivered at two weeks before term by elective caesarean section and weighed slightly above six pounds at birth. Vomiting after meals during the first three months ceased abruptly and did not recur. He was believed to be deaf because he did not respond to the presence of people. He sat up at 8 months and did not try to walk until 2 years, when he "suddenly" began to walk without difficulty. He refused to accept fluids in any but a glass container; once he went for three days without fluid because it was offered in a tin cup. He became upset when there was any change in his accustomed routine.

His parents separated shortly after his birth. The father, a psychiatrist, was described as an intelligent, restless, introspective man, mostly living within himself, at times alcoholic. The mother, a pediatrician, said of herself: "I have little insight into people's problems."

At the time of the first visit, John displayed good motor coordination and determined purposefulness in pursuit of his own goals. He was able to build skillfully a high tower of blocks. He responded to other persons only when they interfered with his privacy; then he shoved them away and screamed. There was no speech whatever. At 5 years, he showed great dexterity with the Seguin form board and kept moving and replacing the pieces all through the examination.

John, now 16 years old, has been living for the past ten years on a farm with simple and accepting country people. He gets along well under the extremely primitive demands of his protective environment. There is no speech and little response to verbal address. He takes walks in the area and always finds his way back to the foster home. On examination, he continues to show the typical signs of inner preoccupation, obsessiveness, perseveration, and lack of affective contact.

This extreme functional limitation is the general picture obtained in the follow-up of 18 of the 19 mute children, except that quite a few of them are more restless and disturbed than John. It is necessary to emphasize that, in this group, the present condition has come about regardless of the manner in which the patients had been handled. In fact, two of them had received intensive psychotherapy in good treatment centers; in both instances, slight apparent progress had given rise to guarded temporary optimism. Only one of the 19 originally mute children has emerged sufficiently to attend public school.

George O. was first seen at 4 years with the complaint that he "behaved very queerly." His mother reported that he did not chew his food, would not feed himself, and did not respond to toilet training. His behavior was markedly obsessive. Frustration resulted in temper tantrums. Interest in people was totally absent. He said only a few single words on very rare occasions. Health history and motor development were satisfactory.

The father, a busy surgeon, was a perfectionist and a detached individual who spent his vacations all by himself and boasted that he never wasted his time talking to his patients and their relatives. When asked specifically, he was not quite sure whether he would recognize any one of his three children if he met them on the street; he did not resent the question and its obvious implication. The mother, a college graduate, looked bedraggled at the time of the first visit. She felt futile about herself, was overwhelmed by her family responsibilities, and gave the impression of drabness and ineffectualness.

George showed no response at the clinic except when he was interfered with in any way. He did well with the Seguin form board and was neat and precise in his activities. When pricked with a pin, he related only to the hand which held the pin, and there was no carry-over of feeling to the person who pricked him. When the mother (upon request) attempted to embrace him, he squirmed away from her.

Therapeutic emphasis was placed on the mother, who came to realize her own latent abilities. The carefully-timed question when she had stopped being "Dorothy" (her first name) brought forth a burst of tears and a spurt of self-appraisal. She became more animated, dressed more attractively, developed an erect posture, and took George over as a challenge. The newly-established symbiotic relationship between her and the child proceeded without disturbance on the part of either. Her ministrations to George were a novel, enriching experience for her. After a year, George began to use language for limited communication. George, now approaching his twelfth birthday, is about to be promoted to the sixth grade in a school connected with a teachers' college. He does fairly well in his studies. His drawings show remarkable artistic ability. Conversation, though limited mostly to a question-and-answer pattern, is fairly adequate. He still has marked obsessive features; he has recently gone through a period when he refused to shake hands with anybody. He has attached himself to a couple of quiet, studious classmates whom he calls his "friends." His latest IQ was 91.

Of the 18 nonspeaking children (not counting George O.), seven are now in institutions for mental defectives, seven are kept at home in a state close to biologic helplessness, two are on farms, and two are in psychiatric state hospitals.

The 23 patients who had used speech in any form and for any purpose from an early age offer a somewhat less disheartening picture. Ten, or less than half, are doing very poorly; of these, five are chronic state hospital patients, three are in schools for retarded children, one is on a farm, and one is at home. Most of them, even at the low ebb to which they have receded, still show remnants which distinguish them from the demented or pseudodemented level of the mute autistic children. This is perhaps illustrated best by the psychologist's report on Barbara M., who is now 20 years old and a resident of a state hospital. It says: "This patient presents a complex and contradictory picture throughout all aspects of her personality. Intellectually, she is a paradox. Her successes and failures range from the very difficult to the very easy material. Verbal capacities are not consistent with a congenital mental deficiency. There is no real power to see herself as a separate entity, to test reality adequately, and to establish some sort of distance between the test material and herself. Her forte comes in abstract, very difficult 'intellectual' material where she can use rather erudite, pedantic words and concepts with ease. Her concept of the world is that of a threatening, overwhelming place, giving her no security. Her affect is for the most part blunted, yet she is capable of, and at the mercy of, explosive, violent feelings of aggressiveness."

Barbara and the other nine patients of this subgroup are much less likely to be mistaken as inherently feebleminded than the 18 mute autistic children of our follow-up series. They have given up much of their earlier ritualism, and the typical features of autism shown in their childhood are much less in evidence. At no stage of their development did they display any delusional content, and there is no certain indication of the existence of any hallucinatory experiences.

Not less than 13 of the 23 speaking children have at this time reached a plateau which allows them to function at home and in the community. One, Robert F., first seen at the age of 8 years in consultation and now 23 years old, has reached a higher pinnacle than the rest. Even at the time of the initial examination, though exhibiting unquestionably the characteristic signs of autism, he had begun to show signs of emergence. He served two years in the Navy as a meteorologist, is married, has a healthy son, and is now studying musical composition. Some of his works have been performed by chamber orchestras.

The other twelve are capable of attending school. They relate well to books and blackboards but have few, if any, real friends, and have retained some of the earlier obsessive-compulsive qualities.

Jay S., now almost 15 years old, presented in the lower grades considerable difficulties to his teachers, who were exceptionally understanding and accepting. He wandered about the classroom, masturbated openly, and staged temper tantrums. He learned to conform, did phenomenally well in mathematics, was sent to an accelerated school, and is now finishing the eleventh grade with top marks. He is a peculiar child, rather obese, who spends his spare time collecting maps and postage stamps and has little more to do with people than is absolutely necessary for the maintenance of a superficial relationship. He achieved a Binet IQ of not less than 150.

All of these twelve children can be said to be markedly schizoid in their make-up and behavior. It is not easy to be particularly optimistic about their adjustment to adult life. For the time being, they maintain a tenuous contact with reality.

We should like to discuss one of these patients in greater detail.

Susan T., an attractive, intelligent looking child, was first seen at 6 years of age. Her mother stated that she had noted "peculiar traits" from the first year of her life, when she displayed an insistence on adherence to routine. She never looked at people nor did she ever address herself to her parents. As an infant, she banged her head and rolled in her crib. She did not play with other children and was content to be alone. Although she spoke distinctly, she did not use language for communication. There were echolalia and pronominal reversals. After one hearing, she could repeat a song or a nursery rhyme. She had a remarkable memory for unimportant details, such as the number of tiles on the bathroom floor.

As soon as she entered the office, she began to ask questions about the objects in the room. She was able to give her name, age, and birth date. She became very angry and struck the physician when a block was taken from her; as soon as it was returned, all traces of anger disappeared. Noticing a crack in the ceiling, she remarked: "Why did this ceiling crack itself? Poor wall and ceiling, cracked all up." She did well on the performance tests, though her Binet responses were erratic. Physical and laboratory examinations showed no abnormalities; there was sensitivity to hyperventilation in the electroencephalogram though the child never presented any clinical dysrhythmic phenomena.

At 16 years, Susan is attending a private boarding school, where she is making satisfactory academic progress. The school noted that she does better in items requiring memory than in those which require reasoning. Susan said of herself: "I am not really a student. I am a plugger. Up to last year, the fundamentals of learning have been easy because of my memory, but this year it's interpretations, and this is difficult for me. I wanted to go to Wellesley but I may be hitching my wagon to a star. Maybe it will be too much pressure." She then sized up her social adjustment: "The girls in school are very nice and I have a good time with them but I don't have any real friends. I am so very sensitive. I feel I am not as mature as I should be and I don't have the interest in boys that I should have." On the Wechsler-Bellevue test, Susan had a verbal IQ of 119, performance of 98, and full scale IQ of 110.

The twelve children of this group have shown marked rises in psychometric rating because of their increased responsiveness.

Robert K., seen in a psychiatric outpatient clinic at 5 years, was diagnosed as a congenital defective, and his parents were urged to send him to a small private place for seriously retarded children. The parents did not "cooperate." After he completed the sixth grade at 13 years, his peculiar behavior caused the school to refer him to our clinic in 1948. He achieved a Binet IQ of 129. But this sample of his "conversation" throws light on his preoccupations: "We had lots of thunderstorms in 1940. Where do you live? (He was told.) Was it windy out there on Friday night? In our section it was still while the rest of Baltimore had plenty of wind. That is very freakish. How can that happen? Do you know Mount Washington? Why don't they get many thunderstorms in Mount Washington?" Robert was hospitalized at the Henry Phipps Psychiatric Clinic for four weeks. He eventually graduated from high school and is in the National Guard Reserve. He is unable to hold a job for any length of time.

It must be pointed out, for whatever this is worth, that only two of these twelve children have had any help which might be regarded as psychiatric treatment, while several of the others had received intensive psychotherapy. This is perhaps also the place to speak of Robert L., who at 4 years presented a picture very much like those shown by our twelve children with the relatively better adjustment. This child was electroshocked (not by us) at 5 years. Immediate deterioration set in. He is now, at 11, in a state hospital, completely out of contact and shows emotional blunting interrupted by periods of excitement.

In summary, the life histories of 42 autistic children at an average age of 14 years indicate that we deal with a distinct syndrome which may well be considered as falling within the broad category of the schizophrenias. As adolescents, they have retained the primary characteristics of the condition and have lost some of the earlier secondary symptoms, such as echolalia and pronominal reversals. At no time did they give evidence of delusions or definitely ascertainable hallucinations. The follow-up survey has led us to the conclusion that the presence or absence of language function in preschool age may serve as a criterion of the severity of the autistic process. All but one of the 19 nonspeaking children have remained in a state of complete isolation and, on superficial observation, can hardly be distinguished from markedly feebleminded persons. None of the varieties of psychiatric treatment employed had any noticeable effect. Of the 23 speaking children, not less than 13 have achieved sufficient emergence to function in more or less schizoid fashion at home and in school, while 10 are now clearly psychotic. These findings force us to believe that, over and above any contributions from external intervention, the child's own psychologic structure, resulting from inherent factors and the dynamics of parent-child relationship, must be regarded as the main determinant of subsequent development. The decisive impact of the early constellation on future destiny is in itself another demonstration of the specificity of early infantile autism. The favorable experience with George O. in connection with his mother's response to treatment introduces a melioristic note. It is true that even in most of the children who have reached a higher plateau, the emergence must be considered as partial, and further follow-up studies of these and other patients will be needed. Hence, this paper is presented as a preliminary report.†

References

Benda, C. E. *Developmental disorders of mentation and cerebral palsies.* New York: Grune & Stratton, 1952.

Cappon, D. Clinical manifestations of autism and schizophrenia in childhood. *Canadian Medical Association Journal,* 1953, **69**, 44–49.

Creak, M. Psychoses in childhood. *Royal Society of Medicine Proceedings,* 1953, **45**, 797–800.

Darr, G. C., & Worden, F. G. Case report twenty-eight years after an infantile autistic disorder. *American Journal of Orthopsychiatry,* 1951, **21**, 559–570.

Despert, J. L. Some considerations relating to the genesis of autistic behavior in children. *American Journal of Orthopsychiatry,* 1951, **21**, 335–350.

Kanner, L. Autistic disturbances of affective contact. *Nervous Child,* 1943, **2**, 217–250.

Kanner, L. Early infantile autism. *Journal of Pediatrics,* 1944, **25**, 211–217.

Kanner, L. Irrelevant and metaphorical language in early infantile autism. *American Journal of Psychiatry*, 1946, **103**, 242–246.

Kanner, L. Problems of nosology and psychodynamics of early infantile autism. *American Journal of Psychiatry*, 1949, **19**, 416–452.

Kanner, L. The conception of wholes and parts in early infantile autism. *American Journal of Psychiatry*, 1951, **108**, 23–26.

Kanner, L. To what extent is early infantile autism determined by constitutional inadequacies? In D. Hooker & C. C. Hare (Eds.), *Genetics and the inheritance of integrated neurological psychiatric patterns.* Baltimore: Williams & Wilkins, 1954.

Mahler, M. S. On child psychosis and schizophrenia. *Psychoanalytic Study of the Child*, 1952, **7**, 286–305.

Mahler, M. S., Ross, J., & DeFries, Z. Clinical studies in benign and malignant cases of childhood psychosis. *American Journal of Orthopsychiatry*, 1949, **19**, 295–305.

Rank, B. Adaptation of the psychoanalytic technique for the treatment of young children with atypical development. *American Journal of Orthopsychiatry*, 1949, **19**, 130–139.

Stern, E. A propos d'un cas d'autisme chez un jeune enfant. *Archives Francaises de Pediatrie*, 1952, **9**, 157.

Stern, E., & Schachter, M. Zum problem des frühkindlichen autismus. *Praxis der Kinderpsychologie und Kinderpsychiatrie*, 1953, **2**, 113–119.

van Krevelen, D. A. Early infantile autism. *Zeitschrift fur Kinderpsychiatrie*, 1952, **19**, 91–97. (a)

van Krevelen, D. A. Een geval van early infantile autism. *Nederlands Tijdschrift voor Geneeskunde*, 1952, **96**, 202–205. (b)

Weil, A. P. Clinical data and dynamic considerations in certain cases of childhood schizophrenia. *American Journal of Orthopsychiatry*, 1953, **23**, 518–529.

Weygandt, W. *Idiotie und imbezillität.* Leipzig: Deuticke, 1915.

†Reset from the original published in *Psychopathology of Childhood*, edited by P. H. Hoch and J. Zubin, pp. 227–239, 1955, by permission of Grune & Stratton, Inc.

EARLY INFANTILE AUTISM,
1943-1955

In 1943, under the title "Autistic Disturbances of Affective Contact," (Kanner, 1943) eleven children were reported whose clinical features appeared to constitute an unique syndrome, later termed "early infantile autism" (Kanner, 1944). Since the publication of the original paper, more than 120 children so diagnosed with reasonable certainty have been observed at the Children's Psychiatric Service of The Johns Hopkins Hospital. The syndrome is now recognized as a clinical entity, as is attested by numerous case reports and discussions of its theoretical and dynamic aspects. Preliminary data from follow-up studies at this clinic have further verified the uniqueness of the syndrome. It seems appropriate at this point to review briefly the nature of the original conception, to consider the modifications necessitated by greater knowledge, and to evaluate the present status of infantile autism.

[1] Co-author: Leon Eisenberg, M.D.

In the original paper, the pathognomonic disorder was seen as "the children's inability to relate themselves in the ordinary way to people and to situations from the beginning of life" (Kanner, 1943). The extreme nature of their detachment from human relationships separated the appearance and behavior of these children in a fundamental fashion from other known behavioral disturbances. It was noted that the process was not one "of withdrawal from formerly existing participation" with others, as is true of the schizophrenic child, but rather "from the start an extreme autistic aloneness" (Kanner, 1943). This could be discerned from the almost universal report by parents that these children, as infants, had failed to assume an anticipatory posture before being picked up, and never displayed the plastic molding which the normal child shows when cradled in his parents' arms. Initially pleased by the child's "goodness"—that is, his ability to occupy himself for long periods without requiring attention—parents later became distressed by the persistence of this self-isolation, and by their observation that their coming or going seemed a matter of complete indifference to the child.

A second distinctive feature was noted as the failure to use language for the purpose of communication. In three of the 11 cases, speech failed to develop altogether. The remaining eight rapidly developed a precocity of articulation which, coupled with unusual facility in rote memory, resulted in the ability to repeat endless numbers of rhymes, catechisms, lists of names, and other semantically useless exercises. The parroting of words intellectually incomprehensible to the child brought into sharp relief the gross failure to use speech to convey meaning or feeling to others. The repetition of stored phrases while failing to recombine words into original and personalized sentences gave rise to the phenomena of delayed echolalia, pronominal reversal, literalness, and affirmation by repetition.

A third characteristic was described as "an anxiously obsessive desire for the maintenence of sameness" (Kanner, 1943), resulting in a marked limitation in the variety of spontaneous activity. Regularly displaying fear of new patterns of activity, these children, once having accepted a new pattern, would incorporate it into the restricted set of rituals which then had to be endlessly iterated. Thus, a walk had always to follow the same prescribed course; bedtime to consist of a particular ritual of words and actions; and repetitive activities like spinning, turning on and off lights and spigots, or flushing toilets would preoccupy the child for long periods. Any attempt to interfere with the pattern would produce bursts of rage or episodes of acute panic.

Fourthly, as distinct from the poor or absent relation to persons, there could be discerned a fascination for objects which were handled with skill in fine motor movements. So intense was this relationship that minor alterations in objects or their arrangement, not ordinarily perceived by the average observer, were at once apparent to these children who might then fly into a rage until the change had been undone, whereupon tranquility was restored.

Finally, it was argued that these children had "good cognitive potentialities" (Kanner, 1943). In the speaking group this could be discerned in the extraordinary, if perverted, use of language, manifesting feats of unusual memory. In the mute children, this was concluded, though with less confidence, from their facility with performance tests, particularly the Seguin form board, at or above their age level.

Thus a syndrome had been delineated which was differentiated from childhood schizophrenia by virtue of detachment present no later than the first year of life, and from oligophrenia by the evidence of good intellectual potentialities. Physical examination failed to reveal any consistent organic abnormality that could be related to the clinical picture. Family background was striking in the universal presence of high intelligence, marked obsessiveness, and coldness. But the extreme aloneness *present from the beginning of life* led to the tentative conclusion that this group of children comprised "pure-culture examples of inborn autistic disturbances of affective contact."

In the light of experience with a tenfold increase in clinical material, we would now isolate these two pathognomonic features, both of which must be present: extreme self-isolation and obsessive insistence on the preservation of sameness, features that may be regarded as primary, employing the term as Bleuler did in grouping the symptoms of schizophrenia (Kanner & Eisenberg, 1954). The vicissitudes of language development, often the most striking and challenging of the presenting phenomena, may be seen as derivatives of the basic disturbance in human relatedness. Preoccupation with simple repetitive activities may be seen at times in severely retarded children and may offer a diagnostic problem, but the presence of elaborately conceived rituals together with the characteristic aloneness serves to differentiate the autistic patients. The case material has expanded to include a number of children who reportedly developed normally through the first 18 to 20 months of life, only to undergo at this point a severe withdrawal of affect, manifested by the loss of language function, failure to progress socially, and the gradual giving up of interest in normal activities. These latter cases have invariably been severe and unresponsive. When seen, they could not be differentiated from the children with the more classical account of detachment apparently present in the neonatal period. But even these cases are much earlier in onset and phenomenologically distinct from cases of childhood schizophrenia.

When this conception was set forth 12 years ago, it met with a reception very similar to that which greeted the reports of childhood schizophrenia advanced in the previous decade. Workers in the field, limiting their thinking to the conventional lines prescribed by the then current notions of adult schizophrenia, had had difficulty in accepting as schizophrenic a clinical picture in children which necessarily had distinctive differences dictated by the much younger age of these patients. Within the past six years confirmatory reports have appeared with increasing frequency, so that now the term infantile autism is rather widely—and often not too accurately—employed. Despert was perhaps the first, in a personal communication, to note the similarities between this group of children and others she had studied (Despert, 1949, 1951). Mahler suggested the useful division between autistic and symbiotic infantile psychoses (Mahler, 1952; Mahler, Ross, & De Fries, 1949). Rank (1949), Weil (1953), Sherwin (1953), Murphy and Preston (1954) in the United States, Cappon (1953) in Canada, Creak (1951, 1953) in England, Stern (1952) and Stern and Schachter (1953) in France, and van Krevelen (1952a, 1952b) in Holland added significant case reports. Recently, the Dutch Society for Child Psychiatry organized a symposium on infantile autism. A number of other workers have discussed the theoretical implications for language and perceptual function of the phenomena shown by the autistic child (Arieti, 1954; Norman, 1954; Ritvo & Provence, 1953). It therefore seems justified to state that the specificity of early infantile autism is now rather commonly accepted, with, of course, inevitable differences in diagnostic allocation; van Krevelen placing it with oligophrenia, most workers in this country with schizophrenia, Stern and Schachter and Grewel regarding it as a syndrome *sui generis*, and so on.

The preliminary results of our follow-up studies are of interest in that they, too, emphasize the phenomenologic uniqueness of the syndrome. Of the some 50 children followed for a mean period of eight years, none is reliably known to have exhibited hallucinations. The major pathology remains in the area of inability to relate in the ordinary fashion to other human beings. Even the relatively "successful" children exhibited a lack of social perceptiveness, perhaps best characterized as a lack of *savoir-faire*. This can be illustrated by the following incident involving one of our patients who has made considerable progress. Attending a football rally of his junior college and called upon to speak, he shocked the assembly by stating that he thought the team was likely to lose—a prediction that was correct but unthinkable in the setting. The ensuing round of booing dismayed this young man, who was totally unable to comprehend why the truth should be unwelcome.

This amazing lack of awareness of the feelings of others, who seem not to be conceived of as persons like the self, runs like a red thread through our case histories. We might cite a 4-year-old boy whose mother came to us with the account that on a crowded beach he would walk straight toward his goal irrespective of whether this involved walking over newspapers, hands, feet, or torsos, much to the discomfiture of their owners. The mother was careful to point out that he did not intentionally deviate from his course in order to walk on others, but neither did he make the slightest attempt to avoid them. It was as if he did not distinguish people from things, or at least did not concern himself about the distinction. This failure to recognize others as entities separate from oneself was exhibited by the 28-year-old patient retrospectively diagnosed as autistic and reported by Darr and Worden (1951). To mention one example of her behavior: "On one occasion she spilled ink on the floor of a dormitory room, dashed out to ask the first person she met to wipe it up, and became angry on being refused." The existence of feelings or wishes in other people that might not accord with the patient's own autistic thoughts and desires seemed beyond recognition.

On clinical grounds, it is now clearly useful to differentiate between the children who have learned to speak by the age of five and those who have no useful language function by that age (Kanner & Eisenberg, 1955). Of the former group, about half have made some sort of scholastic adjustment and participate in a limited way in the social life of the community, though we are none too sanguine about their future. Of the latter group—the nonspeakers—only one out of twenty subsequently developed language and is making at least a mediocre adjustment in a protected school setting. The remainder are either in institutions or remain at home, functionally severely retarded. Interestingly, a number of these emotionally isolated children, though confined to institutions for the feebleminded, are still distinguishable from their fellow patients, as is attested by reports of psychological testing that bewilder the observer in the conjunction of social imbecility with the preservation of isolated areas of unusual intellectual performance.

The information obtained from long term study of these children is beginning to supply us with a natural history of the syndrome, against which therapeutic efforts will have to be evaluated. Thus, it would appear on the basis of current information that, if we consider the cases in aggregate, about one third appear able to achieve at least a minimal social adjustment to school and community. This percentage of improvement without extensive psychiatric treatment is comparable with the data reported on a much larger group of schizophrenic children treated with electric shock by Bender (1953), allowing for differences in diagnostic categories and in indices of improvement. It should be stressed that, insofar as our data permit evaluation, psychotherapy seems in general to be of little avail, with a few apparent exceptions. If one factor is significantly useful, it is a sympathetic and tolerant reception by the school. Those of our children who have improved have been extended extraordinary consideration by their teachers. They constitute a most trying group of pupils. School acceptance of behavior that elsewhere provokes rejection is undoubtedly a therapeutic experience. Obviously, it is feasible only in the case of the less severely psychotic children.

Etiologic investigations have centered about organic, genetic, and psychodynamic factors. Thorough pediatric examination of all the children who have passed through our clinic has failed to reveal any more than occasional and apparently unrelated physical abnormalities, unless one considers relevant the consistent preponderance of boys over girls in a ratio of 4 to 1. Careful medical histories of pregnancy, delivery, and development are negative insofar as any consistent pattern of pathological complications is concerned. Electroencephalographic studies have been carried out only sporadically; of the 28 cases on which reports are available, 21 were stated to be negative, 3 definitely abnormal, and 4 equivocal. It must be recognized, however, that neurologic investigations of the integrity of central function remain as yet in their clinical infancy, and a negative result with current methods cannot be regarded as a conclusive demonstration of the lack of central nervous system pathology.

If we turn to a study of the families, we learn that, of 200 parents, there are only six with clinical psychiatric disorders, only one of whom had a psychotic episode. Among 400 grandparents and among 373 known uncles and aunts, twelve were afflicted with mental illness. This low incidence of psychotic and neurotic relatives, even if we double the figures to allow for the relative youth of these families, contrasts sharply with the high incidence in the families of childhood schizophrenics reported by Bender (1953) and in adult schizophrenics reported by Kallmann (1953). Similarly, of 131 known siblings of 100 autistic children, three can be regarded as probably autistic on the basis of the information supplied and seven others as emotionally disturbed. Thus, if one limits his search for genetic factors to overt psychotic and neurotic episodes in family members, the results would appear to be negative. If one considers the personalities of the parents who have been described as "successfully autistic," the possibility suggests itself that they may represent milder manifestations and that the children show the full emergence of the latent structure. One of the fathers in this group, a physician engaged in research, stressed the mildly schizoid trends of his own grandparents, more strongly evident in his father, fairly marked in himself and to some degree in all of his progeny, and full-blown in his autistic child.

One of the striking features of the clinical histories remains the unusually high percentage of these children who stem from highly intelligent, obsessive, and emotionally frigid backgrounds. Eighty-seven of the fathers and seventy of the mothers had been to college. A large number are professional people who have attained distinction in their fields. A control study of the parents of private patients selected solely by virtue of being next in call number to each of the first 50 autistic cases revealed levels of educational attainment and professional status that were considerably lower. In the control group one does not find the dramatically evident detachment, obsessiveness, and coldness that is almost a universal feature of parents of autistic children. Yet one must admit that some ten percent of the parents do not fit the stereotype, and that those who do have raised other normal, or in any event, nonpsychotic children. Moreover, similarly frigid parents are seen who do not give rise to autistic offspring.

The emotional frigidity in the typical autistic family suggests a dynamic experiential factor in the genesis of the disorder in the child. The mechanization of care and the almost total absence of emotional warmth in child rearing may be exemplified by the case of Brian, who was one of twins born despite contraceptive efforts, much to the distress of his parents: their plans centered about graduate study and had no room for children. Pregnancy was quite upsetting to the mother and caused the father, who was already immersed in study, to withdraw still further from the family. The mother, a psychology graduate student, decided that the children were to be raised "scientifically"—that is, not to be picked up if crying except on schedule. Furthermore, an effort was made to "keep them from infections" by minimizing human contact. What little care was dispensed was centered upon Brian's twin, who was physically weaker and, according to the mother, more responsive. At 5 months of age, the twin was found dead after an evening in which both infants had been crying loudly but had not been visited in accordance with rigid principle. Following this tragedy, the mother withdrew from the remaining child even more completely, and spent her days locked in the study reading. She limited her concern almost exclusively to maintaining bacteriological sterility, so that Brian was isolated from children and almost all adults until he was well over 2. During this period he was content to be alone and to occupy himself, just how the parents rarely bothered to inquire. It was only when he reached the age of 4 without the development of speech and began to display temper tantrums when his routines were interrupted that they began to recognize the fact that he was ill. So distant were the members of this family each from the others that the parents failed to be concerned about, if they did not actually prefer, Brian's indifference to them. One might accurately state that this was an environment that rewarded preoccupation with autistic interests and that provided the barest minimum of human contact compatible with the maintenance of physical health. Stimuli that might have fostered attention to or interest in the human environment were almost entirely absent. This case, an extreme instance chosen for emphasis, can serve as a paradigm of the "emotional refrigeration" that has been the common lot of autistic children.

Psychiatrists are rather widely agreed that emotional deprivation has profound consequences for psychobiological development (Bowlby, 1951). Infants subjected to impersonal care in institutions for prolonged periods in the first year of life display both psychomotor retardation and physiological dysfunction, a syndrome that has been termed hospitalism (Bakwin, 1949; Spitz & Wolf, 1946). Longer periods of exposure are correlated with depression of intellectual function, as measured by scores on "developmental" and "intelligence" tests (Gesell & Amatruda, 1947; Skeels & Dye, 1939). Analogous data are available from controlled animal experiments, in which poverty of environmental stimulation in the neonatal period produces apparently irreversible loss in adaptive ability (Beach & Jaynes, 1954; Thompson, 1954; Thompson & Heron, 1954). Moreover, children exposed to prolonged affective deprivation are likely to display antisocial and psychopathic behavior traits (Bender, 1947; Goldfarb, 1945, 1947). It has been contended that the personality pattern of such children as adolescents is typically "affectionless" (Bowlby, 1944). The most recent study by Lewis casts doubt on the concept of a specific personality pattern in the child who has suffered from lack of mothering, but does confirm the significant correlation between disturbed, usually antisocial behavior, and early separation from the mother without adequate substitution (Lewis, 1954).

Experience in Israel with communally reared children casts cross-cultural light on the nature of the emotional needs of infants and children (Caplan, 1954). From 6 weeks of age, Kibbutz infants live full time in communal nurseries and, though identification with their parents is maintained by frequent visits, the great preponderance of their care is given by permanent nursery workers. They are raised as a group under a common roof until late adolescence. These children grow into mature and capable adults as far as clinical evaluation can determine. Stress should be placed on the fact that the Kibbutz culture is child-oriented, and, while the mother is not the main dispenser of care, the children are reared by warm and demonstrative trained people—as it were, in an atmosphere of affectionate interest.

Thus it is evident that affectionate care and a consistent relationship to one or more adults in the mothering role is a prerequisite for normal growth in infancy and childhood.

The case histories of autistic children reveal that in almost all instances they were raised by their own parents. Obvious mistreatment, overt rejection, or abandonment, usual in the life experience of the children who are classified as emotionally deprived, are the exception. But the formal provision of food and shelter and the absence of neglect as defined by statutory law are insufficient criteria for the adequacy of family care. The role of "parent" is not defined merely by the biological task of giving rise to progeny. In the typical autistic family it is as if the Israeli experiment had been repeated, but in reverse: in having parents, but not a warm, flexible, growth-promoting emotional atmosphere. These children were, in general, conceived, less out of a positive desire, than out of an acceptance of childbearing as part of the marital contract. Physical needs were attended to mechanically and on schedule, according to the rigid precepts of naive behaviorism applied with a vengeance. One can discern relatively few instances of warmth and affection. The usual parental attitude is cold and formal; less commonly it is laden with great anxiety. The child's worth seemed to lie in the extent to which he conformed to predetermined parental expectations: "perfect" behavior, cleverness, "self-sufficiency," and so on. Their parents, who were themselves preoccupied with careers and intellectual pursuits to the exclusion of interest in other people, had little feeling for their own children. It may be a measure of the intellectual aptitude of some of these children that they were able to parrot long and resonant lists of meaningless words, but it even more clearly bespeaks the emphasis placed at home on such useless activities, which were a source of pride to the parents.

It is difficult to escape the conclusion that this emotional configuration in the home plays a dynamic role in the genesis of autism. But it seems to us equally clear that this factor, while important in the development of the syndrome, is not sufficient in itself to result in its appearance. There appears to be some way in which the children are different from the beginning of their extrauterine existence. Indeed, it has been postulated that the aberrant behavior of the children is chiefly responsible for the personality difficulties of their parents, who are pictured as reacting to the undoubtedly trying situation of having an unresponsive child (Rabinovitch, 1949). While we would agree that this is an important consideration, it cannot explain the social and psychological characteristics of the parents, which have a history long anteceding the child.

There is little likelihood that a single etiologic agent is solely responsible for the pathology in behavior. Arguments that counterpose "hereditary" versus "environmental" as antithetical terms are fundamentally in error. Operationally defined, they are interpenetrating concepts. The effects of chromosomal aberrations can be mimicked in the phenotype by environmental pathogens, and genetic factors require for their complete manifestation suitable environmental conditions. It is not possible to distinguish between biochemically mutant microorganisms until we expose them to nutrient media deficient in appropriate metabolites. Conversely, the full effect of environmental agencies cannot be seen unless the genotype is adequate. A culturally rich environment will be little different from a culturally poor one in its influence on the intellectual development of phenylketonuric children.

The dualistic view implicit in a rigid distinction between "organic" and "functional" is no longer tenable. The pharmacologic production of psychosis-like states simulating certain features of schizophrenia (Hoch, Cattell, & Pennes, 1952; Hoch, Pennes, & Cattell, 1953) (and the recent hint that analogue blockade will interfere with chemically induced "model psychoses" (Fabing, 1955)) serves to reassert the obvious fact that biochemical change is accompanied by alterations in thought processes. Nevertheless, the disordered thoughts obey the laws governing psychic processes and lend themselves to psychological analysis. It is equally important to recognize that originally psychogenic forces must by their enduring action transform the physiological substrate, as the conditional reflex so clearly demonstrates. The finding of biochemical or psychological abnormalities is only the starting point in a search for etiology.

Early infantile autism is a total psychobiological disorder. What is needed is a comprehensive study of the dysfunction at each level of integration: biological, psychological, and social. The supposition of an innate difference in the autistic child will mean relatively little until we can specify the nature and meaning of that difference. Currently, research sponsored by the League for Emotionally Disturbed Children is attempting to uncover metabolic and electrophysiologic abnormalities, research that complements the psychodynamic investigations at this and other clinics.

In summary, early infantile autism has been fully established as a clinical syndrome. It is characterized by extreme aloneness and preoccupation with the preservation of sameness, and is manifest within the first two years of life. The history, early onset, and clinical course distinguish it from childhood schizophrenia, to which it is probably related generically. The degree of aloneness constitutes the important prognostic variable, since those children sufficiently related to the human environment to learn to talk have a significantly better outlook for future adjustment. Present knowledge leads to the inference that innate as well as experiential factors conjoin to produce the clinical picture. It remains for future investigation to uncover the precise mode of operation of the pathogenic factors as a basis for rational treatment.†

REFERENCES

Arieti, S. Some aspects of the psychopathology of schizophrenia. *American Journal of Psychotherapy,* 1954, **8**, 396–414.

Bakwin, H. Emotional deprivation in infants. *Journal of Pediatrics,* 1949, **35**, 512.

Beach, F. A., & Janes, J. Effects of early experience on the behavior of animals. *Psychological Bulletin,* 1954, **51**, 239–263.

Bender, L. Psychopathic conduct disorder in children. In R. M. Lindner (Ed.), *A handbook of correctional psychiatry.* New York: Philosophical Library, 1947.

Bender, L. Childhood schizophrenia. *Psychiatric Quarterly,* 1953, **27**, 1–19.

Bowlby, J. Forty-four juvenile thieves: Their characters and home life. *International Journal of Psychoanalysis,* 1944, **25**, 19–53.

Bowlby, J. *Maternal care and mental health.* Geneva: World Health Organization, 1951.

Caplan, G. Clinical observations on the emotional life of children in the communal settlements in Israel. In M. J. E. Senn (Ed.), *Problems of infancy and childhood: seventh conference.* New York: The Josiah Macy, Jr., Foundation, 1954.

Cappon, D. Clinical manifestations of autism and schizophrenia in childhood. *Canadian Medical Association Journal,* 1953, **69**, 44–49.

Creak, M. Psychoses in childhood. *Journal of Mental Science,* 1951, **97**, 545–554.

Creak, M. Psychoses in childhood. *Proceedings of the Royal Society of Medicine,* 1953, **45**, 797–800.

Despert, J. L. Comments on Leo Kanner's "Problems of nosology and psychodynamics of early infantile autism." *American Journal of Orthopsychiatry,* 1949, **19**, 416–452.

Despert, J. L. Some considerations relating to the genesis of autistic behavior in children. *American Journal of Orthopsychiatry,* 1951, **21**, 335–350.

Darr, G. C., & Worden, F. G. Case report twenty-eight years after an autistic disorder. *American Journal of Orthopsychiatry,* 1951, **21**, 559–570.

Fabing, H. D. New blocking agent against the development of LSD-25 psychosis. *Science,* 1955, **121**, 208–210.

Gesell, A., & Amatruda, G. *Developmental diagnosis.* (2nd ed.) New York: Paul B. Hoeber, 1947.

Goldfarb, W. Effects of psychological deprivation in infancy and subsequent stimulation. *American Journal of Psychiatry,* 1945, **102**, 18–33.

Goldfarb, W. Variations in adolescent adjustment of institutionally reared children. *American Journal of Orthopsychiatry*, 1947, **17**, 449–457.

Hoch, P. H., Catell, J. P., & Pennes, H. H. Effects of mescaline and lysergic acid (d. LSD 25). *American Journal of Psychiatry*, 1952, **108**, 579–584.

Hoch, P. H., Pennes, H. H., & Cattell, J. P. Psychoses produced by the administration of drugs. *Publication of Association for Research in Nervous and Mental Diseases*, 1953, **32**, 287–296.

Kallmann, F. J. *Heredity in health and mental disorder.* New York: Norton, 1953.

Kanner, L. Autistic disturbances of affective contact. *Nervous Child*, 1943, **2**, 217–250.

Kanner, L. Early infantile autism. *Journal of Pediatrics*, 1944, **25**, 211–217.

Kanner, L., & Eisenberg, L. Notes on the follow-up studies of autistic children. In P. H. Hoch & I. Zubin (Eds.), *Psychopathology of childhood.* New York: Grune & Stratton, 1955.

Lewis, H. *Deprived children: a social and clinical study.* New York: Oxford University Press, 1954.

Mahler, M. S. On child psychosis and schizophrenia: Autistic and symbiotic infantile psychoses. In R. S. Eissler, et al. (Eds.), *Psychoanalytic study of the child.* Vol. 7. New York: International Universities Press, 1952.

Mahler, M. S., Ross, J. R., Jr., & De Fries, Z. Clinical studies in benign and malignant cases of childhood psychosis. *American Journal of Orthopsychiatry*, 1949, **19**, 295–305.

Murphy, R. C., & Preston, C. E. Three autistic brothers. Paper presented at the annual meeting of the American Orthopsychiatric Association, 1954.

Norman, E. Reality relationships of schizophrenic children. *British Journal of Medical Psychology*, 1954, **27**, 126–141.

Rabinovitch, R. D. A treatment program for parents of schizophrenic children. *American Journal of Orthopsychiatry*, 1949, **19**, 592.

Rank, B. Adaptation of the psychoanalytic technique for the treatment of young children with atypical development. *American Journal of Orthopsychiatry*, 1949, **19**, 130–139.

Ritvo, S., & Provence, S. Form perception and imitation in some autistic children. In R. S. Eissler, et al. (Eds.), *Psychoanalytic study of the child.* Vol. 8. New York: International Universities Press, 1953.

Sherwin, A. C. Reactions to music of autistic (schizophrenic) children. *American Journal of Psychiatry*, 1953, **109**, 823–831.

Skeels, H. M., & Dye, H. B. A study of the effect of differential stimulation on mentally retarded children. *American Association for the Study of Mental Deficiencies Proceedings*, 1939, **44**, 114–136.

Stern, E. A propos d'un cas d'autisme chez un jeune enfant. *Archives Francais de Pediatrie*, 1952, **9**, 157.

Stern, E., & Schachter, M. Zum problem des frühkindlichen autismus. *Praxis der Kinderpsychologie und Kinderpsychiatrie,* 1953, 2, 113-119.

Spitz, R. A., & Wolf, K. M. Anaclitic depression: An inquiry into the genesis of psychiatric conditions in early childhood. In R. S. Eissler, et al. (Eds.), *Psychoanalytic study of the child.* Vol. 2. New York: International Universities Press, 1946.

Thompson, W. R. Exploratory behavior in normal and restricted dogs. *Journal of Comparative and Physiological Psychology,* 1954, **47,** 77-82.

Thompson, W. R., & Heron, W. Effects of restriction early in life on problem solving in dogs. *Canadian Journal of Psychology,* 1954, **8,** 17-31.

van Krevelen, D. A. Early infantile autism. *Zeitschrift fur Kinderpsychiatrie,* 1952, **19,** 91-97. (a)

van Krevelen, D. A. Een geval van early infantile autism. *Nederlands Tijdschrift voor Geneeskunde,* 1952, **96,** 202-205. (b)

Weil, A. P. Clinical data and dynamic considerations in certain cases of childhood schizophrenia. *American Journal of Orthopsychiatry,* 1953, **23,** 518-529.

†Reset from the original published in *American Journal of Orthopsychiatry,* Volume 26, pp. 55-65, 1956.

THE THIRTY-THIRD
MAUDSLEY LECTURE

Too deeply moved to search for originality of expression, I hope that you will allow me to fall back on some of the well-worn phrases in acknowledging the honor conferred on me when I was chosen to be this year's Maudsley lecturer. My reaction was summarized in reply to the notice which reached me in May, 1957. I wrote: "I accept amidst an understandable struggle between pride and humility. The name 'Maudsley Lecture' has an almost hallowed connotation among my professional contemporaries, and this invitation comes to me as a sort of crowning acme of my career." I am delighted to share my laurels with The Johns Hopkins University, which I joined exactly thirty years ago at the call of Adolf Meyer, whose gigantic contributions to psychiatric theory and practice were attested by the Royal Medico-Psychological Association when he was nominated to be the fourteenth Maudsley Lecturer in 1933. In going over the list of my illustrious predecessors in this series of addresses, beginning with Sir James Crichton Browne and Sir Frederick Mott, I find that I am the second United States psychiatrist to receive so great a distinction. I am certain that I voice the sentiments of my university when I say that it considers this event as an added and happily displayed feather in its richly decorated cap. The Johns Hopkins University has recognized the growing importance of child psychiatry by creating a full professorship in this discipline, and I am pleased to be the symbol of this recognition. And now your Association has indicated its desire that I speak as a child psychiatrist "as this specialty has not been covered in a Maudsley Lecture before". To have been selected as the first spokesman for child psychiatry in this group is a thrilling experience laden with heavy responsibilities.

The weight of these responsibilities produced in me quite a bit of anxious stirring from the moment when I began to gear myself for the decision on a suitable topic. Would it, I asked myself, be wise to bracket out a particular issue and elaborate it in some detail? This I and many others have done on frequent occasions, thus carrying together and trying to put in their proper places the numerous bricks which help to make up the total structure. But then it occurred to me that, instead, the occasion might serve me and my audience as a kind of pause for reflection about the nature of the structure itself. I turned for advice to two colleagues for whose wisdom and judgment I have the utmost admiration. John C. Whitehorn felt that a broad review of the field would be in order. Aubrey Lewis thought in terms of emphasis on the historical background of the specialty. Thus strengthened in my ripening preference for an overall discussion, I remembered a presentation which my one-time co-worker, your Kenneth Cameron, gave in 1955 as Chairman of the Child Psychiatry Section of this Association. It was a succinct outline of "past and present trends in child psychiatry". Cameron's brief and meaty address clinched my determination to dwell with you at some length on the evolution and scope of what now is known as child psychiatry.

In the light of present-day usage, it sounds incredible that the term child psychiatry itself had not acquired formal citizenship in the realm of professional or any other parlance until a little less than three decades ago. In the early 1930's, Tramer introduced it in its German form, *Kinderpsychiatrie*, as part of the name of the journal which he founded and which he has so capably edited throughout the years. In 1935, I chose *Child Psychiatry* as the title of my textbook. In 1937, at the initiative of Heuyer, an international congress in Paris, called together under the heading of *Psychiatrie infantile*, voted, not without opposition, to give legitimate status to the term. In 1938, finally, Schröder could proclaim that this name "has apparently become conventional in most civilized countries."

In a way, these baptismal quandaries and their comparatively recent resolution tell the story—a story which goes beyond a mere exercise in semantic niceties—of the origins of a branch of science which has become a respectable ingredient of our contemporary cultural milieu. I venture to say that child psychiatry and the name by which it goes today have arrived on the scene at approximately the same time. I am ready to defend the thesis that prior to the 1920's there was no body of knowledge or of clinical practice integrated enough to merit being set aside as an organized specialty.

Child psychiatry is the result of the convergence of a number of interests which for about half a century have existed alongside each other, with only sporadically and tenuously maintained areas of mutual contact. So long as these interests remained separated and confined to narrowly delimited spheres of activity, they each no doubt afforded highly significant insights which then, however, were applicable solely or principally within the constricted range in which the observations had been made. It was not until they could be brought together in one place that the edifice of child psychiatry could be erected as a comfortable dwelling unit with interconnecting rooms where a family of scientists could indulge in a fruitfully collaborative exchange of ideas and cognitions. Child psychiatry, in brief, is a fusion of what used to be a collection of more or less loosely scattered segments.

With your indulgence, I should like to have some of these segments pass in parade before you. It would seem reasonable to let psychiatry take the lead.

In the second half of the nineteenth century, several texts were published on "psychic disorders", "mental diseases", or "insanity" of children. Behavioral deviations interested Emminghaus (1887), Moreau de Tours (1888), Ireland (1898), and Manheimer (1899) chiefly as they seemed to fit diagnoses in accordance with classifications devised for adults. There was a tendency toward fatalism which saw in the reported disorders the irreversible results of heredity, degeneracy, excessive masturbation, overwork, or religious preoccupation. These texts, nevertheless, offered a wealth of illustrative case material, no matter how sketchily some of it was presented in the form of anecdotal snapshots.

But let it not be said that the psychiatrists of that era were satisfied to be merely the mechanical recorders of observed or quoted instances. In the refreshing vigor of expanded curiosities, we sometimes, paying half-hearted homage to the psychiatric leaders of the past—and not too remote a past at that—are inclined to dismiss their formulations as obsolete relics, of consequence only to the medical historian. Those men certainly did pay attention to, and did try to find explanations for, psychotic manifestations in childhood, the very existence of which was questioned or even denied by many in the early part of this century. No more fitting example can be offered than that of Henry Maudsley in whose honor this series of annual lectures is held. In his *Physiology and Pathology of Mind*, published in 1867, Maudsley included a 34-page chapter on "Insanity of Early Life." In it, he not only attempted to correlate symptomatology with the patient's developmental status at the time of onset but also suggested an elaborate seven-point classification of the infantile psychoses. Anyone superciliously critical of either the terminology or the intrinsic cohesion of the grouping may well be reminded that the classification of the childhood psychoses is to this day a matter of controversial floundering.

Maudsley, as you know, rewrote his book a number of times. I cannot refrain from reproducing the introductory paragraph of the chapter on children in the revision of 1880. He began:

"How unnatural! is an exclamation of pained surprise which some of the more striking instances of insanity in young children are apt to provoke. However, to call a thing unnatural is not to take it out of the domain of natural law, notwithstanding that when it has been so designated it is sometimes thought that no more needs to be said. Anomalies, when rightly studied, yield rare instruction; they witness and attract attention to the operation of hidden laws or of known laws under new and unknown conditions; and so set the inquirer on new and fruitful paths of research. For this reason it will not be amiss to occupy a separate chapter with a consideration of the abnormal phenomena of mental derangement in children."

The "abnormal phenomena of mental derangement" continued for some time to be the almost exclusive interest which academic psychiatry had for children. This type of preoccupation found its culmination in the second edition of Ziehen's treatise on the mental diseases (*Geisteskrankheiten*) of childhood which appeared as late as in 1925. Unparalleled as a reference book and as an exhaustive bibliographic guide, it started out with this categorical statement: "For childhood the same division of psychoses is recommended as for the later ages, namely (a) psychoses *with* intellectual defect and (b) psychoses *without* intellectual defect." Ziehen's book was, indeed, on the whole an almost literal translation of adult psychiatry into terms of how much of it one might find in children. The author must have proceeded in about the following manner: "My readers are, of course, familiar with paranoia, melancholia, hebephrenia, stupor, hysteria, etc., in adults; now let us see how frequently these things are seen in children and how similarly or dissimilarly they manifest themselves." Abnormalities of the cortical structure and constitutional predisposition were considered as the dominant etiological factors.

An avowed emphasis on an organic and genetic background prevailed also in Sancte de Sanctis' *Neuropsichiatria infantile*, published in the same year as Ziehen's book. De Sanctis, scorning the modern direction toward "clinical individualism", complained that "the study of individual differences causes some to lose the aspect of group characteristics" and that "the investigation of intimate psychodynamics distracts the view of others from the inevitable play of its nervous or, more generally, vital partner". He went to the other extreme of losing sight of personality because of his strict adherence to somatic and localizing preoccupations.

This summary completes the psychiatric vanguard of the procession of segments, covering the efforts over a period of about eight decades, partly before and some time after the initial publication of Kraepelin's monumental work. Another segment is represented by the occupation with the problems of mental deficiency. During a long period of stagnation, interrupted only by Paracelsus' discovery of the connection between endemic goitre and intellectual stunting, the feebleminded were regarded as a homogeneous group. The seemingly solid wall believed to be made up of identical material was dented slightly by Langdon Down's description in 1866 of what he first called Kalmuck idiocy and later came to be spoken of as mongolism. From then onwards, ever new entities were singled out and studied separately. Contributions came from various sources. We owe the knowledge of amaurotic family idiocy to the British ophthalmologist-surgeon Tay and the American neurologist Sachs; of dementia infantilis to the Austrian educator Heller; of phenylketonuria to the Norwegian veterinarian Fölling. A compact unit emerged which had its own experts, facilities, journals, and congresses. It sequestered itself from the rest of the concerns about child development and child behavior to the extent that, at least on the North American continent, only a negligible fraction of the medical members of the American Association on Mental Deficiency have found it necessary to affiliate themselves with the American Psychiatric or Orthopsychiatric Association. Exciting things have happened within this unit, especially in the past three decades, owing to advances made in neuropathology, endocrinology, biophysics, biochemistry, psychology, and education.

As the parade of segments marches past, education is next in line. After compulsory school attendance had become an established institution, the educators became increasingly concerned about problems of learning and conduct among their pupils. Psychiatrists, for the most part, kept themselves aloof and thereby forced the teaching profession to look for its own solutions. The movement began in France and was pursued there with remarkable vigor. In Central Europe, a group, under the banner of what was termed *Heilpädagogik* (remedial education), undertook under the leadership of Heller, Hanselmann, Isserlin, and Busemann, to make itself responsible for as much amelioration as was possible in the educational setting. Much was accomplished in this enforced isolation. The second edition of Hanselmann's *Einführung in die Heilpädagogik* (1933) showed a breadth of experience which might well arouse the envy of many a psychiatrist. The labors of these educators resulted in Europe and in America in organized practical arrangements for the special education of the intellectually, sensorily, neuro-orthopedically, and neurotically handicapped children.

A delegation from criminology is next in the procession. In the 1890's a number of civic-spirited men and women found the then existing retaliatory attitude toward young offenders objectionable and detrimental to their development. They exerted all the political influence they could muster. As a result, South Australia in 1895, Illinois and Colorado in 1899 passed statutes establishing juvenile courts in which delinquent children were to be handled separately and differently from adult violators of the law. Since then, juvenile courts have become an established institution. The presiding officers are mostly jurists, assisted often by a staff of social workers, pediatricians, and psychiatrists. In the case of the more severe offenders, re-education and rehabilitation, with or without the aid of psychotherapy, are channelled through special units known as reformatories, correctional or training schools. The names of William Healy, August Aichhorn, Sheldon and Eleanor Gluck are intimately connected with the study of juvenile delinquents.

The procession continues. Psychology joins the ranks. Around the turn of the century, psychologists shifted their emphasis from armchair contemplations to actual attention to real people. Alfred Binet is usually and, I believe, correctly hailed as the great innovator. No longer speculating about the attributes of an abstract soul, he let live children come unto him and, initially for the benefit of French school authorities, inaugurated an era of concrete study and the measured comparison of individuals with regard to certain areas of functioning. There came, after a few earlier examples set by Preyer in Germany, Sully in England, and Compayré in France, a spurt of stage-by-stage examinations and recordings of the gradual emergence of motor, perceptual, conceptual, linguistic, and social behavior. Diaries, interrogations, and a variety of test batteries combined to get together a set of data which, as developmental psychology, has made invaluable contributions. Much information has come—to name but a few—from the work of the Bühlers, William Stern, David Katz, E. Claparède, Jean Piaget, and Kurt Lewin. Following this trend, Arnold Gesell and his co-workers were able to set up a normative scale of infantile development, beginning within a few weeks after birth.

The next marcher in the parade, psychoanalysis, passes by with éclat and fanfare. The awe-inspiring genius of one man created a fascinating system which has had a powerful influence on Western civilization. Freud, on the basis of anthologies of neurotic adults' more or less directly elicited reminiscences, published his theory of infantile sexuality in 1905, three years before he saw any one child professionally. He gave special heed to a set of lawfully progressing centrifugal forces centered around a broadened concept of libido and assumed to govern the development of children's personalities. Freud's profound wisdom and honesty is evident in every one of the 24 pages of the second of the Three Contributions to the Theory of Sex, entitled *Infantile Sexuality*. In this short space, there are not fewer than 55 passages in which the remarks are qualified by "probably", "perhaps", "apparently", "I believe", "it is possible", "as it were", "so to say", "may well be", "it might be supposed", "it may be assumed", "we may gain the impression", etc. This collection of probabilities, possibilities, assumptions, beliefs, opinions, conjectures, impressions and analogies, not as yet validated by dispassionate scrutiny, was somehow transformed into certainties and decreed truths and formed the foundation of an all-embracing credo enveloping all etiology and therapy. This insistence by many, though by no means all, of Freud's followers has threatened to make of psychoanalysis an orthodox all-or-none proposition of the kind which Adolf Meyer liked to characterize as "exclusive salvationism". On the other hand, the excellent accomplishments of Anna Freud are witness to the fact that, with a less dogmatic and more flexible application, psychoanalysis can make significant contributions to the observation and treatment of children.

The column of paraders which next appears on the scene is made up by the child guidance clinics which were inaugurated in the early 1920's. The seeds for their growth were implanted toward the end of the first decade of this century when Clifford Beers, with the encouragement of Adolf Meyer, John Dewey, Stanley Hall, and others, founded the National Committee for Mental Hygiene. Prevention of insanity and delinquency was the key word. The idea of setting up insanity and delinquency as targets to shoot at with the arrows of preventive efforts was laudable enough, to be sure. But it implied an orientation which started out with a vision of calamity, looked upon young nonconformists as wayward youths to be snatched in time from the gates of asylums and prisons, and indulged in the practice of throwing inkwells at devils painted on the wall. Actual work with children taught the workers that proper mental hygiene is not primarily an exercise in trying to prove alarmists wrong, that emotionally upset children deserve treatment of what bothers them because it bothers them *now*, and that the greatest benefit can be derived from dealing effectively with what

Douglas Thom aptly referred to as "the everyday problems of the everyday child". Under Thom's leadership, the Boston Habit Clinic opened its doors in 1921. In 1922, "demonstration child guidance clinics" were established in several cities with the aid of the Commonwealth Fund. They were called so because they were meant to demonstrate their usefulness to the communities in which they were set up. By the end of the decade, there were about 500 such clinics on the North American Continent alone. In 1930, the governments of more than 50 countries sent delegates to the first International Congress of Mental Hygiene, which was held in Washington, D.C.

The greatest contribution made by these clinics to the understanding of children's behavior was the departure from the almost universal tendency to look for explanations one-sidedly in an individual's inherent, genetically, constitutionally, and endopathologically determined, centrifugal propensities for disturbing deviations. The focus of inquiry was broadened, beyond the curiosity about that which goes on *within* a child as he reaches out into his environment, to include the external, centripetal forces which do things *to* him and thereby help to shape his feelings and resulting demeanor. Thus ensued a searching investigation of interpersonal relationships at home and in school as motivating factors. Children's behavior began to be correlated with parents' and teachers' attitudes, which were taken into account as part of the therapeutic strategy. The newly created concept of attitude therapy made it possible to help parents and teachers to examine, discuss, and modify those of their emotional problems which were found to be detrimental to individual children. Simultaneously, through what was called relationship and release therapy, the children themselves were given an opportunity to bring their conflicts to the surface and deal with them in a manner more comfortable and serviceable than theretofore.

The child guidance clinics, aware of the psychological and sociological implications of their job, set up the so-called clinical team of psychiatrist, psychologist, and social worker. This novel and wholesome arrangement, however, was from the beginning allowed to be frozen into a rigid system which came to regard itself as a complete, self-contained unit. Much was made of this "interdisciplinary" collaboration which closed the door to all but three disciplines, and much time, meditation, and printer's ink were spent on trying to figure out and delineate the exact role of each member of what, because of the exhibited air of sacred solemnity, I have sometimes facetiously dubbed "the Holy Trinity". There being no perfection in human enterprise, the great benefit derived from making certain types of children's behavior problems a matter of community concern had in its wake a consciously cultivated estrangement from medicine and an exclusion of all those other types of handicaps which did not fit the clinic's self-imposed limitations. Saying this does not in any way imply a detraction of the historical importance of the work of those clinics. The insights gained from the study of parent-child, sibling-sibling, teacher-pupil, and therapist-patient relationships formed a truly indispensable addition to the sum total of information gathered by the other segments which we have met in the procession.

The parade has come to an end. Psychiatry, the study of mental deficiency, education, criminology, psychology, psychoanalysis, and child guidance have each displayed before you their particular areas of interest, inquiry, and helpfulness. Few of them had more than a nodding acquaintance with one another. I must hasten to add that in every one of those pursuits there were men whose vision went beyond the circumscribed scope of the specific segment. But it was not until 32 years ago that one man, without identifying himself with any one of the segments, managed to blend all of them into a single discipline which viewed the child as the core of psychiatric endeavor—not selectively the psychotic, feebleminded, educationally maladjusted, delinquent, or parentally mismanaged child but every child who needed psychiatric investigation and amelioration.

Such is the nature of public acclaim that the spectacular takes precedence over calm, diligent, unobtrusively persistent labor. It is perhaps because of this that the present generation has lost sight of the merits of him who should be honored as the first all-round, comprehensive child psychiatrist. August Homburger was commissioned in 1917 by his chief, Franz Nissl, to establish a psychiatric outpatient department at the University of Heidelberg. He began to center his interest more and more on the problems of children. It is amazing how much creative work and organizational activity he was able to pack into the 13 years between 1917 and 1930, the time of his death at the age of 57 years. He stepped out of the monastic seclusion of the psychiatric department of his university and got the community at large to participate in the concerns for mental hygiene. He worked in close collaboration with courts, schools, and social agencies. He introduced a series of university lectures on psychotherapy. Mayer-Gross, in his moving obituary, has pointed out how much courage it must have taken to do this "at a time when neither official psychiatry nor official internal medicine paid the slightest attention to the significance and effects of psychogenic factors". In 1926, Homburger published his *Lectures on the Psychopathology of Childhood*. His broad orientation could not abide by the therapeutically sterile and etiologically one-sided categorizing of Ziehen and de Sanctis. His background had given him a mastery of neurology, which served admirably in his work with children, but at the same time made him aware of the fact that cerebral anomalies alone could not account for social, attitudinal and other factors in his young patients' experiences. He set out, with a critical eye and with remarkable fairness, to round up and present to his readers the sum and substance brought together by the various segments as well as the existing theories and hypotheses. Prophetically foreseeing his role as a pacemaker, he wrote in the preface of his book: "The psychopathology of childhood will—of this I am firmly convinced—experience much deepening and enrichment in the years to come. Whatever I may have to say in these chapters bears the nature of transitoriness and is still anchored in tradition." His modesty apparently did not allow him to admit to himself fully that, with all due respect for precedent and while putting up a warehouse of accumulated knowledge and thought, he himself was the originator of a new tradition—that of an inclusive concept of the psychopathology of childhood or child psychiatry.

It was toward the end of 1930, the year of Homburger's death, the year of the first International Congress of Mental Hygiene, the year of the White House Conference on Child Health and Protection, that Adolf Meyer, Edwards A. Park, Stewart Paton, and Ludwig Kast of the Josiah Macy, Jr., Foundation engaged me for an excursion into territory until then neglected by psychiatrists. The preliminary task assigned to me was to consist of "an investigation of the rank and file of patients in the pediatric clinics for the formulation of psychiatric problems, the mastery of which should be made accessible to the pediatrician to serve him as the psychopathological principles in dealing with children".

You have undoubtedly noticed, and possibly been puzzled by, the fact that pediatrics, contrary to logically justified expectation, was conspicuously absent from the procession which has passed before you. Lest the inference be drawn therefrom that the medical child specialists were indifferent about issues involving their patients' intellectual, emotional, and social functioning, it is well to remember that as far back as in 1889 Jacobi, one of the pioneers of American pediatrics, spoke of the desirability of making use of psychiatric knowledge in his specialty. But as no help was offered from psychiatric quarters, a few pediatricians went forth to explore the field for themselves. Rachford's *Neurotic Disorders in Childhood* (New York, 1905), Guthrie's *Functional Nervous Disorders in Childhood* (London, 1907), and Czerny's *Der Artzt als Erzieher des Kindes* (Berlin, 1908) were outstanding efforts in this direction. This essentially homegrown crop was kept from withering by a few members of the pediatric specialty. It is not generally known, for example, that the more recent detailed studies by Goldfarb, Spitz, and Bowlby of the effects of early psychological deprivation were preceded by pertinent observations on the part of two pediatricians. In 1915, Chapin, in an article entitled *Are Institutions for Infants Necessary?* advocated the boarding out of infants so that they might receive individual care and affection. In 1942, just one year before Goldfarb's first report, Bakwin's classical paper, *Loneliness in Infants*, painted a "fairly well defined" clinical picture of the hospitalized infant whose personal needs are neglected aside from the exclusive attention to his somatic illness. Nor should one overlook the fact that in 1919, before the advent of the child guidance clinics, Hector Charles Cameron, physician in charge of the children's department of Guy's Hospital, gave evidence of much sympathetic understanding of emotional features and parent-child relationship in a charming, often reprinted book, *The Nervous Child*, and later in a chapter contained in the 1929 edition of Garrod, Batten and Thursfield's textbook of pediatrics.

But these insights were sporadic and not at all the common property of the pediatrics profession, even though its practitioners, often prodded by the demands of sophisticated parents, became increasingly eager to receive assistance from psychiatry. What did they find? The child guidance clinics, as they came along, ignored them completely; the "team" gave them the cold shoulder. Perusal of the literature resulted in bewilderment. Veeder, shortly before he became editor of the *Journal of Pediatrics*, had this to say at the White House Conference in 1930: "I have a very definite feeling that the psychiatrist and psychologist have contributed somewhat to the pediatric attitude of suspicion, or scepticism. The psychiatrist above all other people with whom I come into close contact has a penchant for obfuscating his thought with a most perplexing, and I feel unnecessarily complicated verbiage."

Such was the situation when in November, 1930, I set foot at the Harriet Lane Home, the children's division of The Johns Hopkins University School of Medicine, as the first pseudopodium stretching out into pediatrics from the psychiatric amoeba. A cautious attempt by von Pirquet in 1911 to have a psychiatric observation station, headed by E. Lazar, at the University Children's Hospital in Vienna was not even locally too successful because at that time child psychiatry and pediatric concern with it were both still in the stage of embryonic incipiency.

Very soon after the assumption of my duties, an anonymous donor, to whom I shall be forever grateful, left on my desk the reprint of an article, just off the press, entitled *The Menace of Psychiatry*. Its author was Joseph Brennemann, an eminent pediatrician known for his long experience and sound judgment, a man whose word had a great resonance among his colleagues. Brennemann declared unequivocally: "There is not only a menace of psychiatry, but it is already seriously in our midst." He castigated the blatant overpopularization and oversentimentalization of child psychology, the overevaluation of certain standardized tests, and the conflicting claims of some of the speculative, aggressively vociferous, and overbearingly dogmatic "schools". Thus Brennemann's blast presented a healthy challenge, the call for a sweeping house-cleaning which deserved to be at least as welcome to psychiatrists as to the pediatric group which he addressed. For here was sound criticism of features which were not so much a menace *of* psychiatry as they were a menace *to* psychiatry.

Brennemann's warning enhanced my already firm resolution to avoid these and many other pitfalls. Coming from a pluricultural and plurilingual background, having emancipated myself from the theological and political absolutism fed me in my youth, falling easily into step with Meyer's practiced advocacy of a scientifically objective, self-scrutinizing, pluralistic and relativistic attitude, I found it impossible to limit myself to any of the segments which have passed before you in the procession. Besides, the setting itself made any such restricted alignment impractical. The children who came to the wards and outpatient department just did not sort themselves in accordance with anybody's preoccupations. They were brought in because they were feverish, coughed, had rashes, lost weight, had fractured a bone, were jaundiced, convulsed, held their breath, stuttered, wet the bed, stole, did poorly in their studies. They came with these and many other complaints. Here, then, was an unprecedented opportunity, offered in no other setting, to study children and their manifold problems in an environment from which no patient was ever kept away for any reason and in which the watchfully and hopefully waiting pediatricians were trying to assess the services rendered by psychiatry and its invited representative. For pediatricians are, as all medical men and all other scientists everywhere should well be, governed by the desire for factual demonstrations, for the careful perception of reality which hesitates to accept even the most beautifully constructed hypotheses unquestionably at their face value.

This psychiatric-pediatric alliance in the daily work with individual children made it possible to utilize all the previously recorded observations and discoveries and to introduce the sum total as the discipline of child psychiatry as a medical concern with psychological, educational, social and cultural ramifications; as a legitimate science within the framework of medical practice, teaching, and research; as a child-centered enterprise engaged in the diagnosis, treatment, and prevention of developmental and behavioral deviations with and without organic involvements. That this trend toward synthesis has more recently spread over the entire field of psychiatry, has been made clear by the publication in 1957 of a volume edited skillfully by H. D. Kruse and entitled *Integrating the Approaches to Mental Disease*. Starting with the deplored awareness of what was referred to as insular grouping, fragmentation, segmentation, and provincialism, an attempt was made by 48 men, including your Hargreaves, Rees, Richter, and Slater, to get together on fundamentals and outline areas of acceptance by all and of nonacceptance by some. It is rather pleasing to know that child psychiatry, under the influence of Adolf Meyer, has gone a long way in striving for this aim over a period of nearly thirty years.

This is not to say that, even though the ranks have been closing, there is complete uniformity of opinion and method. As a matter of fact, I am not sure that such uniformity is a condition to be coveted before that day in the distant future when all the etiological diagnostic, remedial, and prophylactic facts will lie palpably in the palms of our hands. On the contrary, some of us have found it necessary to speak out against a recurrent tendency to impose an inflexible system of thought and action on all patients, regardless of the nature of their difficulties. This tendency seems to have persisted, in one form or another, since the time of Maudsley who, asserting that "whosoever distinguishes well teaches well", felt called upon to militate against uniform procedure. He wrote that for adequate strategy "it would be necessary to have a full and exact knowledge of the construction of the individual mind as well as of the proper remedy: to know the particular character, the special fault of it, the kind of disorder to which the fault was prone to lead, and the exact conditions of life which would be the fit remedy; for different pursuits might wisely be used as so many remedies for different defects of character."

These words, written in 1895, have a peculiarly familiar ring if one considers the still existing controversies about the need for diagnostic accuracy and for investigative as well as therapeutic methodology. The issue, highlighted so well by Maudsley half a century ago and still alive in our midst, is essentially this:

There are those whose medical training has kept in the foreground of their responsibility the obligation to view each patient as—if I may use Meyer's term—a unique experiment of nature. It is the physician's duty to devise and refine means of investigation that would help him to become cognizant of this uniqueness as an indispensable preparation for the regime best adapted to the requirements of the individual. In so doing, whether he be an ophthalmologist, a cardiologist, an orthopedist, or an adult or child psychiatrist, he notices that there are certain combinations of features which, though never completely identical, are similar enough to justify the recognition of specific diagnostic categories. This, after all, has been Kraepelin's great accomplishment, that he perceived, described, and studied these similarities and thus brought order into the thitherto unorganized welter of mental diseases. This search for diagnostic clarity is still going on in the wide area of child psychiatry, with the added awareness that, within each sufficiently defined category, the imperative consideration of genetic, physical, intellectual, situational, and experiential differences presents a fascinating invitation to deal with each child as an exceptional, unduplicated specimen.

This, however, is not a universally established tradition among child psychiatrists. There are those who, rightly dissatisfied with what sometimes, I believe erroneously, has been identified as the only concern of medicine, are inclined to turn their backs to organ pathology, description, and classification. Intrigued, as everybody should be, by the relatively new emphasis on psychodynamics, there has been a tendency to elevate intrapsychic and interpersonal factors to the rank of sole determinants of behavior, or at least as the sole determinants worthy of psychiatric attention. Certain theories have been put forth and certain methods of inquiry and treatment have been laid down which are transmitted from teacher to learner as ultimate, catechistic truths. In the process, theory and method have gained ascendancy over the patient to whom they are applied with little curiosity about his microcosmic uniqueness. If the standard concepts and rules are not suited to his specific problem, then they are either tried out on him for a time anyway or he is sent home unaided. Under these circumstances, with medicine pushed aside, it is not surprising that the door has been opened wide to lay people, with or without a preliminary medical diploma, who have qualified as adept repeaters of the catechism.

A concrete example may serve as an illustration of the manner in which the two groups have approached the problem of diagnosis. During the past two decades, there has been a revival of interest in the infantile psychoses. There has been, especially in the United States, an unprecedented wealth of publications on childhood schizophrenia. In them, two more or less antithetical trends are clearly discernible: one which tries to single out specific, circumscribed, carefully defined syndromes on the basis of precise semeiology, and one which tends to dilute the concept of schizophrenia, with not too much regard for the intricacies of differentiation not only between those syndromes themselves but also between them and conditions of innate mental deficiency. It is true, of course, that, as instances of spontaneous or therapeutically induced improvement have demonstrated, average or better than average original endowment can be dammed up by the psychotic process. It is also true that, as Weygandt pointed out in his monograph written for Aschaffenburg's *Handbuch* in 1915, idiotic and imbecile children can present oddities of behavior reminiscent of schizophrenic phenomena. There is no denying that overlapping symptomatology creates problems in trying to distinguish between different illnesses which have a number of features in common. But the problem is definitely not solved by the decree that the sharing of symptoms makes the conditions identical or that because of the partial resemblance a differentiation is unnecessary.

Nevertheless, on the assumption that lack of adequate mother-child relationship underlies *all* arrest or fragmentation of personality structure at different stages of development, Beata Rank advocated the sweeping notion of the "atypical child". She declared that, in using this term, she referred to "more severe disturbances in early development which have been variously described as Heller's disease, childhood psychosis, childhood schizophrenia, autism, or mental deficiency". Similarly, Szurek, announcing the consensus of his co-workers at the Langley-Porter Clinic in San Francisco, made this statement: "We are beginning to consider it clinically (that is, prognostically) fruitless, or even unnecessary, to draw any sharp dividing lines between a condition that one could call psychoneurotic and another that one could call psychosis, autism, atypical development, or schizophrenia." This is a return to pre-Kraepelinian looseness which throws all the laboriously assembled and refined diagnostic criteria to the winds as irrelevant impediments on the road to treatment. Treatment, under these circumstances, has become a more or less stereotyped method applied to all comers and dispensed as hours of psychotherapy. The therapeutic cart is put before the diagnostic horse and it seems that sometimes the horse is left out altogether.

It is perhaps not out of place if, at this juncture, I beg of you to let me dwell briefly on the role of psychotherapy in child psychiatry. Let me begin with an expression of unreserved admiration for the methods which have been introduced in order to help children to reveal their feelings to themselves and to the therapist. Play, drawing, clay modelling, thematic apperception tests, and other projective tools have proved of inestimable value. Having said this, I wish to add that psychotherapy, no matter how essential it is in the overall remedial strategy, is but a part of the therapist's responsibility. While it aims at an adjustment from within outward, there is ample room for help extended from without inward. I think you will agree with me that, while our professional literature abounds in detailed accounts of excellent observations and more or less realistic interpretations of happenings during therapeutic interviews, the intrinsic goal of psychiatric treatment has never been defined clearly and unequivocally. Is it the purpose to learn and teach specific methods or, as some say, techniques to be employed indiscriminately in every instance, unmindful of the uniqueness of the problems which confront us? I shall never forget the young man just out of training who on a visit to our clinic was stunned by the absence of a sand box and running water in the treatment rooms; it was incomprehensible to him how there could be any child psychiatry without those two implements which, so he had been taught, were absolutely essential parts of the arrangement. Does not this smack too much of an attitude which fosters the rearing of a generation of therapeutic mechanics?

If I may venture a concise statement about the goal of psychiatric treatment, it is this: The sum total of efforts expended in order to help a patient to attain *his* optimal condition of comfort and smoothness of functioning. Such a formulation recognizes that, with the great variety of conditions encountered in the wide realm of child psychiatry, the attainable optimum differs with each individual's somatic, intellectual, and socio-cultural propensities, all of which must therefore be investigated carefully before a plan for treatment is outlined. The plan may, depending on the findings, involve parent counselling, psychotherapy with the child, the correction of impaired vision, adequate classroom placement, the supply of sufficient food and clothes, and any other arrangements in keeping with the patient's specific needs. Patient-centred, individualized programs with concrete aims differ essentially from less goal-defined, method-centered journeys into the unknown with the diffuse hope that somehow this will eventually produce a state of blissful "normalcy" in the image of the therapist's conception of suburbanite propriety.

The children who come streaming to a large pediatric clinic and to its psychiatric station recruit themselves from mansions, middle-class homes, tenement houses, and shacks, from psychometrically intelligent and unintelligent families, from backgrounds of affectionate acceptance, agitated overprotection, perfectionistic disapproval, or overt hostility and neglect. They arrive with healthy bodies, minor physical ailments, and more severe congenital or acquired anomalies and diseases. They are brought with no complaints about their behavior, with everyday problems from which I for sure was not, and possibly some of you were not, totally exempt, with varying degrees of developmentally determined intellectual shortcomings, with anxiety-laden neuroses, and occasionally with major psychotic disturbances. Not one of them deserves to be pushed aside or sent off because he does not fit the preordained requirements of a selectively dosed therapeutic procedure. No physician would, or should, be content with an attitude which makes the choice of patients depend on the method instead of making the choice of methods depend on the needs of the individual patient.

I realize that some of the trends of which I have spoken pertain to psychiatric work with adults as well as with children. I also realize that child psychiatry, being a newcomer among the medical sciences, still experiences enough uncertainty to warrant a great deal of experimentation. I grant that some of the restricted preoccupations with psychodynamic factors can be understood as an overreaction to the earlier disregard of these factors and to earlier satisfaction with the mere description of symptoms and with mere diagnostic labelling with little or no heed to the foundation and meaning of the patient's emotional involvement. But I believe that the time has come when all of us in the field should be willing to submit theories and methods to a sober evaluation of results. It is time for a bit of reality testing. It is time to examine the existing free-floating generalizations in relation to available data of observation and at the same time to build further generalizations on the basis of such data. With this in mind, I can find no more suitable quotation with which to conclude my address than the reiteration of a plea by Henry Maudsley, who said: "Observation should begin with simple instances, ascent being made from them step by step through appropriate generalizations, and no particulars should be neglected."†

†Reset from the original published in *Journal of Mental Science,* Volume 105, pp. 581–593, 1959.

INFANTILE AUTISM AND
THE SCHIZOPHRENIAS

In a paper published in 1943, entitled "Autistic Disturbances of Affective Contact," I reported from the Children's Psychiatric Service of The Johns Hopkins Hospital observations of 11 children (8 boys and 3 girls) who had in common a pattern of behavior not previously considered in its striking uniqueness. The symptoms were viewed as a combination of extreme aloneness from the beginning of life and an anxiously obsessive desire for the preservation of sameness. I concluded the discussion by saying: "We must assume that these children have come into the world with an innate inability to form the usual, biologically provided affective contact with people, just as other children come into the world with innate physical and intellectual handicaps. If this assumption is correct, a further study of our children may help to furnish concrete criteria regarding the still diffuse notions about the constitutional components of emotional reactivity. For here we seem to have pure-culture examples of inborn, autistic disturbances of affective contact."

123

In search for an appropriate designation, I decided in 1944, after much groping, on the term *early infantile autism*, thus accentuating the time of the first manifestations and the children's limited accessibility.

The term autism was introduced by Eugen Bleuler, who wrote: "Naturally some withdrawal from reality is implicit in the wishful thinking of normal people who 'build castles in Spain.' Here, however, it is mainly an act of will by which they surrender themselves to a fantasy. They know that it is just fantasy, and they banish it as soon as reality so demands. I would not call the effects of these mechanisms 'autism' unless they are coupled with a definite withdrawal from the external world."

This definition does not quite account for the status of our patients. For one thing, withdrawal implies a removal of oneself from previous participation. These children have never participated. They have begun their existence without the universal signs of infantile response. This is evidenced in the first months of life by the absence of the usual anticipatory reaction when approached to be picked up and by the lack of postural adaptation to the person who picks them up. Nor are they shutting themselves off from the external world as such. While they are remote from affective and communicative contact with people, they develop a remarkable and not unskillful relationship to the inanimate environment. They can cling to things tenaciously, manipulate them adroitly, go into ecstasies when toys are moved or spun around by them, and become angry when objects do not yield readily to expected performance. Indeed, they are so concerned with the external world that they watch with tense alertness to make sure that their surroundings remain static, that the totality of an experience is reiterated with its constituent details, often in full photographic and phonic identity.

All this does not seem to fit in with Bleuler's criteria for autism. There is no withdrawal in the accepted sense of this word, and a specific kind of contact with the external world is a cardinal feature of the illness. It may therefore appear at first glance that I followed the example of the pseudoetymologists who claimed that the Latin word for dog derives from the animal's inability to sing (*Canis a non canendo*) and the word for grove from the absence of light (*Lucus a non lucendo*). Nevertheless, in full recognition of all this, I was unable to find a concise expression that would be equally or suitably applicable to the condition. After all, these children do start out in a state which, in a way, resembles the end results of later-life withdrawal, and there is a remoteness at least from the human portion of the external world. An identifying designation appeared to me to be definitely desirable because, as later events proved, there was danger of having this distinct syndrome lumped together with a variety of generalized categories.

It can be said in retrospect that the brief history of infantile autism can be separated into three consecutive phases.

1. While the case reports, their phenomenology, and their etiologic implications almost immediately received the attention of the profession, it naturally took some time before similar observations could be made and communicated. For this reason, the earliest reactions dealing with the issue did not appear in print for several years. Meanwhile, studies were continued and intensified at The Johns Hopkins Hospital. For a period of approximately one year a special ward was set aside at the Henry Phipps Psychiatric Clinic for close investigation and therapeutic experimentation. In a 1946 paper, I discussed the peculiarities of metaphorical and seemingly irrelevant language of autistic children, and in a 1949 article, having by that time become acquainted with 55 patients who could be so diagnosed with reasonable certainty, I tried to set forth my ideas about the problems of nosology and psychodynamics of early infantile autism.

2. This state of affairs changed abruptly in 1951. No fewer than 52 articles and one book were concerned specifically with the subject between then and 1959. The first European confirmations of the existence of the syndrome came in 1952 from van Krevelen in Holland and from Stern in France. In the same year, Clemens Benda included in his book, *Developmental Disorders of Mentation and Cerebral Palsies*, a brief chapter with four illustrations, entitled "The Autistic Child." In it, he wrote: "The great question is whether autism is a part of the schizophrenic syndrome complex or should be considered a separate entity. A decision of this question cannot be made without a more thorough discussion of what constitutes childhood schizophrenia."

This sage advice was not heeded by many authors. While the majority of the Europeans were satisfied with a sharp delineation of infantile autism as an illness *sui generis,* there was a tendency in this country to view it as a developmental anomaly ascribed exclusively to maternal emotional determinants. Moreover, it became a habit to dilute the original concept of infantile autism by diagnosing it in many disparate conditions which show one or another isolated symptom found as a part feature of the overall syndrome. Almost overnight, the country seemed to be populated by a multitude of autistic children, and somehow this trend became noticeable overseas as well. Mentally defective children who displayed bizarre behavior were promptly labeled autistic and, in accordance with preconceived notions, both parents were urged to undergo protracted psychotherapy in addition to treatment directed toward the defective child's own supposedly underlying emotional problem.

By 1953 van Krevelen rightly became impatient with the confused and confusing use of the term infantile autism as a slogan indiscriminately applied with cavalier abandonment of the criteria outlined rather succinctly and unmistakably from the beginning. He warned against the prevailing "abuse of the diagnosis of autism," declaring that it "threatens to become a fashion." A little slower to anger, I waited until 1957 before I made a similar plea for the acknowledgment of the specificity of the illness and for adherence to the established criteria.

To complicate things further, Grewel, in the hope of avoiding confusion between true autism and other conditions with autistic-like features, suggested the term pseudo-autism for the latter. Even this term came to be employed haphazardly, and conditions variously described as hospitalism, anaclitic depression, and separation anxiety were put under the heading of pseudo-autism.

All this resulted in the need for a careful evaluation of the reports of cases presented as samples of autism. A sifting of the literature of the 1950's compels one to eliminate many alleged illustrations as descriptive of something other than that which they were intended to portray.

3. The 1960's have witnessed a considerable sobering up. The fashion deplored by van Krevelen has gradually subsided. This is perhaps caused in part by the fact that those who go in for the summary adoption of diagnostic clichés have now found another handy label for a variety of abnormalities. Instead of the many would-be autistic children who are not autistic, we have the ever-ready rubber stamp of "the brain-injured child." While this certainly is regretable, it has at least driven the acrobatic jumpers onto another bandwagon and has left the serious study of autism to those pledged to diagnostic accuracy. Hence, it is easier to single out properly designated cases, not lost in the shuffle of a peculiarly miscellaneous deck, for an investigation of their pathognomonic characteristics. And indeed, in the past few years, the diagnoses made have been more uniformly reliable and the discussion has been considerably less obfuscated by the smuggling in of irrelevant materials.

However, the question of nosological allocation of infantile autism has continued to be a matter of puzzlement. This is especially true of the formulations regarding its relation to schizophrenia.

Anyone attempting such a formulation ought to bear in mind Clemens Benda's quoted suggestion that a decision will have to depend on a discussion of what constitutes schizophrenia. One cannot get away from the need for semantic clarification and for a historical and ideological review of the meaning attached to all that is involved when this term is used. Has the meaning been stationary since the word was coined or have there been fluctuations and modifications? Is schizophrenia to be conceived as a unitary disease or as a generic noun encompassing a variety of kindred entities? Would all psychiatrists respond to these questions with unanimity?

In the 1890's, Kraepelin undertook the magnificent architectural job of erecting a solid structure of psychiatry from the many building stones lying around in disarray. Guided by the search for basic similarities and dissimilarities, he found a common denominator in a number of psychotic conditions which impressed him as sharing a "deteriorating process." Among them he included the catatonia of Kahlbaum (1863), the hebephrenia of Hecker (1871), the simple deterioration of Pick (1891) and Sommer (1894), and paranoid states associated with disorganization. He subsumed the whole deteriorating group under the term dementia praecox. As soon as this was accomplished, Kraepelin found it necessary to retain the above syndromes, not as the separate units as which they had been previously presented but as subdivisions of the *specific* disease dementia praecox.

Before we proceed, it is important to pause for an examination of the meaning of the word "specific." Some of the dictionaries offer among their definitions two which, if used interchangeably, are apt to produce—and are indeed producing—semantic quandaries. One says: "Designating a definitely distinguishable disease." The other says: "Of or pertaining to a species, or group, of which the members have common characteristics and are called by a common name."

Kraepelin viewed dementia praecox with its subdivisions essentially as specific in the sense of the first-quoted definition. When Bleuler suggested the term schizophrenia in 1911, he announced that he looked upon it as a common name for a species and emphasized his point by speaking not of schizophrenia in the singular but of the "group of the schizophrenias." He declared significantly: "This concept may be only of temporary value inasmuch as it may later have to be reduced," adding parenthetically, "(in the same sense as the discoveries in bacteriology necessitated the subdivision of the pneumonias in terms of various etiologic agents)."

This prediction indicates a profound grasp of medical history and may prove to be prophetic in the long run. For much of the progress of medicine has been characterized by the singling out of circumscribed diseases from a welter of ill-defined generalities, by the gradual transition from the assumption of the homogeneity to the recognition of the heterogeneity of conditions which have certain broad aspects in common. We are far removed from the time when learned treatises were published, entitled *De febribus* or *De pestibus*, dealing with febrile illnesses and contagious diseases as if they were all of them identical in nature and origin. The falling sickness, once regarded as a single entity, is now divided into a variety of dysrhythmic conditions of different provenances. Before Langdon Down's description of mongolism in 1866, mental defectives were thought of as if, to paraphrase Gertrude Stein, the feebleminded were the feebleminded were the feebleminded; since then, neuropathologic, metabolic, genetic, and psychological studies have managed to do away with the illusion of the sameness of all mental deficiency.

There is at present cause to believe that similar developments are in store for the concept of schizophrenia, resulting in the "reduction" envisioned by Bleuler. Moreover, concrete demonstrations of this trend are beginning to be supplied in the area of child psychiatry.

When Kraepelin created the concept of dementia praecox, he did so entirely on the basis of his work with adults. At no time was there any reference to its occurrence in children. He mentioned once, as a hunch rather than on grounds of careful statistics, that of 1,054 patients 3½ percent had shown signs of "psychic weakness" before 10 years of age. All that Bleuler had to say about this in his sizable monograph is contained in a footnote, which reads: "The disease rarely becomes manifest in childhood. Yet there are cases in which a primary schizophrenia can be traced back to the earliest years of life." On the page above this footnote Bleuler reported an estimate according to which the onset of schizophrenia could be found in 4 percent of the case histories to go back to the age of "before 15 years." Obviously, when any thought was given to children at all in connection with dementia praecox or schizophrenia, it was done so largely in terms of retrospect and not as a result of direct examination at the time of the anamnestically recorded incipiency. Childhood schizophrenia was not something seen and clinically investigated as such but rather merely hinted at as an occasional prelude remembered by the relatives of adolescent and adult patients.

Between 1905 and 1908, Sante de Sanctis tried to accomplish for children what Kraepelin had done for adults. He gathered a number of cases which had in common symptoms of lack of affect, negativism, stereotypy, talkativeness, delirium, hallucinations, and catatonic features. As etiologic factors he enumerated hereditary predisposition, acute or chronic toxic diseases, and "factors inherent in child development." He combined all cases under the name dementia praecocissima, a sort of miniature version of dementia praecox. His reports were followed by additional illustrations of his own and other Italian investigators, and a few cases were published under this caption by German, French, and Swiss authors. De Sanctis felt that the clinical picture was indistinguishable from dementia praecox but he was not sure that the adult and the infantile forms had the same causative background.

A review of the contemporary and subsequent literature shows that the notion of dementia praecocissima proved to be of limited viability and has now been discarded altogether as a valid collective designation. Most of the patients turned out to be specimens of an assortment of neuropathologically identifiable, more or less progressive, congenital or acquired anomalies of the central nervous system. Some of them (e.g., Schilder's disease) could not have been known to De Sanctis because they were not isolated until after the time when he incorporated them in his classification. Clinical neurological tests, biopsies, or autopsies removed them from the category; the concept of dementia praecocissima continued to be "reduced" to a point where it lost its justification altogether. In view of later attitudes it is significant to note that the finding of a clearly definable organic disorder automatically excluded an ailment from the diagnosis of childhood schizophrenia.

This became evident again when the Viennese educator (*Heilpädagoge*) Heller described in 1908 a group of children presenting "an almost photographic identity of course" with the following features: After normal development during the first two or three years of life, there was a rapid change of behavior with anxiety, motor restlessness, loss of speech and of sphincter control, and general regression, leading in a short time to complete dementia, while the children showed no clinical signs of physical disturbance and retained an intelligent facial expression. Heller's disease or dementia infantilis (a term coined by Weygandt), though extremely rare, was observed by others as well and was entered in the textbooks as the earliest form of childhood schizophrenia. It remained there until Corberi in 1931 discovered in four brain biopsies "acute diffuse degeneration of the ganglion cells." Schilder averred categorically in 1935: "I assume as a matter of course that dementia infantilis has nothing to do with schizophrenia but is an organic process."

This is a pivotal statement around which hinges the whole philosophy of the distinction between organic and functional psychoses. Schizophrenia was classed as a functional psychosis by definition. Ergo, if you find in a patient signs of an organic process his condition logically has nothing to do with schizophrenia.

Two departures are possible from here. One goes in the direction of viewing the term functional as a temporary, perhaps even a bit embarrassing admission of the inability to find an organic substratum; this spurs a search for one so that, if it is discovered, the adjective functional can be dropped. This is, after all, the gist of Kraepelin's postulate of a metabolic disorder, of Bleuler's prophecy, and of much that is happening today in the realm of schizophrenia research. The other departure goes in the direction of regarding "functional" as synonymous with nonorganic; this has encouraged a search for environmental, psychogenic noxa as the explanation of schizophrenic phenomena. The one focuses on the quest for internal, centrifugal springs of psychotic behavior; the other on the shaping influence of external, centripetal forces. Until recently, the twain did not meet and were bogged down in an irreconcilable antithesis.

This antithesis did not become conspicuous until the early 1940's. Until that time, when there was talk of childhood schizophrenia, curiosity was extended mainly to patterns resembling adult syndromes. Strohmayer's treatise on the psychopathology of childhood, which appeared in 1910, and the 1926 (second) edition of Ziehen's textbook of the mental diseases of children discussed juvenile (hardly ever infantile) schizophrenia in Kraepelinian terms. Strohmayer did not hesitate to say that, except for senile, arteriosclerotic, and true paranoid psychoses, all mental illnesses known in adults can be encountered in children with the same symptomatology. Ziehen viewed schizophrenia as an "acquired defect psychosis," together with paralytic, epileptic, traumatic, meningitic, and toxic dementia, in contrast to diseases not resulting in intellectual defect. He spoke of the latter (e.g., mania, melancholia, delirious states, paranoia, and obsessive psychosis) as "functional." This runs counter to the usual inclusion of schizophrenia among the functional psychoses.

However, in the late 1920's and in the 1930's more and more voices were raised in favor of a distinction between adult and childhood schizophrenia, attributable to maturational and experiential factors. There was growing agreement that the Kraepelinian subdivision was not suited for the preadolescent years, and efforts were made to find a grouping more in harmony with direct observations. In Germany, Homburger, one of the pioneers of child psychiatry, decided to use the type of onset and course of illness as a starting point, rather than the symptoms noted at any given time. He thus suggested two different groups, one with acute onset and another with insidious onset. Partly in consequence of Homburger's lead and in part independently, Ssucharewa in Russia, Lutz and Tramer in Switzerland, and Despert in this country underlined this grouping in their discussions of childhood schizophrenia. Patients of the first group, mostly older children, have seemed to make a good adjustment prior to the appearance of recognizable psychotic symptoms. In the second group, there is a gradual withdrawal from contact with reality, a progressive loss of interest in play, an increasing tendency to brood, a preoccupation with abstractions, and obsessively repetitious ruminations. It was deemed essential for the diagnosis in both groups that a period of relative normalcy had preceded the beginning of the illness.

This was the situation around the start of the 1940's, at the time when I published the first cases and introduced the concept of infantile autism. One year earlier Bender had summed up the general professional attitude in a few sentences which deserve to be quoted because of their clarity and succinctness.

Bender

She wrote: "There are those who do not believe in childhood schizophrenia, not having seen a case. At the best, none of us has seen very many cases in which we could make a definite diagnosis, not knowing the acceptable criteria. There are others who, having seen certain types of mental disorders in children, prefer to call them schizophrenia-like psychoses of childhood."

While Bender and others began to look for acceptable criteria, a sizable group of workers, temporarily influential especially in this country, joined in a chorus chanting the refrain, *Cherchez la mère* (which I tried in vain to silence in 1941 in my book, *In Defense of Mothers*). Poohpoohing description as an obsolete pastime of atavistic nosographers, they started out with interpretations in which the mother-child relationship was put on the pedestal as the only valid etiologic consideration. The underlying idea was: Why bother about questions of genetics, organicity, metabolism, or anything else if we can proceed promptly with the psychogenic denominator common to all disturbances of the ego? Thus arose a tendency to set up a pseudodiagnostic waste basket into which an assortment of heterogeneous conditions were thrown indiscriminately. Infantile autism was stuffed into this basket along with everything else. On the East Coast, Beata Rank, creator of the notion of "the atypical child," comprised in this hodgepodge "all more severe disturbances in early development which have been variously described as Heller's disease, childhood psychoses, childhood schizophrenia, autism, or mental defect." On the West Coast, Szurek announced: "We are beginning to consider it clinically fruitless, or even unnecessary, to draw any sharp dividing lines between a condition that one could call psychoneurotic and another that one could call psychosis, autism, atypical development, or schizophrenia." Such looseness threw all curiosity about diagnostic criteria to the winds as irrelevant impediments on the road to therapy which was applied to all comers as if their problems were identical. The therapeutic cart was put before the diagnostic horse and, more often than not, the horse was left out altogether. With a perfunctory bow in the direction of "heredity and biology," we were urged to give up the concern for the differentiation of any kind of behavioral deviation. By decree, mother-infant involvement was to be accepted as the sole key to everything that goes on within and around the neonate; it alone was supposed to determine his destiny. Modify it therapeutically by using the right technique, and the child has a chance to become adapted to the requirements of suburban propriety.

In contrast to this summary disavowal of biological factors, Bender, assuming the possibility of an underlying diffuse encephalopathy, defined childhood schizophrenia as follows: "A disorder in the regulation of maturation of all the basic behavior processes, represented in children by a maturation lag at the embryonic level, characterized by a primitive plasticity in all patterned behavior, determined before birth and activated by a physiological crisis, such as birth." With anxiety as the organismic response to such crises, secondary symptoms were called forth as defense mechanisms which served Bender as a basis for the grouping of childhood schizophrenia into three types: (1) the pseudodefective or autistic type; (2) the pseudoneurotic or phobic, obsessive, compulsive, hypochondriacal type; (3) the pseudopsychopathic or paranoid, acting-out, aggressive, antisocial type.

This formulation accomplished a number of things. It managed to dispose of the idea that childhood schizophrenia must be viewed as *either* functional *or* organic. It implied that at the present state of our knowledge one can—and must—take into consideration the likelihood of a fusion of innate physiological and postnatal emotional factors. It suggested a grouping based on observed phenomena differing in character and in course.

Questions have arisen, however, with regard to the ease with which the diagnosis was suddenly bestowed upon a relatively vast contingent of patients. Bender, who in 1942 had, as she said, "not seen very many cases in which we could make a definite diagnosis," announced later that by 1951 "over 600" schizophrenic children had been studied in one single psychiatric unit, that of the Bellevue Hospital in New York. By 1954, she had as many as 850 cases on her list, which means an addition of about 250 in the short span of three years. It is highly improbable that all of them would be acknowledged as being schizophrenic by many other experienced child psychiatrists, and yet it cannot be denied that Bender has made careful investigations and has conscientiously adhered to her established criteria.

Out of this emerges a rather disturbing dilemma. We seem to have reached a point where a clinician, after the full study of a given child, can say honestly: He is schizophrenic because in my scheme I must call him so. Another clinician, equally honest, can say: He is not schizophrenic because according to my scheme I cannot call him so. This is not a reflection on anyone in particular. The whole concept has obviously become a matter of semantics.

It is not unreasonable to hope that the bracketing out of the syndrome of infantile autism portends a way out of the dilemma. Returning to the two definitions of the word "specific," we can state unreservedly that, whether or not autism is viewed as a member of the species schizophrenia, it does represent a "definitely distinguishable disease." This disease, specific—that is, unique, unduplicated—in its manifestations, can be explored per se. Unimpeded by the perplexities of nosological assignment, investigators can agree on its own phenomenology, search for its own etiology, and follow its own course in ordinary and experimental settings.

This is in keeping with the trend to which Eugen Bleuler's son, Manfred, referred when in a comprehensive review of theory and research between 1941 and 1950, he wrote: "The formulation of schizophrenia has rid itself during the past ten years of the hypothetical idea that a disease termed schizophrenia is available for investigation; instead, it has turned its focus on the study of separate diseases within the group of the schizophrenias."

Once it is acknowledged that infantile autism is a separate disease (and then only), the controversy about its rightful position in any hierarchic nomenclature becomes a matter of personal preference and will remain so until we have acquired more substantial knowledge of fundamentals and depend less on speculation and dialectics.

There are those who insist that infantile autism is one of the schizophrenias, even though this means giving up the original idea that childhood schizophrenia develops after a period of relative normalcy. There are some who, because of the poor response by many patients to psychometric assessment, want it placed among the mental deficiencies. And there are those who refuse it a domicile in either group.

Rimland (1964) believes "that there is sufficient information at hand to demonstrate clearly that early infantile autism is *not* the same disease or cluster of diseases which has come to be called childhood schizophrenia, and that autism can and should be distinguished from it at all levels of discourse." Further, he states that "it is clearly accurate and desirable to treat infantile autism and childhood schizophrenias as separate and quite unrelated disease entities." But is childhood schizophrenia a separate disease entity?

The singling out of autism has been followed by a number of other attempts to describe specific conditions lifted out of the schizophrenic package. Mahler reported in 1949 a syndrome which she named "symbiotic infantile psychosis," distinguished by a symptomatology which she thought to be centered around a desperate effort to avert the catastrophic anxiety of separation. In the same year, Bergman and Escalona discussed "children with unusual sensitivity to sensory stimulation." In 1954, Robinson and Vitale introduced a number of "children with circumscribed interest patterns." It may well turn out that this is just a beginning and that other syndromes will be detected and studied on their own merit.

There is, indeed, no "disease entity" called childhood schizophrenia, just as there is no disease entity called mental deficiency. It would not occur now to anybody to look for a uniform background for such anomalies as phenylketonuria, galactosemia, and familial oligoencephaly. By the same token, it is hardly feasible to house together an assortment of dissimilar phenomenologic conditions grouped loosely as childhood schizophrenia, be that on the basis of genetics, neuropathology, biochemistry, psychoanalysis, existentialism, or what have you.

Infantile autism serves as a paradigm. Unfortunately, cause and effect are not as easily ascertainable as Fölling has been able to make them for phenylketonuria. But we have at least a well-defined clinical picture of beginnings, symptoms, and course which in their totality are unmatched and therefore specific in the same sense as phenylketonuria is specific—that is, "a definitely distinguishable disease." Efforts have been made recently by Polan and Spencer and particularly by Rimland (1964) to refine the diagnostic criteria and to compile a check list of symptoms as a guide for differential diagnosis. Since my own publication in 1946, valuable studies have been made of the language peculiarities of autistic children, especially in the German monograph by Bosch, *Der frühkindliche Autismus*, which appeared in 1962. In 1951, I reported observations on the conception of wholes and parts in early infantile autism. In 1954, I attempted to review autism from the point of view of genetics or at least genealogy. Others have investigated the effects of drugs on autistic children. There have been a number of follow-up studies through, and some beyond, adolescence. A valuable contribution was made in 1953 by Ritvo and Provence about form perception and imitation. The occurrence of autism in twins has been reported.

I was greatly impressed from the start by an observation which stood out prominently and that I made a point of in my first report. Among the first 11 cases, the parents of my patients were for the most part strongly preoccupied with abstractions of a scientific, literary, or artistic nature, and limited in genuine interest in people. Even some of the happiest marriages were rather cold and formal affairs. I remarked: "The question arises whether and to what extent this fact has contributed to the condition of the children. The children's aloneness from the beginning of life makes it difficult to attribute the whole picture exclusively to the type of the early parental relations with our patients." As time went on and more autistic children were seen, the coincidence of infantile autism and the parents' mechanized form of living was startling. This was confirmed by most observers. These were realities which were impossible to ignore. Yet there were some exceptions. Approximately 10 percent of the parents did not fit the stereotype. Besides, those who did reared other normal or, at any rate, nonpsychotic offspring. Moreover, similarly frigid parents are often seen whose children are not autistic.

Aspects of interplay between patients and their parents have been studied by various investigators, and on the basis of these studies four viewpoints have emerged. One theory regards parental behavior as a reaction to the children's peculiarities and of no etiologic significance; this would be justified if it were not for the established fact that the parents' personalities had displayed the characteristic traits long before the arrival of their autistic children. At the other extreme, parents, particularly mothers, are considered the basic cause of pathogenicity; the assumption is that a healthier maternal attitude would have precluded the disorder. A third group feels that the patient, endowed with an innate disability to relate to people, is further influenced adversely by the parents' emotional detachment and the resulting manner of handling him; this in no way discounts the possibility of a reciprocal awkwardness of living together. A fourth theory looks upon the children's psychoses and the antecedents' emotional aloofness as stemming from a common, biologic, genetically determined source; some of the parents indeed give one the impression of autism that has escaped psychotic propensities.

Without going into further details, all of which are fascinating and instructive, the following points can be made with regard to the present state of affairs.

1. It is now generally agreed that a unitary disease entity, schizophrenia, does not exist. Analogously, there is no such unit as childhood schizophrenia.

2. For the time being, however, this caption cannot be discarded. It is "specific" only in the sense that it "pertains to a species, or group, of which the members have common characteristics and are called by a common name." After all, we still speak of mental deficiency, knowing well that the term, a semantic convenience, includes etiologically and clinically heterogeneous conditions.

3. Bender's pioneering work has helped do away with the either-or antithesis of functional and organic by recognizing the fusion of innate as well as experiential components.

4. Attempts have been made to subdivide clinical varieties comprised under the term childhood schizophrenia: cases with acute and insidious onset; "organic and nonorganic" (Goldfard & Dorsen, 1956); pseudodefective, pseudoneurotic, and pseudodelinquent types. These, I believe, have important though only temporary value in that we may anticipate a splitting off of specific syndromes—"specific" in the sense of a "definitely distinguishable disease."

5. Infantile autism has been split off from the cluster and offers itself for investigation of its unique features. It has an identity of its own.

6. Some of the remaining controversies are based more on semantics than on intrinsic essentials.

In closing, I would like to quote from a paper, entitled "Schizophrenia as a Concept," which I presented at a symposium in 1959. I said there: "Child psychiatry is showing the way to the practical application of Bleuler's vision of the plurality of the schizophrenias. It is encouraging to note that similar attempts are beginning to be made with regard to the adult schizophrenias. The smug certainty about a disease schizophrenia has been definitely sloughed off. For the time being, there is still much groping and more or less emotionally tinted clinging to cherished opinions. But so long as facts are scarce, it is inevitable that there be differences of opinion about the delineation of the concept itself, about etiology, and about therapeutic procedures. It is my opinion that in the foreseeable future the same thing will happen to the schizophrenias as has happened to the hyperpyrexias, the insanities, and the amentias and that, when we stop searching for an identical cause and treatment of different ailments tied together in the schizophrenia bundle, we may expect the opening up of new and clearer vistas. But this, also, is only an opinion."†

References

Rather than list the voluminous literature on infantile autism and childhood schizophrenia, I would like to call the reader's attention to three good bibliographic sources on the topic:

Bradley, C. *Schizophrenia in childhood.* New York: Macmillan, 1941.
Goldfarb, W., & Dorsen, M. M. *Annotated bibliography of childhood schizophrenia.* New York: Basic Books, 1956.
Rimland, B. *Infantile autism.* New York: Appleton-Century-Crofts, 1964.

†Reset from the original published in *Behavioral Science,* Volume 10, pp. 412–420, 1965.

10

EARLY INFANTILE AUTISM REVISITED

The year 1968 marks the first quarter-century anniversary of a publication in which this author reported a pattern of child behavior which had not previously been considered in its striking uniqueness. The paper, appearing in 1943 in the now extinct journal, *The Nervous Child*, dealt in some detail with 11 children (eight boys and three girls) who presented a combination of extreme aloneness from the beginning of life and an anxiously obsessive insistence on the preservation of sameness. In searching for an appropriate designation, I decided, after much groping, on the term "early infantile autism," which described time of the first manifestations and accentuated the children's limited accessibility. Beyond the descriptive nosographic account, I ventured this opinion: *We must assume that these children have come into the world with an innate inability to form the usual, biologically-provided affective contact with people, just as other children come into the world with innate physical and intellectual handicaps .... Here, we seem to have pure-culture examples of inborn autistic disturbances of affective contact.*

137

From the start I was greatly impressed with one observation which stood out prominently: The parents of these patients were, for the most part, strongly preoccupied with abstractions of a scientific, literary, or artistic nature, and limited in genuine interest in people. As time went on and more autistic children were studied, the coincidence of infantile autism and the parents' mechanized form of living was really startling. This was confirmed by many other observers. I noted then, however: *These children's aloneness from the beginning of life makes it difficult to attribute the whole picture exclusively to the type of early parental relationships that they have experienced.*

At no time have I pointed to the parents as the primary, postnatal sources of pathogenicity.

The publication of the case findings of the first 11 patients was prompted merely by a wish to communicate to my colleagues a number of experiences for which I could find no reference in the literature. It did not, and could not, occur to me at the time that we were on the threshold of creating, unexpectedly and unintentionally, a great deal of excitement in the field of child psychiatry. This was, in fact, a piece of serendipity, an unpremeditated "discovery" which was not the result of a specific search. Of course, I was interested in the peculiarities of the illness; more such children came to my attention, and I made and reported several studies on the irrelevant and metaphoric language of some of these patients, on their conception of wholes and parts, and on their family backgrounds. These findings and assumptions were cautiously summarized in a paper entitled, "Problems of Nosology and Psychodynamics of Early Infantile Autism" (Kanner, 1949).

By now, thanks to several efforts at diagnostic refinement, the existence of the syndrome, as such, has been universally acknowledged. Several books and hundreds of articles attest to the interest which it has aroused in many quarters, especially on this continent, in Western and Central Europe, and in Japan, but there is still much speculation and understandable confusion concerning etiology and therapy. Notions expounded on this subject have ranged all the way from the assumption of basic organicity to the idea proffered recently, which ascribes the illness to the effects of profound parental psychopathology. There are conflicting opinions about the relation between autism and childhood schizophrenia. The concept of operant conditioning occasionally has been misapplied; in precipitous zeal, this approach to therapy has been championed as a foregone success on the basis of what are, in fact, fragmentary attainments. Various groups have exhibited an attitude of monopolistic ownership of anything pertaining to autism and from time to time have awed the lay press with "evidence" of miraculous-sounding cures.

Fortunately, parents in this and a few other countries have recently banded together into special associations, and these groups are making an organized effort to obtain whatever clarification is possible at this time about the nature and prognosis of their children's autism.

Where, then, do we stand at present with regard to our knowledge of early infantile autism? What progress has been made since the first report 25 years ago? What lies ahead of us in the near future? Here are a few points for consideration:

The existence of early infantile autism is generally accepted as a syndrome known to have specific and typical symptomatology and well-defined diagnostic criteria, but it matters little whether autism be regarded as a form of schizophrenia or looked upon as a disease *sui generis.* Since Bleuler's (1950) courageous—and as time has proved, correct—refusal to view schizophrenia as a disease entity, and his insistence that there is a "group of schizophrenias," there should be no quarrel with those who wish to retain for autism a place within the "group." Nor should there be any objection to those who would maintain that "Kanner's syndrome" is so clearly delineated that it stands apart in its uniqueness. The issue is more semantic than basic. The illness has been, in either case, split off from the cluster of "the schizophrenias" and has been singled out for investigation of its specific features; it has (and is dealt with by most authors as having) an identity of its own.

It is recognized by all observers, except for the dwindling number of those impeded by doctrinaire allegiances, that autism is not primarily an acquired, or "man-made" disease. The fact that many of the parents are rather detached people has been confirmed frequently enough, but this observation cannot be translated summarily into a direct cause-and-effect etiologic relationship, an assumption sometimes ascribed to me via pathways of gross misquotation. Making parents feel guilty of responsibility for their child's autism is not only erroneous, but cruelly adds insult to injury.

Considerable research has so far failed to produce evidence of any consistent neurologic, metabolic, or chromosomal pathology which can be connected with the origin of autism. Infantile autism is a relatively rare illness; hence, many pediatricians and psychiatrists have had little opportunity to become acquainted with it, and diagnostic uncertainties are to be expected. Even the most experienced know that in some instances differential diagnosis may present difficulties, but it is hoped that there are at least a few professionals in each population center who are familiar with the conditions with which autism could be confused. There are still parents driven to despair by the differing "diagnoses" given out by the various physicians consulted: On the one hand, children who are severely retarded, children with Heller's disease, or who are aphasic, have been miscalled "autistic"; on the other hand, autistic children have been miscalled mentally retarded or aphasic. Valid diagnostic criteria are now available (and have been since 1943), and adherence to these is important. We are still in the dark about the true etiology; it is one thing to speculate about "impairment of the reticular formation" and to philosophize about its role by inference, analogy, and deduction, and still another to have established concrete facts.

The futility of such speculation is illustrated by a recent publication, *The Empty Fortress* (Bettelheim, 1967). Its intrepid dust jacket promised the reader that it "sheds new light on the nature, origin and treatment of infantile autism," but the author of the book, being perhaps somewhat more hampered by actual fact than the author of the dust jacket, felt called upon to employ such qualifications as "maybe," "perhaps," "probably," "possibly," "as if," "as it were," "seemed to," "suggests," 146 times in 48 pages of the report of the first case, and he cautions his readers further within the text, "This, like other interpretations of Laurie's behavior, is highly speculative. ..."

Realistically, we must at present accept the fact that our knowledge of the etiology of autism is still extremely limited, and when facts are not available, there is, to be sure, room for theory and hypothesis which lend themselves to sober validation; modesty, however, and the discipline integral to all proper scientific investigation, should protect us from lapses in which we are moved to forget that, however tempting, a theory, unproved, is only that.

This modesty, humility and caution must be applied to therapy as well as to etiology, and this is the keynote at certain centers where efforts continue to be made, consistently and patiently, to help these children find their way into a world which is threatening to them. Other techniques are also being practiced which are founded on theories which have been so dogmatically pronounced and pursued that one must wonder if the earnest "believers" do not hope to elevate their speculative philosophy to the realm of proven fact by dint of pure zeal and enthusiasm—but so far, no better results have been obtained with these theoretically-based techniques than have been obtained with the calm, persistent, nonspectacular attempts to wean the autistic child away from his self-isolation.

This is where we stand at present, approximately 25 years after the first report of 11 autistic children. Much research, much curiosity, is still needed, but so, also, is the kind of sobriety which shies away from fancy-born, pseudo-scientific and premature shouts of *Eureka!*†

References

Bettelheim, B. *The empty fortress.* New York: Free Press, 1967.

Bleuler, E. *Dementia praecox or the group of schizophrenias.* New York: International Universities Press, 1950.

Kanner, L. Autistic disturbances of affective contact. *Nervous Child,* 1943, 2, 217–250.

Kanner, L. Problems of nosology and psychodynamics of early infantile autism. *American Journal of Orthopsychiatry,* 1949, **19**, 416–426.

†Revised from the original published in *Psychiatry Digest*, Volume 29, pp. 17–28, 1968.

11

THE CHILDREN HAVEN'T READ THOSE BOOKS

Even the most sketchy review of the history of science leads one to the conclusion that all progress has been marked by a gradual transition from the general to the specific, from the massive to the minute, from the ill-defined to the ever more concise and delineated. This is certainly true of medicine and of that section of it which has eventually become known as the specialty of psychiatry.

At the time of the emergence from the Middle Ages, there still were learned treatises, entitled *De febribus* or *De pestibus*, in which all febrile illnesses were dealt with as if they were a unitary phenomenon and ascribed to an undifferentiated miasma as the implied source. The advent of bacteriology made it possible to identify specific microorganisms which produced characteristic forms of disease. If you wished to know, cure, and try to prevent an infection, you were obliged to study the properties of the invader, its mode of propagation, its habitat, its path of entry, its behavior inside the victim, and the means which might destroy or reduce its pathogenicity. By adding to, enlarging, and refining the investigative facilities, many diseases, previously lumped together rather diffusely, were singled out and sufficiently identified to establish reliable criteria for differential diagnosis.

The bulk of this process took place in the course of the nineteenth century, which inaugurated a period of reexamining vague concepts and exploding the fallacy of their assumed universality. Thus the notion of amentia or feeblemindedness, nowadays couched more euphemistically in the term mental retardation, was striped of the connotation of nondescript sameness. The sudden spurt of interest in endemic cretinism, Langdon Down's description of so-called mongolism, the etiologic classification of Ireland, the study of amaurotic family idiocy by Tay and Sachs, Fölling's "breakthrough" discovery of phenylpyruvic acid oligophrenia, and numerous other delimitations gave consecutive proof that the one common denominator of cognitive deficiency does not justify the assumption of etiologic and pathologic identity. Old statistics about the heredity of "feeblemindedness" have become meaningless because of the great variety of genetic implications in the different syndromes. A diversity of yardsticks had to be applied to conditions brought about by chromosomal anomalies, metabolic deviations, congenital or acquired structural disorders of the central nervous system, or nutritional and cultural deprivation.

As for the psychoses, it is customary to refer to the chaotic state in the pre-Kraepelinian era. This was the kind of chaos in which generic terms, such as madness, lunacy, or insanity, constituted an ideational cobweb covering up the distinctive features of basic dissimilarities. It is true that since Hippocrates and Aretaeus sporadic attempts were made to outline some forms of psychotic behavior. It is true that in the second half of the past century a few symptom combinations were sequestered out as deserving designations of their own. But it was not until the 1890's that Kraepelin managed to work out a systematic grouping which, in essence, still governs our nosologic nomenclature. Yet at present the walls of Kraepelin's magnificent structure are beginning to show signs of crumbling. He himself had pulled together catatonic, hebephrenic, simple deteriorating, and certain paranoid states, considered separately in the preceding decades, under the unifying name of dementia praecox. Not long afterwards, after renaming it, Bleuler became skeptical of the supposed oneness and prophetically called his book not Schizophrenia but *The Group of the Schizophrenias*, declaring in the introduction that he foresaw an eventual breaking up of "schizophrenia" into a number of similar, but by no means identical, diseases. This has happened in the last quarter century especially in the field of child psychiatry. Early infantile autism, symbiotic psychosis, the syndrome of the child with circumscribed interest patterns were set apart as such and, even though retained in the cluster of the childhood schizophrenias, have been defined and discussed as existences *sui generis*. In a like manner, early problems of communication, no longer tied together collectively in a package named "aphasia," have been recognized, and are being dealt with, as representing conditions of pathogenic and clinical disparity.

It would seem, then, that there has been a growing tendency to get away from sweeping, all-inclusive generalizations in search of compact behavioral patterns which could be observed, described, and ameliorated in terms of their unduplicated uniqueness. Theoretically, if this could be pursued to its logical conclusion, it would seem possible, with the help of even finer tools for research, to discard amorphous generalities, much as the medieval notion of the fevers and the plagues was discarded. This could, indeed, be anticipated *if—if* the child patients had read all those books and articles which in the past few decades have so painstakingly set forth the criteria for exact diagnostic formulations of specific syndromes and, having read them, had endeavored to live up precisely to those criteria. Since, as is to be expected, they have not done so, a major dilemma has arisen.

One substantial cause of the dilemma lies in the fact that, throughout the centuries, along with the diagnostic looseness, there was also a recurring need for uniform etiologic explanations of all behavior. For nearly two millennia, the four humors of the body were made responsible for four—not two, not three, not five—different temperaments and their consequences. When this was found untenable, the notion of the somatic configurations and their psychological correlates took over. Some of the patients, not having read the published anthropometric tables, became manic-depressive even though they had the narrow intercostal angles of the asthenic, or became schizophrenic even though they had the wide intercostal angles of the pyknic. Without further ado, they were decreed to be "mixed types." This took care of things rather neatly, and no sleep had to be lost by anybody.

The quest for something akin to the miasma before the coming of bacteriology had its heyday in the twentieth century. The focal infection theory led to the summary removal of teeth, tonsils, gallbladders, appendices, and parts of the colon. Others elevated the endocrines to the status of "the glands of destiny" or "the glands regulating personality." The central nervous system served some, dubbed by Adolf Meyer as "neurologizing tautologists," as the one and only cradle of behavioral deviations. One group, using Pavlov's work as a starting point and parading under the banner of "behaviorism," saw all mental disorders rooted in faulty conditioning.

Still others allowed themselves to become fixated in the concept of infantile sexuality as the sole explanation of anything that went wrong. It is fascinating to recall how this came about. Freud, in the second of his *Three Contributions to the Theory of Sex*, honestly and wisely presented a hypothetical construction as just this—a hypothetical construction. In 24 pages there were as many as 55 qualifying remarks, such as "perhaps," "probably," "apparently," "so to say," "as it were," "possibly," "it may be supposed," "it may be assumed," "may well be," "I believe that. . .," "we may gain the impression that. . .," etc. Out of these probabilities, assumptions, beliefs, conjectures, and impressions emerged a credo which transformed them into professed certainties and decreed verities, and nonbelievers were burned by the "orthodox" on the stake of red-hot contempt. There was no need for differential diagnosis based on clinical observation. Melanie Klein, asserting not less than 9 times how "very clear" and "very obvious" it all was, could decide in an *unfinished* play analysis of 575 hours spread over 2½ years that 6-year-old Erna suffered from megalomania, paranoia, pseudologia, severe depression, sadistic and cannibalistic impulses, masochism, homosexual tendencies, anal love desires, and a desire to be seduced, all this held together by a "clearly" insatiable appetite for her father's penis and her mother's breasts.

Meanwhile, a new dimension was added to child psychiatry. Until about the teens of this century, most of the occupation with child development and behavior was centered around intraorganismal phenomena, around happenings which had their origin *within* the individual. Much indeed was learned from the stage-by-stage examinations and recordings of the gradual emergence of motor, perceptual, conceptual, linguistic, and adaptive behavior. But the focus of inquiry began to be broadened to include also the outer, attitudinal forces which do things *to* the child and thereby help to shape his feelings and resulting demeanor. This brought about a curiosity about interpersonal relationships as motivating factors. Infantile behavior began to be correlated with parents' attitudes. Children were no longer viewed merely as something like amebas sending out their constitutional pseudopodia into an unconcerned environment. A child's emotional needs began to be seen not only as derived from instinctual drives alone but also as they were satisfied or frustrated by those around him. The external influences were studied in terms of parental, especially maternal, affection, rejection, overprotection, neglect, and exploitation as outgrowth of the parents' own emotional needs. The fusion of the centrifugal propensities which a child brings with him and the centripetal impacts which are helping to mold his personality is being recognized as an indispensable necessity for the understanding of any one child's individual make-up.

The recognition of this fusion, however, has been, and still is, slow in asserting itself. No sooner did the news of the significance of the mother-child relationship get around than a new group arose which elevated it to the status of the *only* feature worth considering etiologically, clinically, and therapeutically. If anything went astray, the ready-made answer was: *Cherchez la mère.* Diagnosis, under these circumstances, was regarded as a secondary, if not altogether superfluous, by-product. There was, as it were, the ubiquitous miasma of noxious mothering, and differences in infant pathology were seen merely as variants of the same misadventure. Thus arose Beata Rank's notion of "the atypical child" which, in her own words, referred to the "more severe disturbances in early development which have been variously described as Heller's disease, childhood psychosis, childhood schizophrenia, autism, or mental deficiency." Some went even further than Rank; Stanislaus Szurek declared emphatically: "We are beginning to consider it clinically fruitless, or even unnecessary, to draw any sharp dividing lines between a condition that one could call psychoneurosis and another that one could call psychosis, autism, atypical development, or schizophrenia." Are these different designations really nothing more than pseudo-semantic extravagances? Is this kind of relinquishment of all diagnostic differentiations really far removed from the haziness underlying the old treatises on the fevers and the plagues?

Nevertheless, I should like to plead for a sympathetic leniency toward the impatience which has made some people despair of what seemed to be the hopeless task of looking for neatly packaged bundles, each and everyone labeled accurately and unmistakably and identified promptly as soon as the wrappers were taken off. Most of us had children brought to us whose parents had been told in turn by a succession of competent, well-trained experts that the little patients were severely retarded, brain-damaged, schizophrenic, autistic, aphasic, or "emotionally blocked." Severe mental disorders of young children often *are* protean in their manifestations and may present the elements of any of these conditions in a variety of combinations. Before we are too superciliously critical of the advisers who happened to precede us in the understandably confused parents' groping tour of consultations, it well behooves us to remember that not infrequently, after a careful review of all our findings, the diagnosis arrived at may still have to be regarded as tentative for some time.

All this is reflected in the many attempts that have been made to find a suitable classification of the psychopathological disorders in childhood. One of the latest such efforts was published in June 1966 by the Committee of Child Psychiatry of the American Psychiatric Association (Volume VI, Report No. 62 of the Group for the Advancement of Psychiatry). A statement in the short introduction deserves being quoted verbatim. It says: "The task has been a challenging and a humbling one. As yet, no all-encompassing, unequivocally accepted conceptual framework exists within which the intricate interrelationships among somatic, intellectual, emotional and social processes and phenomena in the developing child can be comprehended and organized in a thoroughly logical, all-inclusive fashion. Nevertheless, the Committee still felt that sufficient understanding and knowledge are available at this time for the development of a workable if not ideal classification. The marked discrepancies among current nosological approaches to childhood disorders and the disparities among nomenclatural terms employed underline the need for a classification based upon explicit and clearly defined categories that can be employed by clinicians from varying conceptual backgrounds. Such categories are important for the purposes of ready communication in work and teaching, the collection of comparable data, the study of the natural history of disease pictures, the assessment of treatment outcome and prognostic outlook, and the investigation of epidemiologic factors."

The appendix to this report of the Committee of Child Psychiatry offers not less than 23 samples of other groupings suggested between 1920 and 1964. I am certain that there will be others to follow in the future. As more and more distinctive categories will be delineated and allocated in the nosological chest of drawers, there will be a continuing need for regrouping.

After all, what is the historical basis for differential diagnosis? Now and then, out of the welter of diagnostic diffuseness, a symptom constellation has been isolated and named in accordance with its intrinsic character or after the person or group of persons first on the scene to call attention to it. It is then, after analogous observations have been made by other investigators, incorporated in the check-list of similar, related, specific constellations and is available for comparison or contrast. Some such units are more easily identified and more permanently established than others, depending on the simpler or more complex link between phenomenon and ascertainable etiology or on the incontestable singularity of the phenomenon itself. It has become relatively easy, through definite biochemical tests, to point to phenylketonuria, galactosemia, or lead encephalopathy. It is not difficult, with the aid of ophthalmoscopy, to determine the presence of Tay-Sachs disease. Cerebral palsy can be diagnosed as a result of thorough neurologic exploration. A brain biopsy can help decisively in clinching the diagnosis of Heller's disease, especially in conjunction with the typically distinguishing anamnestic peculiarities. Inspection alone often leads the expert to the thought of Down's disease or gargoylism. All that is required in these instances is a sufficient acquaintance with the conditions presenting themselves and with the means available for the removal of any existing doubt. With this as a premise, it becomes a matter of *res ipsa loquitur*—the thing speaks for itself. The patients, even though they have not read those books, somehow act as if they had; they comply with the requisites essential for a clearcut diagnosis.

But there is a host of clinical pictures which do not offer themselves so conveniently for a diagnostic aha-response. The issues are so much more blurred; the range is so much more widespread; there is so much more overlapping of symptoms; there is no such easy reference to cause and effect. Indeed, there is a plurality of possible causes, and the effect itself is perplexingly equivocal. The thing just would not speak for itself. How does one go on from here?

You can, as has been done, unperturbedly invent a common matrix for all infantile disorders, be this inside the cranium, a metabolic vagary, faulty conditioning, early fixation, an unhealthy mother-child relationship, or what have you. Then you can proclaim, for instance, that an epithet, such as "atypical" or "emotionally disturbed" or "brain-damaged," takes care of the whole gamut of behavioral deviations. Thus fortified, you need not be bothered by any sense of obligation to join the other branches of medicine where, because of the possibility of greater precision, such summarizing adjectives are no longer accepted as the last word in diagnostic certitude.

You can, on the other hand, more in keeping with reality, admit that there are indeed many children whose conditions are enigmatic in terms of their exact origin and of their nosology. Such awareness enhances the desire to see what additional syndromes can be bracketed out and set apart as specific entities. This is so very much more difficult than is the contentment with overall would-be diagnostic epithets. You can start out with the assuring knowledge that such entities have been described, even though you know that even some of those have eventually been found to be collections rather than units.

One can think, for example, of the courageous work of Sante De Sanctis who a decade or so after Kraepelin's introduction of the dementia praecox concept, came forth with the corresponding concept of dementia praecocissima as a specific infantile psychosis. Soon the Italian and Central European literature abounded with case reports and discussions of this "disease." In the course of time, the concept lost its validity because the group, after all, was found to consist of a mixture of such things as postencephalitic problems, dementia infantilis, Schilder's encephalitis periaxialis diffusa, and forms of behavior which to this day impress most of us as belonging to the schizophrenic cluster.

De Sanctis, nevertheless, did a pioneering job, insofar as his careful descriptions and observations led others to compare and contrast and, through their own discoveries, to take out a growing number of clearly specified units from the originally supposed oneness. Dementia praecocissima was, if I may say so, like an onion from which more and more layers were peeled off, leaving a core of syndromes still viewed as schizophrenic in the sense of the boundaries set later by Homburger, Lutz, Ssucharewa, Despert, and others.

When, in 1943, early infantile autism was further peeled off on the basis of definite criteria, the ensuing events tended to pinpoint the old nosological dilemma. In the 1950's, it seemed of a sudden as though the world was swarming with a great multitude of autistic children. It became a habit to dilute the concept of diagnosing autism in many discrepant conditions which showed one or more symptoms encountered as a part feature of the overall syndrome. Mentally defective children who displayed bizarre behavior were promptly labeled autistic and, in accordance with preconceived notions, both parents were urged to undergo protracted psychotherapy, in addition to treatment directed toward the defective child's own supposedly underlying emotional problems rooted in pathological mother-child relationship. By 1953, van Krevelen, rightly impatient with the cavalier abandon of the criteria outlined rather succinctly from the beginning, warned against the prevailing "abuse of the diagnosis of autism," declaring that it "threatens to become a fashion." In the first book on autism, which was published in Holland, the term "pseudo-autism" was suggested, and promptly conditions variously described as hospitalism, anaclitic depression, and separation anxiety were made to sail under this banner. Since then, numerous volumes and a plethora of articles on "autism" have appeared. More often than not the term is still being used far too loosely. Many of the case illustrations bear little resemblance to that which they purport to illustrate. The authoritatively decreed causes range all the way from anomalies of the reticular system to disorders of communication or pathogenic mother-child relationship.

On the other hand, elaborate attempts were made to refine the diagnostic criteria so that the thing could really speak for itself to anybody bound by an established set of pathognomonic features. But even then, some of those who had conscientiously labored at this task have become uneasy and reverted to shoving different conditions under a common etiologic umbrella. This is evident in a recent study by Ornitz and Ritvo (1968), who declare that "early infantile autism, atypical development, symbiotic psychosis, and certain cases of childhood schizophrenia" are "essentially variants of the same disease."

So here we stand. Where do all these reflections on differential diagnosis leave us at the present time? I think that we can make the following points:

1. We have always been—and still are—under the obligation to study each individual child with his own unequalled profile as we find him developmentally,

somatically, intellectually, emotionally, and in the framework of the centripetal (environmental) forces that may have contributed to the situation with which we are confronted. Henry Maudsley wisely urged about a century ago: "Observation should begin with simple instances, ascent being made from them step by step through appropriate generalizations, and no particulars should be neglected."

2. While it is true that each child patient is, by virtue of being none other than himself, not like anybody else to the point of complete identity, his profile may closely resemble that of other child patients. If we find a sufficient number of such similar profiles, we try, as has been customary throughout the ages, to subsume them under a joint heading, or diagnosis. The closer the resemblance is, the more certain are we that a fitting diagnosis has been made and can be confirmed by all colleagues. Many such profiles have been singled out and the mere mention of the heading is enough to give one a reasonably clear idea of the gist of the problem.

3. When, however, the profile contains features found also in one or several profiles combined under different headings, then the question of differentiation arises. A review of the history tells us that, with the growing improvement of the facilities for observation, there has been a continuum of new discoveries, chiseling off chip after chip from what were imagined to be monolithic edifices. We are now far removed from the bland ascription of commonness to the fevers and plagues, to amentia, or to madness. The emphasis has shifted, instead, to ever finer differentiation. This has yielded everywhere in the medical specialties a body of knowledge to which something new is added constantly by the introduction of previously unknown specifically itemized pathologic existences.

4. In our own specialty, we are still confronted with many child patients whose profiles cannot be easily matched with those for which a joint heading already exists. This is true especially of the more severe disturbances in the first years of life. The children, unfamiliar with those books and articles, simply do not have their symptoms arranged to indicate which are basic and dominant and which are incidental and derivative.

5. This indisputable fact has led some to an anachronistic reversal to the medieval and earlier diffuseness and an a priori insistence on somthing like the all-pervading miasma. Since several groups have insisted on different "miasmas," we have been confronted with the sectarianism of different so-called approaches. The term "approach" ought to be viewed with some misgivings. It implies that it is we who march toward the patient with a ready-made set of convictions and techniques applicable to all. To the contrary, it is the patient who comes or is brought to us and, in his various ways, approaches us with whatever it is that ails him.

6. We do, indeed, have general joint headings, such as mental retardation, delinquency, psychosis, aphasia, or minimal brain damage, which lend themselves for book titles or periodic reviews of the pertinent literature. We have such general joint headings elsewhere in medicine, such as cardiac ailments, infectious diseases, or neurodermatoses, but it would not occur to anybody to view those as diagnostic categories.

7. As things stand now, we have gradually been able to observe and describe a number of profiles with characteristic syndromes that *do* speak for themselves. Beyond this, we have many combinations, overlaps, and fluctuations for which there is no provision in the more clearly defined profiles. The children, not having read those books, do not, for the sake of our convenience, merge into any of the well-known, clear-cut patterns. It is then up to us to go on studying those children as individuals with their own unique peculiarities patiently and pluralistically from every angle, without the air of feigned omniscience, without pressing them into any preconceived diagnostic and etiologic dogma, and with the hope that thus we shall from time to time discover more profiles which speak for themselves.†

REFERENCES

Ornitz, E. M., & Ritvo, E. R. Perceptual inconstancy in early infantile autism. *Archives of General Psychiatry,* 1968, **18**, 76–98.

†Reset from the original published in *Acta Paedopsychiatrica,* Volume 36, pp. 2–11, 1969.

12

CHILDHOOD PSYCHOSIS:
A HISTORICAL OVERVIEW

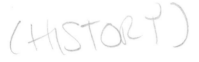

In 1867 Maudsley, the noted British psychiatrist, included in his textbook, *Physiology and Pathology of Mind*, a 34-page chapter on "Insanity of Early Life." In it he not only tried to correlate symptoms with developmental status but also suggested an elaborate seven-point classification, which went as follows:

1. Monomania
2. Choreic mania
3. Cataleptoid insanity
4. Epileptoid insanity
5. Mania
6. Melancholia
7. Affective insanity

Anyone superciliously critical either of the terminology based on the then circulating coinage or of the cohesion of the grouping may be reminded that the differentiation of the childhood psychoses has to this day not gone far beyond a degree of controversial floundering.

Maudsley was severely taken to task by his colleagues for daring to acknowledge the existence of "insanity" in childhood. Undaunted, he retained the chapter in the 1880 edition but deemed it necessary to lead off with an introductory paragraph that masterfully combined a seeming apology with a forceful affirmation. He wrote:

> "How unnatural!" is an exclamation of pained surprise which some of the more striking instances of insanity in young children are apt to provoke. However, to call a thing unnatural is not to take it out of the domain of natural law, notwithstanding that when it has been so designated it is sometimes thought that no more needs to be said. Anomalies, when rightly studied, yield rare instruction; they witness and attract attention to the operation of hidden laws or of known laws under new and unknown conditions, and to set the inquirer on new and fruitful paths of research. *For this reason it will not be amiss to occupy a separate chapter with a consideration of the abnormal phenomena of mental derangement in children.*

There have been earlier sporadic anecdotal reports about misdeeds of "mentally deranged" children. Rarely does one come upon an effort to look for explanations on other than pseudomoralistic grounds. All that even the great Esquirol had to say in 1838 about a "little homicidal maniac" was that the 11-year-old girl who had pushed two infants into a well "was known for her evil habits." Maudsley himself, searching for an etiologic common denominator, stated that "neurotic parents" implant a genetic predisposition for the fulminant effects of fright, chorea, convulsions, or cerebral trauma; he raised the question whether all "insanities" of children could be forms of "larvated epilepsy."

Maudsley's chapter is a major landmark in the history of childhood psychoses, which soon became a legitimate topic of psychiatric curiosity. It is worthy of note that in the first 45 volumes of the *American Journal of Insanity* (1844-1889) there was not a single article pertaining to children. In 1883 Clevenger, compiling a review of the world literature on mental illness in childhood, got together 55 references. In the same year, Spitzka devoted considerable space in his *Treatment of Insanity* to infantile psychoses, which he declared to be rare and caused by heredity, fright, sudden changes of temperature, or masturbation.

Thus, a little less than a century ago, after some initial reluctance, the doors of academic psychiatry were opened to the childhood psychoses. In the subsequent two decades, the number of case reports in the periodicals increased perceptibly. Four textbooks appeared which dealt exclusively with the subject—

one by a German (Emminghaus, 1887), two by Frenchmen (Moreau de Tours, 1888; Manheimer, 1899), and one by a Scotsman (Ireland, 1898).

All this happened at a time when a newly introduced classification of adult psychoses, which to this day still governs our nosologic nomenclature, was creating a stir in the profession. It is customary to refer to the chaotic state in the pre-Kraepelinian era when genetic terms, such as madness, lunacy, or insanity, constituted an ideational cobweb covering up the distinctive features of basic dissimilarities. A few disease patterns had already been singled out. Kraepelin pulled together catatonic, hebephrenic, simple deteriorating, and certain paranoid states, considered separately before then, under the unifying name dementia praecox. Once this was generally accepted, the question inevitably arose whether and to what extent the new concept could be applied to children.

De Sanctis in Italy noticed among "phrenasthenic" (retarded) children some whose "vesanic" (psychotic) symptoms caused him to study the relationship between mental deficiency and dementia praecox. In 1906, he concluded that, while primarily feebleminded children can display psychotic behavior, others, though neurologically intact and intellectually well endowed, deserve the term dementia praecocissima because of the very early age at which dementia praecox becomes manifest. Soon the Italian and Central European literature abounded with case illustrations and discussions of this "disease." In the course of time, the term lost its validity because the group thus designated was found to be made up of an assortment of disparate, etiologically unrelated conditions.

Nevertheless, De Sanctis did a pioneering job. His careful descriptions and observations led others to compare and contrast and, through their own discoveries, to take a growing number of clearly specified units out of the originally assumed homogeneity.

In 1908, the Austrian educator Heller reported six cases of an infantile affliction that took an unusual course: Onset in the third or fourth year of life after normal development; increasing malaise; rapid diminution of interests with loss of speech and sphincter control; final complete idiotic regression, with retention of an intelligent physiognomy and of adequate motor functioning.

The story of this extremely rare condition highlights a dual and intertwined dilemma of psychiatric nosology—that of generalization versus specification and of assumed nonorganicity ("functional" psychosis) versus demonstrated organicity. Heller's disease was first regarded as the earliest form of dementia praecox and hence "functional." It was evicted from this location when in 1931 brain biopsies revealed "acute diffuse degeneration of the ganglion cells" in the lower layers of the cortex; it was moved to the category of a specific ailment *sui generis*, "organic" in nature.

Bleuler announced in 1911 that he looked on schizophrenia (his term for what until then was known as dementia praecox) as a common name for a cluster of related conditions. He spoke not of schizophrenia in the singular but of the "group of the schizophrenias." He wrote: "This concept may be only of temporary value inasmuch as it may later have to be reduced, in the same sense as the discoveries in bacteriology necessitated the subdivision of the pneumonias in terms of various etiologic agents."

In retrospect, it is indeed easy to stand in admiration of Bleuler's prophetic vision. He himself had next to nothing to say about children. Having made the above-quoted reservation, he gave a brilliant general summary of adult and adolescent schizophrenia (in the singular) with its Kraepelinian varieties. Meyer, stressing the significance of constitutional factors as well as life experiences, saw schizophrenia as "still definitely an entity with nosologic pretense," as "an abnormal reaction which certain individuals develop as an inadequate adaptation to the total life situation," as "a habit disorganization on constitutional ground."

It took more than two decades before a sufficient overall grasp could develop to allow a similar characterization of infantile schizophrenia. In 1933, Potter formulated a set of criteria that could be applicable to children: To justify the diagnosis, there must be (a) a generalized retraction of interests from the environment; (b) dereistic thinking, feeling, and acting; (c) disturbances of thought, manifested through blocking, symbolization, condensation, perseveration, incoherence, and diminution, sometimes to the extent of mutism; (d) defect of emotional rapport; (e) diminution, rigidity, and distortion of affect; (f) alteration of behavior with either an increase of motility, leading to incessant activity, or a diminution of motility, leading to complete immobility or bizarre behavior with a tendency to perseveration or stereotypy.

By the middle of the 1930's infantile schizophrenia was plainly on the map. It was placed there differently from the manner in which its adult counterpart had been placed. Kraepelin had assembled several previously described syndromes under one common nosologic roof. The observers of children at first took over the same structure in toto. Eventually, looking under the roof, they noticed that their patients displayed some obvious dissimilarities of incipiency and clinical course. Independently of each other, Homburger in Germany, Sukhareva in Russia, Lutz in Switzerland, and Despert in this country recognized two distinct varieties—those with acute onset and those with insidious onset. Bender, widening the roof beyond the Kraepelinian boundaries, distinguished under it three clinical types: pseudodefective, pseudoneurotic, and pseudopsychopathic. In 1943 Kanner reported the syndrome of early infantile autism as "a pure culture sample of inborn autistic disturbance of affective contact." In 1949 Mahler and Furer introduced the concept of symbiotic psychosis occurring in "constitutionally vulnerable infants." In 1956 Goldfarb described a contrast between "organic" and "non-organic" infantile schizophrenia.

For quite some time, "constitutionality" or "innateness" was spoken of diffusely as an absolute prerequisite. Bender went beyond this generality by stating more specifically that schizophrenia is

> a psychobiologic entity determined by an inherited predisposition, an early physiologic or organic crisis, and a failure in adequate defense mechanism; schizophrenia persists for the lifetime of the individual but exhibits different clinical or behavioral or psychiatric features at different epochs in the individual's development and in relationship to compensating or decompensating defenses which can be influenced by environmental factors.

This formulation reduced the major dilemma still floating about as a leftover from the old body-mind dualism. It helped to lay at rest the either-or antithesis of functional and organic by pointing to the fusion of innate as well as experiential components.

In the early 1950's, Rank created the concept of the "atypical child" as an overall designation for children presenting signs of "ego fragmentation" in close connection with maternal psychopathology. The underlying idea was: Why bother about questions of genetics, organicity, metabolism, or anything else if we can proceed promptly with the psychogenic denominator common to all disturbances of the ego? Thus a pseudodiagnostic waste basket was set up into which went "all more severe disturbances in early development which have been variously described as Heller's disease, childhood psychosis, childhood schizophrenia, autism, or mental defect." With a perfunctory bow in the direction of "heredity and biology," mother-infant involvement was decreed to be the sole key to everything that goes on within or around the neonate.

On the whole, however, there has been a tendency in the past three decades to study infantile psychoses with close attention to all their variations and to investigate all conceivable etiologic and developmental factors. The scientific refinements in the past half century have made this increasingly possible. One may enlarge a bit on Bleuler's bacteriologic analogy. There was a time when all "fevers" and "plagues" were referred to a nondescript "miasma"; the discoveries of the microbes broke it up into specific pathogens producing specific diseases and suggesting specific methods of treatment and prevention. We have entered on a similar stage with regard to the childhood psychoses. We have been moving away from miasma-like summary explanations based on opinions, wholesale postulates, and armchair play with semantics in search of factual data of origin, phenomenology, pathology, epidemiology, and psychodynamics. What is more, the accumulated findings, fractional though they still be, led to a manifold array of experimental and heuristic therapeutic endeavors, beginning to be checked by controlled followup studies.

Exactly 90 years ago, Maudsley felt called upon to apologize for so much as making childhood psychoses mentionable. At present we are witnessing a veritable avalanche of publications with thousands of articles and hundreds of monographs crowding the international literature. A helpful incentive has come from groups of parents who had become impatient with the laissez-faire preoccupation of earlier academicians with generalities, speculations, and satisfaction with would-be diagnostic name-calling. By far the greatest incentive is coming from child patients themselves who, not having read those articles and monographs and unconcerned about existing nomenclature, present themselves as they are and thus, as individuals, continue inviting further refinements of criteria for differential diagnosis.

So acute has been the understandable excitement about trying to solve the riddles of infantile autism and schizophrenia that other psychotic conditions of childhood have received relatively little attention. Of late, there have been serious considerations of manic-depressive episodes. There has been, regrettably, a reduction of interest, stimulated by Weygandt in 1915, in psychotic phenomena observed in children with basic mental deficiency. Moreover, the psychotic behavior associated with clearly demonstrated cerebral and metabolic disorders has, at least in this country, been dealt with rather sparingly; Stutte in Germany and Bollea in Italy have become the principal exponents of these much-needed investigations.

This brings to a conclusion the admittedly sketchy outline of the history of childhood psychosis. A complete chronicle remains to be written and would best be reserved for a future date. For, after the preliminary events sketched above, the history is at present in its vigorous incipiency.

Hence, the time has now become ripe for a central depository for the variegated clinical and research activities in many related sciences and in many countries. We are still far from knowing all there is to be known but we are learning how to ask pertinent questions and how to go about looking for the answers. Luckily, the leading contributors, many of whom are well-known pioneers, have readily agreed to join an integral task force of collaborators in forming the editorial board of this new multidisciplinary journal "devoted to all psychoses and severe disorders of behavior in childhood."

REFERENCES

Bender, L. The nature of childhood psychosis. In J. G. Howells (Ed.), *Modern perspectives in international child psychiatry.* Edinburgh: Oliver and Boyd, 1969 (210 references).

Despert, J. L. *The emotionally disturbed child, then and now.* New York: Vantage Press, 1965.

Goldfarb, W., & Dorssen, M. M. *Annotated bibliography of childhood schizophrenia.* New York: Basic Books, 1956.

13

FOLLOW-UP STUDY OF ELEVEN AUTISTIC CHILDREN ORIGINALLY REPORTED IN 1943

The June 1943 issue of the now extinct journal *The Nervous Child* carried a paper entitled "Autistic disturbances of affective contact"; the first 24 pages told about 11 children who had in common a pattern of behavior not previously considered in its startling uniqueness; this was followed by 9 pages of discussion and comment. An introductory paragraph concluded with the sentence: "Since none of the children of this group has as yet attained an age beyond 11 years, this must be considered a preliminary report, to be enlarged upon as the patients grow older and further observation of their development is made."

Twenty-eight years have elapsed since then. The periodical in which the article was printed has been out of circulation for a long time.

The patients were between 2 and 8 years old when first seen at the Children's Psychiatric Clinic of the Johns Hopkins Hospital. What has become of them? What is their present status?

Under the auspices of Dr. Alejandro Rodriguez, the present director of the Clinic, Miss Barbara Ashenden, head social worker since 1931, undertook the task of learning about their whereabouts, functioning levels, and interim destinies. The results will be presented in the sequence of the original presentation, preceded in each instance by a synopsis of the status found at first acquaintance.

Case I

Donald T.'s arrival on October 14, 1938, was heralded by a 30-page history in which the father gave an excellent account of the child's background. Donald was born normally at term on September 8, 1933. Breastfeeding until the eighth month was followed by frequent changes of formulas. He walked alone at 13 months. Dentition proceeded satisfactorily.

"At one year, he could hum and sing many tunes accurately. . . . He was encouraged by his family in reciting short poems and even learned the 23rd Psalm and 25 questions and answers of the Presbyterian Catechism. . . . He very soon knew an inordinate number of pictures in a set of *Compton's Encyclopedia*. . . . He quickly learned the whole alphabet backwards and as well as forwards and to count to 100. But he was not learning to ask questions or answer questions unless they pertained to rhymes or things of that nature. . . . He seems to be self-satisfied. He has no apparent affection when petted. He does not notice when anyone comes or goes. He seems to draw into his shell and live within himself. He seldom comes when called but has to be picked up and carried or led wherever he has to go. When interfered with, he has temper tantrums during which he is destructive. . . . At 2 years, he developed a mania for spinning blocks and pans and other round objects, but at the same time he had a dislike for self-propelling vehicles. He is still fearful of tricycles and seems to have almost a horror of them when he is forced to ride."

In August 1937, he was placed in a preventorium (State Institution for the Prevention and Care of Tuberculosis) "in order to provide for him a change of environment." While there, "he displayed an abstraction which made him oblivious to everything about him. He seems to be always thinking and to get his attention almost requires one to break down a mental barrier between his inner conscience and the outside world." The family physician suggested an appointment at our Clinic. The director of the preventorium was against it, stating that Donald "is getting along nicely" and "it looks that now he is going to be perfectly all right"; his advice was "to let him alone." When the parents insisted and asked him to send us a report, he did so on less than half a page, referring to Donald as "a concentrated child mentally" and surmised that "he might have some glandular disease."

The father, whom Donald resembled physically, was "a successful, meticulous, hardworking lawyer, who takes everything very seriously.... When he walks down the street, he is so absorbed in thinking that he sees nothing and nobody and cannot remember anything about the walk." The mother, a college graduate, was a calm, capable person to whom her husband felt superior. A second child, a boy, was born on May 22, 1938.

At the Clinic, Donald was found to be in good physical condition. He was placed for 2 weeks at the Child Study Home of Maryland for an intensive observation by Drs. Eugenia S. Cameron and George Frankl. After this, Donald came back three times for a checkup. Space does not allow our even coming close to the minutely recorded data in the Clinic files and in the frequent letters sent by and to the mother who, while her husband had functioned as a reliable historian, became the active participant in the child's management. Suffice it to say that the father's description could be confirmed. Donald wandered about smiling, making stereotyped movements with his fingers, shaking his head from side to side, humming the same three-note tune. He spun with great pleasure anything he could seize upon to spin. Most of his actions were repetitious, carried out the same way each time. He kept parroting what he had heard said to him, using the personal pronouns for the persons quoted, even to the point of imitating their intonation.

In 1942, his parents placed him on a tenant farm about 10 miles from their home. When I visited there in May 1945, I was amazed at the wisdom of the couple who took care of him. They managed to give him goals for his stereotypies. They made him use his preoccupation with measurements by having him dig a well and report on its depth. When he kept collecting dead birds and bugs, they gave him a spot for a "graveyard" and had him put up markers; on each he wrote a first name, the type of animal as a middle name, and the farmer's last name, e.g.: "John Snail Lewis. Born, date unknown. Died, (date on which he found the animal)." When he kept counting rows of corn over and over, they had him count the rows while plowing them. On my visit, he plowed six long rows; it was remarkable how well he handled the horse and plow and turned the horse around. It was obvious that Mr. and Mrs. Lewis were very fond of him and just as obvious that they were gently firm. He attended a country school where his peculiarities were accepted and where he made good scholastic progress.

The rest of the story is contained in a letter from the mother, dated April 6, 1970:

"Don is now 36 years old, a bachelor living at home with us. He had an acute attack of rheumatoid arthritis in 1955. Fortunately, this lasted only a few weeks. Physically, since that time, he has been in perfect health. . . . Since receiving his A.B. degree in 1958, he has worked in the local bank as a teller. He is satisfied to remain a teller, having no real desire for promotion. He meets the public there real well. His chief hobby is golf, playing four or five times a week at the local country club. While he is no pro, he has six trophies won in local competition. . . . Other interests are Kiwanis Club (served as president one term), Jaycees, Investment Club, Secretary of Presbyterian Sunday School. He is dependable, accurate, shows originality in editing the Jaycee program information, is even-tempered but has a mind of his own. . . . He owns his second car, likes his independence. His room includes his own TV, record player, and many books. In College his major was French and he showed a particular aptitude for languages. Don is a fair bridge player but never initiates a game. Lack of initiative seems to be his most serious drawback. He takes very little part in social conversation and shows no interest in the opposite sex.

"While Don is not completely normal, he has taken his place in society very well, so much better than we ever hoped for. If he can maintain status quo, I think he has adjusted sufficiently to take care of himself. For this much progress, we are truly grateful. . . . Please give Dr. Kanner our kindest regards. Tell him the couple Don lived with for 4 years, Mr. and Mrs. Lewis, are still our friends. We see them quite often. Don has never had any medication for his emotional trouble. I wish I knew what his inner feelings really are. As long as he continues as he is now, we can continue to be thankful."

Case 2

Frederick Creighton ("Wikky") W. was seen on May 29, 1942, one week before his sixth birthday. This is an abstract of his mother's complaint statement:

"He has always been self-sufficient, I have never known him to cry demanding attention. He was never very good with cooperative play. Until last year, he acted as if people weren't there. About a year ago, he began showing more interest in observing them, but usually people are an interference. To a certain extent he likes to stick to the same thing. On one of the bookshelves we had three pieces of a certain arrangement. Whenever this was changed, he always rearranged it in the same pattern. . . . He had said at least two words before he was 2 years old. Between 2 and 3 years, he would say words that seemed to come as a surprise to himself. One of the first words he said was 'overalls'. . . . At about 2½ years, he began to sing. He sang about 20 or 30 songs, including a little French lullaby. In his fourth year, I tried to make him ask for things before he'd get them. He was stronger willed than I was and held out longer; he would not get it but he would never give in. . . . Now he can count up to into the hundreds and can read numbers, but he is not interested in numbers as they apply to objects. He has great difficulty in learning the proper use of personal pronouns. When receiving a gift, he would say to himself: "You say, 'Thank you.' "

He was delivered by elective Caesarean section 2 weeks before term because the mother had "some kidney trouble." He was well at birth. Feeding presented no problem. His mother never saw him assume an anticipatory posture when she came to pick him up. He sat up at 7 months and walked along at 18 months.

Wikky was an only child. His father, a plant pathologist, was "a patient, even-tempered man" who as a child did not talk "until late" and was "delicate." The mother, "healthy and even-tempered," had been a secretary, a purchasing agent, and at one time a teacher of history. She was 34 and her husband was 38 years old when their son was born.

The paternal grandfather, whose autobiography (published in 1943) was dedicated "to my family of 11 children and grandchildren," had disappeared in 1911, his whereabouts remaining obscure for 25 years, during which he had married a British novelist (without obtaining a divorce from his wife). He had two listings in Who's Who—one under his real name and one under an assumed name. He has had several careers on four continents, which include manganese mining, directorship of an art museum, deanship of a medical school, and organization of medical missions. His (legal) wife was a "dyed-in-the-wool missionary." He had five children, of whom Wikky's father was the second. One son was a newspaper man, one a science fiction writer, one worked for a TV network; a daughter was a singer. Of the maternal relatives the mother said: "Mine are very ordinary people."

Wikky was well-nourished; occiput and frontal region were prominent. He had a supernumerary nipple in the left axilla. X-ray of the skull was normal. Tonsils were large and ragged.

In the office, he wandered aimlessly about for a few moments, then sat down, uttering unintelligible sounds, and abruptly lay down, smiling. Questions and requests, if reacted to at all, were repeated in echolalia fashion. Objects absorbed him, and he showed good attention in handling them. He seemed to regard people as unwelcome intruders. When a hand was held out before him so that he could not possibly ignore it, he played with it as if it were a detached object. He promptly noticed the wooden form boards and worked at them spontaneously, interestedly, and skillfully.

In September 1942, he was enrolled at the Devereux Schools, where he remained until August 1965. A close contact was maintained between the

Schools and our Clinic. In 1962, a report from Devereux stated: "He is, at 26 years, a passive, likeable boy whose chief interest is music. He is able to follow the routine and, though he lives chiefly within his own world, he enjoys those group activities which are of particular interest to him." He was a member of the chorus in the Parents' Day program and was in charge of the loud speaker at the annual carnival. He went on weekend trips to town unaccompanied and made necessary purchases independently.

Wikky, now addressed as Creighton, has been with his parents for the past 5 years. He is now 34 years old. After leaving Devereux, the family spent a year in Puerto Rico where "he picked up a lot of Spanish and worked out a schedule of studying language lessons on records at 4 o'clock every afternoon." The family then moved to Raleigh. The parents report: "We settled into a new home and he did his part in it. He has become acquainted with the neighbors and sometimes makes calls on them. We tried him out in the County Sheltered Workshop and Vocational Training Center. He took right to it, made friends with the teachers, and helped with some of the trainees. Through his relationship there, he took up bowling and he does pretty well. . . . Creighton was suggested by the Workshop for a routine job in connection with running duplicating machines. Since November 25, 1969, he has been working in the office of the National Air Pollution Administration (HEW) every day, and all day." A letter from the Acting Director, dated April 29, 1970, says, "Creighton is an outstanding employee by any standard. Outstanding to me means dependability, reliability, thoroughness, and thoughtfulness toward fellow workers. In each case Creighton is notable."

Case 3

Richard M. was 39 months old when admitted to the Johns Hopkins Hospital on February 5, 1941, with the complaint of deafness "because he did not talk and did not respond to questions." The pediatrician who examined him reported: "The child seems quite intelligent, playing with the toys in his bed and being adequately curious about instruments used in the examination. He seems quite self-sufficient in his play. He will obey commands, such as 'Sit up' or 'Lie down', even when he does not see the speaker. He does not pay attention to conversation going on around him, and although he does make noises, he says no recognizable words."

Richard's father was a professor of forestry, very much immersed in his work, almost to the exclusion of social contacts. The mother was a college graduate. The family, in both branches, consisted of professional people. Richard's younger brother was described as normal and well-developed.

Richard was born normally. He sat up at 8 months and walked at 1 year. His mother began to "train" him at the age of 3 weeks, giving him a suppository every morning "so his bowels would move by the clock." Nutrition and physical growth proceeded satisfactorily.

In September 1940, the mother wrote: "I can't be sure just when he stopped the imitation of word sounds. It seems that he has gone backward mentally. We have thought it was because he did not disclose what was in his head, that it was there all right. Now that he is making so many sounds, it is disconcerting because it is evident that he can't talk. Before, I thought he could if he only would. He gave the impression of silent wisdom to me. . . . One puzzling and discouraging thing is the great difficulty one has in getting his attention."

Richard was found to be healthy except for large tonsils and adenoids, which were removed on February 8, 1941. His EEG was normal.

He had himself led willingly to the office and engaged at once in active play with the toys, paying no attention to the persons in the room. Occasionally, he looked up at the walls, smiled and uttered short staccato sounds. He complied with a spoken and gestural command to take off his slippers. When the command was changed to another, this time without gestures, he again took off his slippers (which had been put on again).

Richard was again seen at 4½ years. He had grown considerably and gained weight. He immediately turned the lights on and off. He showed no interest in the examiner or any other person but was attracted to a small box that he threw as if it were a ball.

At near 5 years, his first move on entering the office was to turn the lights on and off. He climbed on a chair, and from the chair to the desk in order to reach the switch of the wall lamp. He had no contact with people, whom he definitely regarded as an interference when they talked to him or otherwise tried to gain his attention.

The mother felt that she was no longer capable of handling him, and he was placed in a foster home with a woman who had shown a remarkable talent for dealing with difficult children. After two changes of foster homes, he was placed at a State School for Exceptional Children in his home State in May 1946. A report, dated June 23, 1954, said: "The institution accepted him as essentially a custodial problem; therefore, he was placed with a group of similar charges."

Richard is now 33 years old. In 1965, he was transferred to another institution in the same State. The Superintendent wrote on September 29, 1970: "At the time of admission, tranquilizers were pushed to the point of toxicity. After about 3 months, he showed some awareness of his environment and began feeding himself and going to the toilet. He is now being maintained on

Compazine, 45 milligrams t.i.d. . . . He now resides in a cottage for older residents who can meet their own personal needs. He responds to his name and to simple commands and there is some non-verbal communication with the cottage staff. He continues to be withdrawn and cannot be involved in any structured activities."

Case 4

Paul G. was 5 years old when he was brought to the Clinic on March 21, 1941, "for determination of his degree of feeblemindedness." He had a history of normal birth. Early development milestones had progressed satisfactorily. His enunciation was clear, and he had a good vocabulary.

The father, a mining engineer, had left the family in 1939 "after an unhappy marriage." The mother, a "restless, unstable, irritable woman," who moved from London to the United States, gave a conflicting story of her efforts to make Paul clever by teaching him to memorize poems and songs. At 3 years, "he knew the words of not less than 37 songs and many nursery rhymes."

Paul was a slender, attractive child. He had good manual dexterity. He rarely responded to any form of address, even to the calling of his name. Sometimes an energetic "Don't!" caused him to interrupt his activity but usually, when spoken to, he went on with whatever he was doing. He was always vivaciously occupied with something and seemed to be highly satisfied, unless someone made a persistent attempt to interfere. Then he first tried to get out of the way and, when this met with no success, screamed and kicked in a full-fledged tantrum. . . . There was a marked contrast between his relations to people and to objects. Upon entering the room, he instantly went after objects and used them correctly. He opened a box, took out a toy telephone, singing again and again: "He wants the telephone," and went around the room with the mouthpiece and receiver in proper position. He got hold of a pair of scissors and cut a sheet of paper into small bits, singing "cutting paper" many times. He helped himself to a toy engine, ran around the room holding it up high and singing over and over again: "The engine is flying." Some of his utterances could not be linked up with immediate situations. These are a few examples: "The people in the hotel"; "Did you hurt your leg?" "Candy is all gone, candy is empty." Reproductions of warnings about bodily injury constituted a major portion of his utterances. . . . All statements pertaining to himself were made in the second person, as literal repetitions of things said to him before. He would express his desire for candy by saying: "You want candy." He would put his hand away from a hot radiator and say: "You get hurt."

When the mother came to this country, she deposited Paul with a lady who ran a small home for retarded children. She removed him some time at the end of 1941, wrote friendly sounding letters to the Clinic but did not keep return appointments. She consulted Dr. Walter Klingman in 1941, Dr. Samuel Orton in 1943, applied for Paul's admission to the Devereux Schools in 1945 but decided that this was not the proper place for him. This is where the trail ends. Mother and child could not be located since then.

Case 5

Barbara K. was first seen at the Clinic on February 7, 1942, at the age of 8 years. Her father, a noted physician, stated in a written note:

"First child, born normally October 30, 1933. She nursed poorly and was put on bottle after a week. She quit taking any nourishment at 3 months. She was tube-fed five times daily up to 1 year of age. She began to eat then, though there was much difficulty until she was 18 months old. Since then she had been a good eater, likes to experiment with food, tasting, and now fond of cooking. . . . Ordinary vocabulary at 2 years, but always slow at putting words into sentences. Phenomenal ability to spell, read, and a good writer, but still has difficulty with verbal expression. Can't get arithmetic except as a memory feat. . . . Repetitious as a baby, and obsessive now; holds things in hands, takes things to bed with her, repeats phreases, gets stuck on an idea or game and rides it hard, then goes to something else. She used to say 'you' for herself and 'I' for her mother or me, as if she were saying things we would in talking to her. . . . Very timid, fearful of changing things, wind, large animals, etc. Mostly passive, but passively stubborn at times. Inattentive to the point where one wonders if she hears. (She does!) No competitive spirit, no desire to please her teacher. If she knew more than any member in the class about something, she would give no hint of it, just keep quiet, maybe not even listen. . . . In Camp last summer she was liked, learned to swim, is graceful in water (had always appeared awkward in her motility before), overcame fear of ponies, played best with children of 5 years of age. At camp she slid into avitaminosis and malnutrition but offered almost no verbal complaints."

Barbara's mother is a well-educated, kindly woman. A younger brother, born in 1937, was healthy, alert, and well-developed.

Barbara "shook hands" upon request (offering the left upon coming, the right upon leaving) by merely raising a limp hand in the approximate direction of the examiner's proffered hand; the motion lacked the implication of greeting. During the entire interview, there was no indication of any kind of affective contact. A pin prick resulted in withdrawal of her arm, a fearful glace at the pin (not the examiner), and utterance of the word "Hurt," not addressed to anyone in particular.

She read excellently, finishing the 10-year Binet fire story in 33 seconds and with no errors, but was unable to reproduce from memory anything she had read. In the Binet pictures, she saw (or at least reported) no action or relatedness between the single items, which she had no difficulty enumerating. Her handwriting was legible. Her drawing was unimaginative and stereotyped. She used her right hand for writing, her left for everything else; she was left-footed and right-eyed.

She knew the days of the week. She began to name them: "Saturday, Sunday, Monday," then said, "You go to school" (meaning, "on Monday"), then stopped as if the performance were completed.

Throughout all these procedures, she scribbled words spontaneously: "oranges," "lemons," "bananas," "grapes," "cherries," "apples," "apricots," "tangerine," "grapefruits," "watermelon"; the words sometimes ran into each other and were obviously not meant for others to read.

Her mother remarked: "Appendages fascinate her, like a smoke stack or a pendulum." Her father had previously stated: "Recent interest in sexual matters, hanging about when we take a bath, and obsessive interest in toilets."

Barbara was placed at the Devereux Schools in the summer of 1942 and remained there until June 1952, when she was admitted to the Springfield State Hospital (Maryland) where she is still residing. She is now 37 years old. A note written by her ward physician October 8, 1970, has this to say, "She still has the stereotyped smile, the little girl-like facial expression with a placid grin, the child-like voice when uttering her parrot-like repetitions. Whenever I pass the ward, she greets me as follows: 'Doctor, do you know I socked you once?' She then usually gets very close to the writer following her to the office. . . . She still shows a total absence of spontaneous sentence production; the same phrases are used over and over again with the same intonation. Her mind is fixed to the same subjects, which vary to some degree with the person she is communicating with. Besides all of this she is childish, impulsive, subject to temper outbursts with stamping her feet, crying loudly and upsetting other patients. Her memory is completely intact. She likes to hum some melodies montonously; whenever she feels like it she bangs the piano with well-known songs."

Case 6

Virginia S., born September 13, 1931, had resided in a State Training School for retarded children since 1936. Dr. Esther L. Richards, who saw her there wrote in May 1941: "Virginia stands out from other children because she is absolutely different from any of the others. She is neat and tidy, does not play with other children, and does not seem to be deaf but does not talk. The child will amuse herself by the hour putting picture puzzles together, sticking to them until they are done. I have seen her with a box filled with the parts of two puzzles gradually work out the pieces for each. All findings seem to be in the nature of a congenital abnormality."

Virginia was the daughter of a psychiatrist, who said of himself: "I have never liked children, probably a reaction on my part to the restraint from movement, the minor interruptions, and commotions." Of his wife he said: "She is not by any means the mother type. Her attitude (toward a child) is more like toward a doll or pet than anything else." Virginia's brother, 5 years her senior, when referred to us because of severe stuttering at 15 years of age, burst out in tears when asked how things were at home and he sobbed: "The only time my father has ever had anything to do with me was when he scolded me for doing something wrong." His mother did not contribute even that much. He felt that all his life he had lived in "a frosty atmosphere" with two inapproachable strangers.

In August 1938, the psychologist at the training school observed that Virginia "pays no attention to what is said to her but quickly comprehends whatever is expected. Her performance reflects discrimination, care, and precision." With the non-language test items, she achieved an IQ of 94. "Without a doubt, her intelligence is superior to this. . . . She is quiet, solemn, composed. Not once have I seen her smile. She retires within herself, segregating herself from others. She seems to be in a world of her own, oblivious to all but the center of interest in the presiding situation. She is mostly self-sufficient and independent. When others encroach upon her integrity, she tolerates them with indifference. There was no manifestation of friendliness or interest in persons. On the other hand, she finds pleasure in dealing with things, about which she shows imagination and initiative."

When seen on October 11, 1942, Virginia was a tall, slender, neatly dressed girl. She responded when called by getting up and coming nearer without ever looking up to the person who called her. She just stood listlessly, looking into space. Occasionally, in answer to questions, she muttered: "Mamma, baby." When a group was formed around the piano, one child playing and the others singing, she sat among the children, seemingly not even noticing what went on, and gave the impression of being self-absorbed. She did not seem to notice when the children stopped singing. When the group dispersed, she did not change her position and appeared not to be aware of the change of scene. She had an intelligent physiognomy, though her eyes had a black expression.

Virginia will be 40 years old next September. She has been transferred to the Henryton State Hospital. "She is," the report from there, dated November 2, 1970, says, "in a program for adult retardates, with her primary rehabilitation center being the Home Economics Section. She can hear and is able to follow instructions and directions. She can identify colors and can tell time. She can care for her basic needs, but has to be told to do so. Virginia likes to work jigsaw puzzles and does so very well, preferring to do this alone. She can iron clothes. She does not talk, uses noises and gestures, but seems to understand when related to. She desires to keep to herself rather than associate with other residents."

Case 7

Herbert B. was brought to the Clinic by his mother on February 5, 1941.

Born November 18, 1937, 2 weeks before term by elective Caesarean section, he vomited all food from birth through the third month; then feeding proceeded satisfactorily. He sat up at 8 months but did not try to walk until 2 years old, when he "suddenly got up and walked without any preliminary crawling or assistance by chair." He persistently refused to take fluid in any but an all-glass container. For a time he was believed to be deaf because "he did not register any change of expression when spoken to and made no attempt to speak." He became upset by any change of accustomed pattern: "When he notices change, he is fussy and cries but he himself likes to pull blinds up and down, open and close doors, and tear cardboard boxes into small pieces and play with them for hours."

His parents separated shortly after his birth. The father, a psychiatrist, was described as "unusually intelligent, sensitive, restless, serious-minded, not interested in people, mostly living within himself." The mother, a pediatrician, spoke of herself as "energetic and outgoing, fond of people but having little insight into their problems, finding it easier to accept people rather than try to understand them." Herbert was the youngest of three children. The mother kept voluminous diaries for each of them, especially for her daughter who, born in 1934, for the first few years "wanted to be left alone, ignored persons, reversed personal pronouns, was first declared to be feebleminded, then schizophrenic, but blossomed out after the parents' separation." At the time when Herbert was seen at the Clinic, she attended school, had an IQ of 108, and "though sensitive and moderately apprehensive, was interested in people and got along well with them."

Herbert showed remarkably intelligent physiognomy and good motor coordination. He displayed astounding purposefulness in the pursuit of self-selected goals. Among a group of blocks, he instantly recognized those that were glued to a board and those that were detachable. He could build a tower of blocks as skillfully and as high as any child of his age or even older. He was annoyed by any interference, shoving intruders away (without ever looking at them), or screaming when the shoving had no effect.

He was again seen at 4½ and at 5 years of age. Both times he entered the office without paying the slightest attention to the people present. He went after the form board and busied himself putting the figures into their proper spaces and taking them out again adroitly and quickly. When interfered with, he whined impatiently. When one figure was stealthily removed, he noticed its absence, became disturbed, but promptly forgot all about it when it was put back. At times, after he had finally quieted down following the upset caused by the removal of the form board, he jumped up and down with an ecstatic expression. He was completely absorbed in whatever he did. He never smiled. He sometimes uttered inarticulate sounds in a monotonous singsong. At one time, he gently stroked his mother's leg and touched it with his lips. He often brought blocks and other objects to his lips. There was an almost photographic likeness of his behavior during the two visits.

After a short stay at the Emma Pendleton Bradley Home in Rhode Island, and another at Twin Maples ("a school of adjustment for the problem child") in Baltimore, he was placed by his mother with Mr. and Mrs. Moreland who had a farm in Maryland. He seemed happy there from the beginning. He followed the farmer around on his chores and helped him "making things in the barn." Mrs. Moreland reported in October 1950: "He knows his way around the area near the farm and can go for miles and come back without getting lost. He had learned to cut wood, uses the power mower, rakes the lawn, sets the table perfectly, and in his spare time works jigsaw puzzles. He is a manageable and nice child. Occasionally he get upset if there is a sudden change in plans. . . . When his mother comes to visit, he gets himself absorbed and does not come toward her." After Mr. Moreland's death, the widow opened a nursing home for elderly people. Herbert remained with her, took the old ladies out for walks, brought them their trays to their rooms but never talked.

His mother, after serving as a public health officer in Maryland, spent several years (1953-1958) abroad—in Iraq and in Greece. On her return, she took a position in Atlanta, Georgia. She died in 1965.

Herbert is now 33 years. His father wrote on January 5, 1971: "He is still with the people in Maryland. It is several years since I have seen him but I have word that he is essentially unchanged. More than anything else, he seems to enjoy doing jigsaw puzzles which he can do with the utmost skill."

A letter from his mother, written shortly before her death, contained this lament: "Our marriage seems to have produced three emotionally crippled children. Dorothy, after a disastrous marriage, is at home with her little baby girl and is trying to get on her feet working part time as a nurse in a local hospital. Dave is on the West Coast and has cost me $450.00 monthly as he gets intensive psychiatric treatment."

Dorothy is Herbert's legally appointed guardian.

Case 8

Alfred L. was brought to the Clinic by his mother in November 1935, at 3½ years with this complaint: "He has gradually shown a marked tendency toward developing one special interest which will dominate his day's activities. He talks of little else while the interest exists, he frets when he is not able to indulge in it and it is difficult to get his attention because of his preoccupation. . . . There has also been the problem of an overattachment to the world of objects and failure to develop the usual amount of social awareness. . . . Language developed slowly; he seemed to have no interest in it. He seldom tells experiences. He still confuses pronouns. He never asks questions in the form of questions (with the appropriate inflection). Since he talked, there has been a tendency to repeat over and over one word or statement. He almost never says a sentence without repeating it. Yesterday, when looking at a picture, he said many times, 'Some cows standing in the water.' We counted 50 repetitions, then he stopped after several more and began over and over. . . . He frets when the bread is put in the oven to be made into toast and is afraid it will get burned and be hurt. He is upset when the sun sets or because the moon does not always appear in the sky at night. He prefers to play alone; he will get down from a piece of apparatus as soon as another child approaches. He like to work out some project with large boxes (make a trolley, for instance) and does not want anyone to interfere."

Alfred was born June 20, 1932. For the first 2 months, "the feeding formula caused much concern but then he gained rapidly and became unusually large and vigorous." He sat up at 5 months and walked at 14 months. First words at one year. At 22 months, he swallowed cotton from an Easter rabbit, some of which lodged in the windpipe; a tracheotomy was performed under local anesthesia.

He was an only child. The father, a chemist and a law school graduate, was described as "suspicious, easily angered, spends his spare time reading, gardening, and fishing, has to be dragged out to visit friends." The mother, a clinical psychologist, "very obsessive and excitable," was the only parent in the Clinic's experience who did not allow notes to be taken when she gave the history. She left her husband 2 months after Alfred's birth; both lived with the maternal grandparents in a home in which the mother ran a nursery school and kindergarten. The grandfather, a psychologist, was severely obsessive-compulsive and had numerous tics.

Alfred, upon entering the office, immediately spotted a train in the toy cabinet, took it out, and connected and disconnected the cars in a slow, monotonous manner. He kept saying many times: "More train—more train—more train." He "counted" the car windows: "One, two windows, four windows, eight windows." He could not be distracted from the trains. A Binet test was attempted in a room in which there were no trains. It was possible with much difficulty to pierce through his preoccupations. He finally complied in a manner that clearly indicated that he wanted to get through with the particular intrusion. Finally, he achieved an IQ of 140.

The mother did not bring him back after his first visit because of "his continued distress when confronted with a member of the medical profession." In August 1938, she sent upon request a written report from which the following lines are quoted: "He is called a lone wolf. He prefers to play alone and avoids groups of children at play. He does not pay attention to adults except when demanding stories. He avoids competition. He reads simple stories to himself. He is very fearful of being hurt; he talks a great deal about the use of the electric chair."

He was again seen in June 1941. His parents had decided to live together. Prior to that he had been in 11 different schools. He had been kept in bed often because of colds, bronchitis, chickenpox, impetigo, and a vaguely described condition that the mother insisted was rheumatoid fever.

Alfred was extremely tense and serious-minded; had it not been for his juvenile voice, he might have given the impression of a worried little old man. At the same time, he was restless and showed considerable pressure of talk, which consisted of obsessive questions about windows, shades, dark rooms, especially the X-ray room. He never smiled. In between he answered questions, which often had to be repeated. He was painstakingly specific in his definitions. A balloon "is made out of lined rubber and has air in it and some have gas and sometimes they go up and sometimes they can hold up and when they got a hole in it they'll bust up; if people squeeze they'll bust. Isn't it right?" A tiger "is a thing, animal, striped, like a cat, can scratch, eats people up, wild, lives in the jungle sometimes and in the forests, mostly in the jungle. Isn't it right?" He once stopped and asked, very much perplexed, why "The Johns Hopkins Hospital" was printed on the history sheets: "Why do they have to say it?" Since the histories were taken at the hospital, why should it be necessary to have the name on every sheet, though the person writing on it knew where he was writing? The examiner, whom he remembered from his visit 6 years previously, was to him nothing more nor less than a person who was expected to answer his obsessive questions about darkness and light.

This ended the Clinic's contact with Alfred. The mother started him out on a tour of schools and hospitals, not informing them about preceding evaluations and taking him out after a time, not disclosing the next step she planned to take. We do know that he was at the V.V. Anderson School in Stratsburg-on-Hudson, N.Y. (1948-1950); the Taylor Manor in Ellicott City, Md. (July to October 1954); and the Philadelphia Hospital Department for Mental and Nervous Diseases (March 3 to April 20, 1955). Some time between the last two, he was for a time on Thorazine; then at a "school for brain damaged children" founded by his mother in October 1954.

Alfred is now 38 years old. So far as can be determined, he is at his mother's "school." Both at Sheppard-Pratt and Philadelphia Hospitals he was interested in the occupational therapy materials and did well with them. When this was brought to the mother's attention, she decided to take him out.

Case 9

Charles N. was brought by his mother on February 2, 1943, with the chief complaint: "The thing that upsets me most is that I can't reach my baby."

Charles was born on August 9, 1938. He was a planned and wanted child. He sat up at 6 months; at 14 months "he stood up and walked one day." As a baby, he was "slow and phlegmatic." He would lie in his crib "almost as if hypnotized." Thyroid extract medication had no effect.

He was the oldest of three children. Mr. N., a high school graduate clothing merchant, was described as a "self-made, gentle, and placid person"; his relatives were said to be "ordinary, simple people." Mrs. N., "of remarkable equanimity," had a successful business record, running a theatrical booking office. Her "dynamic and forceful" mother had done some writing and composing. Mrs. N. had a brother, a psychiatrist, who had great musical talent, a sister who was "very brilliant and psychoneurotic," and a sister who was referred to as "the Amazon of the family."

The mother prefaced her story thus: "I am trying hard not to govern my remarks by professional knowledge which has intruded in my own way of thinking now." In this she succeeded. This is a brief abstract of her report: "His enjoyment and appreciation of music encouraged me to play records. When he was 1½ years old, he could discriminate between symphonies. He recognized the composer as soon as the first movement started. He would say 'Beethoven.' At about the same age, he began to spin toys and lids of bottles and jars by the hour. He would watch it and get excited and jump up and down in ecstasy. Now he is interested in reflecting light from mirrors and catching reflections. When he is interested in a thing, you cannot change it. . . . The most impressive thing is his detachment and his inaccessibility. He lives in a world of his own where he cannot be reached. No sense of relationship to persons. He went through a period of quoting another person; never offers anything himself. His entire conversation is a replica of whatever has been said to him. He used to speak of himself in the second person, now he uses the third person at times. . . . He is destructive; the furniture in his room looks like it has hunks out of it. He will break a purple crayon into two parts and say, 'You had a beautiful purple crayon and now it's two pieces. Look what you did.'. . . . He developed an obsession about feces, would hide it anywhere (for instance, in drawers), would tease me if I walked into the room: 'You soiled your pants, now you can't have your crayons!. . . . As a result, he is still not toilet trained. He never soils himself in the nursery school, always does it when he comes home. The same is true of wetting. He is proud of wetting, jumps up and down with ecstasy, says; 'Look at the big puddle he made.' "

Charles was a well-developed, intelligent looking boy, who was in good physical health. When he entered the office, he paid no attention to the people present. Without looking at anyone, he said: "Give me a pencil," took a piece of paper from the desk and wrote something resembling a figure 2 (a large desk calendar prominently displayed a figure 2, the day was February 2). He had brought with him a copy of *Readers Digest* and was fascinated by a picture of a baby. He said: "Look at the funny baby," innumerable times, occasionally adding: "Is he not funny? Is he not sweet?" When the book was taken away from him, he struggled with the hand that held it, without looking at the person who had taken the book. When he was pricked with a pin, he said: "What's this?" and answered his own question: "It is a needle." He looked timidly at the pin, shrank from further pricks, but at no time did he seem to connect the pricking with the person who held the pin. When the *Readers Digest* was put on the floor and a foot placed over it, he tried to remove the foot as if it were a detached and interfering object, with no concern for the person to whom the foot belonged.

When confronted with the Seguin form board, he was interested in the names of the forms before putting them into their appropriate holes. He often spun the forms around, jumping up and down excitedly while they were in motion. He knew names, such as "octagon," "diamond," "oblong block," but nevertheless kept asking: "What is this?"

He did not respond to being called and did not look at his mother when she spoke to him. When the blocks were removed, he screamed, stamped his feet, and cried: "I give it to you!" (meaning: "You give it to me").

Charles was placed at the Devereux Schools on February 10, 1943. Early in 1944, he was removed, spent 3 months (from March to June) at Bellevue Hospital; was admitted on June 22, 1944, to New Jersey State Hospital at Marlboro; transferred to Arthur Brisbane Child Treatment Center on November 1, 1946; transferred to Atlantic County Hospital, February 1, 1951; transferred to the State Hospital at Ancora on October 14, 1955. He is still there, now 32 years old. This means that he has been a State Hospital resident from the age of 5 years and 10 months. Inquiries by the Clinic, if responded to at all, yielded meager general statements about continuing deterioration. One note of December 1953, said something about "intensive psychotherapy." The last note, dated December 23, 1970, said: "This patient is very unpredictable in his behavior. He has a small vocabulary and spends most of the time singing to himself. He is under close observation and is in need of indefinite hospitalization."

Case 10

John F. was first seen at the Clinic on February 13, 1940, at 28 months of age.

His father said: "The main thing that worries me is the difficulty in feeding. That is the essential thing, and secondly his slowness in development. During the first days of life he did not take the breast satisfactorily. After 15 days he was changed from breast to bottle. There is a long story of trying to get food down. We have tried everything under the sun. He has been immature all along. At 20 months he first started to walk. He sucks his thumb and grinds his teeth quite frequently and rolls from side to side before sleeping. If we don't do what he wants, he will scream and yell."

John was born September 19, 1937. There was frequent hospitalization because of the feeding problem. The anterior fontanelle did not close until he was 2½ years of age. He suffered from repeated colds and otitis media, which necessitated bilateral myringotomy.

John was an only child until February 1943. The father, a psychiatrist, was "a very calm, placid, emotionally stable person, who is the soothing element in the family." The mother, a high-school graduate, worked as a secretary in a pathology laboratory before marriage; she "saw everything as a pathological specimen; throughout the pregnancy, she was afraid she would not live through the labor."

John was brought to the office by both parents. He wandered about the room constantly and aimlessly. Except for spontaneous scribbling, he never brought two objects into relation to each other. He did not respond to the simplest commands.

At the end of his fourth year, he was able to form a limited kind of affective contact. Once a relationship was established, it had to continue in exactly the same channels. He formed grammatically correct sentences but used the pronoun of the second person when referring to himself. Language was mainly a repetition of things he heard, without alteration of the personal pronoun. There was marked obsessiveness. Daily routine must be adhered to rigidly; any change called forth outbursts of panic. He had an excellent rote memory and could recite many prayers, nursery rhymes, and songs; the mother did a great deal of stuffing in this respect and was very proud of these "achievements": "He can tell victrola records by their color, and if one side of the record is identified, he remembers what is on the other side."

At 4½ years, he began to use pronouns adequately. He wanted to make sure of the sameness of the environment literally by keeping doors and windows closed. When his mother opened the door, he became violent in closing it again and finally, when again interfered with, burst helplessly into tears, utterly frustrated.

He was extremely upset upon seeing anything broken or incomplete. He noticed two dolls to which he had paid no attention before. He saw that one of them had no hat and became very much agitated, wandering about the room to look for the hat. When the hat was retrieved from another room, he instantly lost all interest in the dolls.

At 5½ years, he had good mastery of the use of pronouns. He had begun to feed himself satisfactorily. He saw a group photograph in the office and asked his father: "When are they coming out of the picture and coming in here?" He was serious about this. His father said something about the pictures they have at home on the wall. John corrected his father: "We have them *near* the wall." (*On* meant to him "above" or "on top"). His father whistled a tune and John instantly and correctly identified it as "Mendelssohn's Violin Concerto." Though he could speak of things as big or pretty, he was incapable of making comparisons. ("Which is the bigger line? Prettier face?")

In December 1942, and January 1943, he had two series of predominantly right-sided convulsions, with conjugate deviation of the eyes to the right and transient paresis of the right arm. Neurologic examination showed no abnormalities. His eyegrounds were normal. An EEG indicated "focal disturbances in the left occipital region."

After attending a private nursery school, John was at the Devereux Schools (1945-1949), then at the Woods Schools, then at Children's House (June 1950), and attended Town and Country School in Washington, D.C. An inquiry about him came from Georgetown Hospital in 1956.

Dr. Hilde Bruch, who saw him in 1953, remarked on his "exuberant emotional expression with no depth and variation and with immediate turnoff when the other person withdraws the interest."

John died suddenly in 1966 at 29 years of age.

Case 11

Elaine C. was brought by her parents on April 12, 1939, at the age of 7 years because of "unusual development." She doesn't adjust. She stops at all abstractions. She doesn't understand other children's games, doesn't retain interest in stories read to her, wanders off and walks by herself, is especially fond of animals of all kinds, occasionally mimics them by walking on all fours and making strange noises."

Elaine was born on February 3, 1932. She appeared healthy, took feedings well, stood up at 7 months and walked at less than a year. She could say 4 words at the end of her first year but made no progress in speech for the following 4 years. Deafness was suspected but ruled out. Because of a febrile illness at 13 months, her increasing difficulties were interpreted as possible postencephalitic behavior disorder. Others blamed the mother, who was accused of inadequate handling of the child. Feeblemindedness was another diagnosis. For 18 months, she was given anterior pituitary and thyroid preparations. "Some doctors thought she was a normal child and said that she would outgrow this."

At 2 years, she was sent to a nursery school, where "she independently went her way, not doing what the others did. She, for instance, drank the water and ate the plant when they were being taught to handle flowers." She developed an early interest in pictures of animals. Though generally restless, she could for hours concentrate on looking at such pictures.

When she began to speak at 5 years, she started out with complete, though simple sentences that were "mechanical phrases" and knew especially the names and "classifications" of animals. She did not use pronouns correctly, but used plurals and tenses well. "She could not use negatives but recognized their meaning when others used them. . . . She could count by rote. She could set the table for numbers of people if the names were given her but she could not set the table 'for three.' If sent for a specific object in a certain place, she could not bring it if it was somewhere else but still visible. . . . She was frightened by noises and anything moving toward here. She was so afraid of the vacuum cleaner that she would not even go near the closet where it was kept, and when it was used, ran out into the garage, covering her ears with her hands."

Elaine was the older of two children. Her father had studied law and the liberal arts in three universities (including the Sorbonne), was an advertising copy writer, "one of those chronically thin persons, nervous energy readily expended." The mother, a "self-controlled, placid, logical person," had done editorial work for a magazine before marriage.

Physically Elaine was in good health. Her EEG was normal. When examined in April 1939, she shook hands with the physician upon request, without looking at him, then ran to the window and looked out. She automatically heeded the invitation to sit down. Her reaction to questions—after several repetitions—was an echolalia-type reproduction of the whole question or, if it was too lengthy, of the end portion. Her expression was blank, though not unintelligent, and there were no communicative gestures. At one time, without changing her physiognomy, she said suddenly: "Fishes don't cry."

She was placed at the Child Study Home of Maryland, where she remained for 3 weeks. She soon learned the names of all the children, knew the color of their eyes, the bed in which each slept, but never entered into relationship with them. When taken to the playground, she was upset and ran back to her room. She was restless, but when she was allowed to look at pictures, play alone with blocks, draw, or string beads, she could entertain herself for hours. She frequently ejaculated stereotyped phrases, such as, "Dinosaurs don't cry"; "Crayfish and frogs live in children's tummies"; "Butterflies live in children's tummies and in their panties too"; "Fish have sharp teeth and bite little children"; "There is war in the sky"; "Gargoyles bite children and drink oil"; "Needle head, Pink wee-wee. Has a yellow leg. Cutting the dead deer. Poison deer. Poor Elaine. No tadpoles in the house. Men broke deer's leg" (while cutting the picture of a deer from a book).

Elaine was placed in a private school. The father reported "rather amazing changes: She is a tall, husky girl with clear eyes that have long since lost any trace of that wildness they periodically showed in the time you knew her. She speaks well on almost any subject, though with something of an odd intonation. Her conversation is still rambling, frequently with an amusing point, and it is only occasional, deliberate, and announced. She reads very well, jumbling words, not pronouncing clearly, and not making proper emphases. Her range of information is really quite wide, and her memory almost infallible."

On September 7, 1950, Elaine was admitted to Letchworth Village, N.Y. State School. While there, "she was distractible, assaultive, and talked in an irrational manner with a flat affect. She ran through wards without clothing, threw furniture about, banged her head on the wall, had episodes of banging and screaming, and imitated various animal sounds. She showed a good choice of vocabulary but could not maintain a conversation along a given topic. EEG did not show any definite abnormality." She was found to have an IQ of 83.

On February 28, 1951, she was transferred to the Hudson River State Hospital. She is still there. A report, dated September 25, 1970, says: "She is up and about daily, eats and sleeps well and is acting quite independent. She is able to take care of her personal needs and is fairly neat and clean. Her speech is slow and occasionally unintelligible and she is manneristic. She is in only fair contact and fairly well oriented. She cannot participate in a conversation, however, except for the immediate needs. If things do not go her way, she becomes acutely disturbed, yelling, hitting her chest with her fist, and her head against the wall. In her lucid periods, however, she is cooperative, pleasant, childish, and affectionate. She has epileptic seizures occasionally of grand mal type and is receiving antiepileptics and tranquilizers. Her general physical condition is satisfactory." She is now 39 years old.

Discussion

Those were the 11 children who were designated in 1943 as having "autistic disturbances of affective contact." They were reported as representing a "syndrome, rare enough, yet probably more frequent than is indicated by the paucity of observed cases." The outstanding pathognomonic characteristics were viewed as (a) the children's inability from the beginning of life to relate themselves to people and situations in the ordinary way, and (b) an anxiously obsessive desire for the preservation of sameness. A year after the first publication, the term early infantile autism was added to psychiatric nomenclature.

Now, 28 years later, after early infantile autism has become a matter of intensive study, after dozens of books and thousands of articles, after active stimulation by concerned parent groups in many countries, after the creation of special educational, therapeutic, and research units, it may be of interest to look back and see how these few children have contributed to the introduction of a concept that has since then stirred professional and lay curiosity.

For quite some time, there was considerable preoccupation with the nosological allocation of the syndrome. The 1943 report had this to say: "The combination of extreme autism, obsessiveness, stereotypy, and echolalia brings the total picture into relationship with some of the basic schizophrenic phenomena. Some of the children have indeed been diagnosed as of this type at one time or another. In spite of the remarkable similarities, however, the condition differs in many respects from all known instances of childhood schizophrenia." The "uniqueness" or "unduplicated nature" of autism was emphasized strongly then and in subsequent publications. Nevertheless, it has been just recently that this view has been generally accepted. The ultimate concession has come in 1967 from Russian investigators who had the courage to break through the officially sanctioned "line," according to which autism had been assigned the status of "schizoid psychopathy." The message, however, has not quite percolated to the framers of the 1968 Diagnostic and Statistical Manual of Mental Disorders (DSM II) adapted by the American Psychiatric Association. This is a widely used code system in which autism is not included, and children so afflicted are offered item 295.80 ("Schizophrenia, childhood type") as the only available legitimate port of entry.

As for the all-important matter of etiology, the early development of the 11 children left no other choice than the assumption that they had "come into the world with an *innate* disability to form the usual, biologically provided contact with people." The concluding sentence of the 1943 article said, "here we seem to have pure-culture examples of *inborn* autistic disturbances of affective contact." One can say now unhesitatingly that this assumption has become a certainty. Some people seem to have completely overlooked this statement, however, as well as the passages leading up to it and have referred to the author erroneously as an advocate of postnatal "psychogenicity."

This is largely to be ascribed to the observation, duly incorporated in the report, that all 11 children had come from highly intelligent parents. Attention was called to the fact that there was a great deal of obsessiveness in the family background. The very detailed diaries and the recall, after several years, that the children had learned to recite 25 questions and answers of the Presbyterian catechism, to sing 37 nursery songs, or to discriminate between 18 symphonies, furnish a telling illustration. It was noticed that many of the parents, grandparents, and collaterals were persons strongly preoccupied with abstractions of a scientific, literary, or artistic nature and limited in genuine interest in people. But at no time was this undeniable and repeatedly confirmed phenomenon oversimplified as warranting the postulate of a direct cause-and-effect connection. To the contrary, it was stated expressly that the aloneness from the beginning of life makes it difficult to attribute the whole picture one-sidedly to the manner of early parent-child relationship.

The one thing that the 1943 paper could neither acquire nor offer was a hint about the future. Everywhere in medicine, prognosis can be arrived at only through retrognosis. No empirical data were available at the time; the whole syndrome as such was a novelty as far as anybody was aware. Now we have information about the fate of the 11 children in the ensuing three decades.

We must keep in mind that they were studied before the days when a variety of therapeutic methods were inaugurated, based on a variety of theoretical premises: psychoanalytically oriented, based on operant conditioning, psychopharmacological, educational, via psychotherapy of parents, and combinations of some of them. Sufficient time has not elapsed to allow meaningful long-range followup evaluations. At any rate, no accounts are as yet available that would afford a reasonably reliable idea about the more than temporary or fragmentary effects of any of these procedures intended for amelioration.

Of the 11 children, 8 were boys and 3 (cases 5, 6, and 11) were girls. It was, of course, impossible at the time to say whether or not this was merely a chance occurrence. A later review of the first 100 autistic children seen at the Johns Hopkins Hospital showed a ratio of 4 boys to 1 girl. The predominance of boys has indeed been affirmed by all authors since then. It may be added that the boys were brought to the Clinic at an earlier age (between 2 and 6 years) than the girls (between 6 and 8 years).

Nine of the children were Anglo-Saxon descent, two (cases 9 and 10) were Jewish. Three were only children, 5 were the first-born of two, one was the oldest of three, one the younger of two, and one the youngest of three. Order of birth was therefore not regarded as being of major significance *per se*.

On clinical pediatric examination, all 11 children were found to be in satisfactory health physically. Two had large tonsils and adenoids, which were soon removed. Five had relatively large head circumferences. Several of the children were somewhat clumsy in gait and gross motor performances but all were remarkably skillful with regard to finer muscular coordination. Electroencephalograms were normal in all except John (case 10), whose anterior fontanelle had not closed until he was 2½ years old and who, 3 years after his first visit to the Clinic, began having perdominantly right-sided convulsions. Frederick (case 2) had a supernumerary nipple in the left axilla. There were in the group no other instances of congenital somatic anomalies. All had intelligent physiognomies, giving at times—especially in the presence of others—the impression of serious-mindedness or anxious tenseness, at other times, when left alone with objects and with no anticipation of being interfered with, a picture of beatific serenity.

While there were, as is to be expected, individual nuances in the manifestation of some of the specific features, the degree of the disturbance, and in the step-by-step succession of incidental occurrences, it is evident that in the first 4 or 5 years of life the overall behavioral pattern was astoundingly similar, almost to the point of identity in terms of the two cardinal characteristics of aloneness and sterotype. Now, after 30 or more years, it is also evident that from then on, notwithstanding the basic retention of these two features, major differences have developed in the shaping of the children's destinies.

We do not know about the present status of Paul A. (Case 4) and of Alfred N. (Case 8). Paul's mother went shopping around to a number of specialists, dropping out each time after one or two appointments, and could not be located since 1945, despite many efforts worthy of a competent detective agency. Alfred's mother had him at first in rapid succession in 11 different public and private schools and then in several residential settings. He responded well to occupational therapy but the mother, not considering this adequate, took him out and kept him with her in a "school" founded and run by herself.

Two of the children, John and Elaine (Cases 10 and 11) developed epileptic seizures. John's began about 3 years after his first visit to the Clinic; after sojourns in several residential places, he died in 1966. Elaine's convulsions started in her middle to late twenties and she is now, at 39 years, still "on anti-epileptics and tranquilizers"; her EEG was reported normal in 1950, when she was admitted to the Letchworth Village, N.Y. State School. She was later transferred to the Hudson River, N.Y. State Hospital, where she still resides.

Richard M., Barbara K., Virginia S., and Charles N. (Cases 3, 5, 6, and 9), who spent most of their lives in institutional care, have all lost their luster early after their admission. Originally fighting for their aloneness and basking in the contentment that it gave them, originally alert to unwelcome changes and, in their own way, struggling for the status quo, originally astounding the observer with their phenomenal feats of memory, they yielded readily to the uninterrupted self-isolation and soon settled down in a life not too remote from a nirvana-like existence. If at all responsive to psychological testing, their IQ's dropped down to figures usually referred to as low-grade moron or imbecile.

This fortunately did not happen to the remaining three children. Herbert B. (Case 7), still mute, has not attained a mode of living that one can be jubilant about but has reached a state of limited but positive usefulness. He was placed on a farm, where, following the farmer around on his chores, he learned to participate in some of them. When the farmer died and the widow established a nursing home for elderly people, he learned to perform the functions of a kind, helpful, competent orderly, using his routine-consciousness in a goal-directed, dependable manner.

Donald T. (Case 1) and Frederick W. (Case 2) represent the two real success stories. Donald, because of the intuitive wisdom of a tenant farmer couple, who knew how to make him utilize his futile preoccupations for practical purposes and at the same time helped him to maintain contact with his family, is a regularly employed bank teller; while living at home, he takes part in a variety of community activities and has the respect of his fellow townspeople. Frederick had the benefit of a similarly oriented arrangement in the framework of the Devereux Schools, where he slowly was introduced to socialized pursuits via his aptitude for music and photography. In 1966, his parents took over. He was enrolled in a sheltered workshop and received vocational training, learning to run duplicating machines. He has now a regular job and is reported by his chief as "outstandingly dependable, reliable, thorough, and thoughtful toward fellow workers."

COMMENT

Such was the fate of the 11 children whose behavior pattern in preschool age was so very much alike as to suggest the delineation of a specific syndrome. The results of the followup after about 30 years do not lend themselves for statistical considerations because of the small number involved. They do, however, invite serious curiosities about the departures from the initial likeness ranging all the way from complete deterioration to a combination of occupational adequacy with limited, though superficially smooth social adjustment.

One cannot help but gain the impression that State Hospital admission was tantamount to a life sentence, with evanescence of the astounding facts of rote memory, abandonment of the earlier pathological yet active struggle for the maintenance of sameness, and loss of the interest in objects added to the basically poor relation to people—in other words, a total retreat to near-nothingness. These children were entered in institutions in which they were herded together with severely retarded coevals or kept in places in which they were housed with psychotic adults; two were eventually transferred from the former to the latter because of their advancing age. One superintendent was realistic enough to state outright that he was accepting the patient "for custodial care." Let it be said, though, that recently a few, very few, State Hospitals have managed to open separate children's units with properly trained and treatment-oriented personnel.

The question arises whether these children might have fared better in a different setting or whether Donald and Frederick, the able bank teller and the duplicating machine operator, would have shared the dismal fate of Richard and Charles in a State Hospital environment. Even though an affirmative answer would most likely be correct, one cannot get away from wondering whether another element, not as yet determinable, may have an influence on the future of autistic children. It is well known in medicine that any illness may appear in different degrees of severity, all the way from the so-called *forme fruste* to the most fulminant manifestation. Does this possibly apply also to early infantile autism?

After its nearly 30-year history and many bona fide efforts, no one as yet has succeeded in finding a therapeutic setting, drug, method, or technique that has yielded the same or similar ameliorative and lasting results for all children subjected to it. What is it that explains all these differences? Are there any conceivable clues for their eventual predictability?

At long last, there is reason to believe that some answers to these questions seem to be around the corner. Biochemical explorations, pursued vigorously in the very recent past, may open a new vista about the fundamental nature of the autistic syndrome. At long last, there is, in addition, an increasing tendency to tackle the whole problem through a multidisciplinary collaboration. Genetic investigations are barely beginning to be conducted. Insights may be gained from ethological experiences. Parents are beginning to be dealt with from the point of view of mutuality, rather than as people standing at one end of a parent-child bipolarity; they have of late been included in the therapeutic efforts, not as etiological culprits, nor merely as recipients of drug prescriptions and of thou-shalt and thou-shalt-not rules, but as actively contributing cotherapists.

This 30-year followup has not indicated too much concrete progress from the time of the original report, beyond the refinement of diagnostic criteria. There has been a hodge-podge of theories, hypotheses, and speculations, and there have been many valiant, well-motivated attempts at alleviation awaiting eventual evaluation. It is expected, with good justification, that a next 30- or 20-year followup of other groups of autistic children will be able to present a report of newly obtained factual knowledge and material for a more hopeful prognosis than the present chronicle has proved to be.

14

HOW FAR CAN AUTISTIC
CHILDREN GO IN MATTERS
OF SOCIAL ADAPTATION?

In a long-range follow-up study of eleven autistic children, it could be ascertained that two of them, not differing essentially from the others in their basic initial symptoms, had in their childhood attained a modus vivendi which allowed them to function gainfully in society (Kanner, 1971a, 1971b). One, Donald T., is a regularly employed bank teller who takes part in a variety of community activities and has the respect of his fellow townspeople. The other, Frederick W., has a full time job running duplicating machines; he has been described by his chief as "outstandingly dependable, reliable, thorough, and thoughtful toward fellow workers."

It cannot be emphasized strongly enough that—even with the full knowledge of family background, parents' personalities, prenatal, paranatal and neonatal data, developmental milestones and complete physical and psychological assessments—it would have been impossible for anyone to predict this outcome. There was nothing in the detailed observations of the patients' childhood development and behavior, nor is there anything in the documented experiences with psychotic children generally, that would offer reasonably sure indicators of prognostic value.

It has occurred to us that an expansion of up-to-date follow-ups beyond the first eleven cases might contribute to the scope of information about the "natural history" of the autistic illness. In this investigation, we have limited ourselves to those who have by now passed the age of adolescence and we have tried to trace their destinies until the present time (January 1972). Out of the 96 patients diagnosed as autistic at the Children's Psychiatric Clinic of The Johns Hopkins Hospital before 1953, we singled out for special consideration those whom we have found to be sufficiently integrated into the texture of society to be employable, move among people without obvious behavior problems, and be acceptable to those around them at home, at work, and in other modes of interaction.

In addition to Donald T. and Frederick W., mentioned above, we came upon nine other such persons. They will be reported in the order of the age which they have now attained.*

CASE MATERIAL

Case 1

Thomas G., born September 11, 1936, was brought to the Clinic by his maternal grandmother on April 19, 1943. The complaint story began as follows:

> He acts so silly. First he kissed shoes and now it's watches and clocks.
> He is awful smart for his age. He is not a bad child, more of a girl, quiet.
> He does not play with children. He comes in the house and shuts the
> door when the neighborhood school is let out.

Thomas was born at term. His mother, 17 years old at the time, had "kidney trouble" during pregnancy. Delivery was normal and birth weight was 7 pounds. Thomas sat up at 6 months and walked at 18. He had measles at 2 and a T&A at 3 years of age. There was no history of severe illness.

---

*For the sake of accuracy, we must point out that we have so far been unable to trace the whereabouts of one patient since 1962, at which time he was doing exceptionally well in college; we have not given up the search but cannot include him in this report. Another patient, who excelled in mathematical physics on a scholarship at Columbia University, might well have figured in our account had he not been run over by a truck on New York's Broadway and killed several years ago.

The father, an upholsterer of Italian extraction, the son of a municipal band conductor and nephew of a composer, died in 1941 at 31 years of age in a tuberculosis sanitarium. The two parents had lived together only from January to December 1936. The mother gave Thomas little attention because "she feared he would give her tuberculosis" (which he did not have), touched him "as little as possible" and frequently went off leaving the child long periods to be cared for by the paternal grandmother who was "on relief" in New York. When the maternal grandmother finally took full charge of Thomas, who was then close to 4 years old, he still had no sphincter control and did not talk. The boy improved quickly and remained with her until he attained school age and rejoined his mother, who had remarried. He was entered in the first grade but soon had to be taken out because of his "peculiar behavior"—paying little heed to directions and insisting on kissing other children's shoes. Thomas was returned to his maternal grandmother who, sensing that he was not well, brought him to our Clinic.

He was in good physical health. At times he answered the examiner's questions and at other times stared ahead or giggled to himself. He was very preoccupied with watches, for which he had a special name: "I like to fool with *dishnishes*—they go tick-tick . . . watches get me excited. It makes me *embarranness*." He referred to his two grandmothers in terms of their ages: "One is 64 and one is 55. I like 55 best." Generally fascinated by numbers, the boy had to make sure how many pages a dictionary or a Sears Roebuck's catalog had, when he spotted them in a room.

Thomas was followed at the Clinic for several years by the social worker to whom he took a liking. For a time it was difficult to get him away from his engrossment with watches and numbers. Obsessions, after running their course, shifted consecutively to measuring cups, maps, and astronomy. He did quite a bit of drawing, was very serious-minded, never cried and became upset by sad pictures or stores. There was some slowness in the boy's response. Before giving details about what went on in school, he would say: "Wait, I have to get it in my mind first." With other children, he never took the initiative but joined in their games. Thomas took piano lessons, won a scholarship and always enjoyed playing.

At 12 years of age, he was at the top of his class in the sixth grade. The school considered him "adjusted," though he was still looked upon as a "queer fellow." Thomas' marks were excellent. He spent one term each in the school's athletic association, art club, and newspaper, and helped the librarian after school. He also took on a central part in a demonstration during a folk dance. Teachers liked him because of his good academic performance: "He works slowly but what he turns in is excellent." Schoolmates neither accepted nor entirely rejected him. He was the butt of much teasing finding it best to ignore because, if he teased back, "it got worse."

After graduation from high school, Thomas got a Johns Hopkins University Scholarship, which was discontinued after 2 years because his marks were not good enough. He then enlisted in the military service. Because of the slowness of his responses, Thomas was after 5 months directed to undergo medical examination. While at the hospital, he suddenly had a *grand mal* seizure and received a medical discharge. Thomas managed to go back to evening school and earn his college diploma. He continued to experience seizures when neglecting to take his medication regularly.

Interests in astronomy and music provided much personal satisfaction and some social contact. Thomas was a scout leader in demand to teach astronomy and also play the piano. He belongs to a swimming and athletic club and likes to read about science and astronomy, but not fiction.

Among his several jobs was that of a file clerk at a Government agency for a period of five years. He changed this position for work in a military test center focused on electronics and science.

In 1969, the grandmother, now 83 years old, had to be placed in a nursing home. Due to negligence in taking medication, Thomas had another seizure and lost his job. Rather resourceful in rapidly securing other employment, he now works for a charitable organization. Thomas owns a house which he bought several years ago, drives his own car, and plays the piano and tape recorder when at home. He is not interested in girls: "They cost too much money."

Case 2

Sally S., born May 6, 1937, was first seen at the Clinic on March 8, 1943. There were the typical pronominal reversals. An excerpt of the summary states:

> Sally is a well-developed, attractive, intelligent-looking girl. Physical examination showed no noticeable abnormalities. Her main difficulty lies in disability to relate to persons and situations. Aloneness and a marked degree of obsessiveness are the outstanding features, combined with a phenomenal memory and unusual dexterity in solving puzzles considerably beyond her age level.

Both parents were college graduates. The father, an advertising copywriter, was described by his wife as "devoted to his family, not a particularly warm person but everybody likes him; he does not put himself out for people, as I do." The mother, a librarian, spoke of herself as "extremely democratic, a high-strung person; I cross the bridge before I get there." The paternal grandfather, a "brillant lawyer, who got himself involved with women and alcohol," committed suicide; his widow ran a home for old people. The maternal grandfather, a surgeon, died of cancer; the grandmother taught school for some time. A brother, three years older than Sally, was described as rebellious and defiant.

Sally was born normally at term. Reported to be "an exceedingly healthy child," she stood up at 10 months but did not walk until 22 months. "Since a time when she was less than one year old, the girl would scream when members of the family would fail to sit down in their usual chairs, if the routine of the daily walk was changed, if the order of the dishes on the tray was altered, or when she was hindered in going through one special door leading into the garden." She was obsessively interested in all processes which had to do with body functions.

Sally went regularly to school in her home town. At 13 years of age, while in the sixth grade, she had a full scale WISC score of 110 (verbal 119 and performance 98). Among her school marks were A's in Spelling and French, B's in Geography, Mathematics, Bible, and Art, and C in English. She was reported by the school psychologist to have "difficulty with relationship aspects of adjustment."

Seen again at the Clinic on December 6, 1953, the girl was characterized by her mother as follows: "Since you saw her in 1943, Sally has learned to adjust socially. She is now in the eleventh grade. Her records show her depending too much on her memory instead of any power of reasoning." Sally spoke of herself as "a plugger," indicating that she put considerable pressure on herself in order to do well: "Up to last year, the fundamentals of learning have been easy because of my good memory but this year it is the interpretations, and this is difficult for me." Sally had the ambition to go to college but added: "I may be hitching my wagon to a star." About her relationship with schoolmates she said: "The girls are very nice and friendly. There are some points in which I am not close to them. I don't have the interest in boys that most girls of my age have." She expressed concern about her brother who was expelled from school because of drinking and misconduct and had a job at a gasoline station. Sally called him "a strong victim of adolescence—he needs real psychiatric help."

After finishing high school, Sally was successfully enrolled in a woman's college, graduating with a B average. She decided to go into nurses' training and tried to live up to the rules and regulations. Rotation through the different departments, prompted difficulties in adjustment at the beginning of a new service: "Maybe I was anxious to do too well." While on the obstetrical ward,

Sally was asked by the dean to reconsider her plans. Having been told that 20 minutes were the usual time for breastfeeding, she entered the room at the exact moment and took the babies away without saying a word; there were many complaints from the mothers.

Sally readily accepted the suggestion to take up laboratory work and has done well in this field since then. In 1968, the family moved to Chicago and the young woman secured a regular job in one of the hospitals in that city. She is appreciated "because of her excellent facility in chemistry." A psychiatrist consulted in August 1970 writes: "She struggled for a long time to expand her social life . . . . Currently she has been dating a man for the past six months but it is clear that Sally is frightened by any intimacies. She has, with some encouragement, used her interest in music to establish herself in a church-affiliated singing group."

Her father committed suicide in 1969 and her brother is an alcoholic. Sally remains interested and proficient in her work and persistent in efforts to sustain relations with friends and acquaintances. The young woman and her mother remain on good terms and are in contact with each other.

Case 3

Edward F., born October 11, 1939, was first seen on November 15, 1943. His mother said that he was a retarded child who had always appeared very withdrawn:

> He is happy in his own world. He was about 3 years old before he knew members of the family. He has certain stereotypes, has to touch telephone poles, will lay sticks against the pole and walk round and round. He talks better than he understands.

Edward was the younger of two boys and two additional brothers were born later. The father, a lawyer "of worrisome disposition," who was 34 years old at the time of Edward's birth, consulted a psychiatrist in 1939 because of "anxiety about work, fear about making mistakes, panic at night." He had always been "interested in things political, world events, hiking and mountain climbing." The mother, two years younger and also a college graduate, worked as a social worker until marriage at 26 years of age, "always interested in people, fairly well balanced, perhaps extremely logical, always has 4 or 5 reasons for or against." An older sibling was described as healthy and well adjusted.

Edward was an attractive, slender, intelligent-looking boy with vivid dark eyes. Immediately after entering the office, he went after crayons and paper and became absorbed in them. At his mother's insistence, he "read" from a book which he had brought along by repeating remembered passages and interspersing them with neologisms of his own coinage. The boy then tried to jab the point of a pencil into the secretary's leg; when diverted, he attacked a paper bag. He could be engaged in games usually used with very young children.

Edward was born about three weeks before term, weighing 5 pounds and 14 ounces; his "finger nails were not quite developed." He was a planned and wanted child, "never very active." Apathetic as an infant who did not nurse vigorously, Edward did not appear to be aware of his surroundings. The difference from other children was noted when he was 4 months old: "When you picked him up, he relaxed in your arms rather supinely. Almost from the beginning he seems to have had no desire to grow up."

The child sat up at 7 months and walked at 20. "He preferred to crawl even after he learned to walk, had flat feet, wore corrective shoes, and walked like a drunken sailor." Fine muscular coordination developed better than gross motility. Speech development was "slow and unusual." When he finally started to talk, his speech consisted mainly of repetition of what he had heard. Bowel control was acquired at an early age. Wetting by day stopped when he was past the age of three.

When Edward was still an infant, his mother resumed work and he was cared for by the maternal grandmother and a maid, both described as patient with him. When seen at the Clinic, the mother had ceased to work as a result of increasing concern about her son. He was beginning to develop an attachment to her.

At five, Edward was admitted to the Henry Phipps Psychiatric Clinic where a ward had been set up for a few months to study autistic children. He seemed unaware of his environment; however, his later memory of this experience was an unhappy one as he was afraid of the other children.

At six, the boy attended a kindergarten with an understanding teacher who let him participate in group activities or keep him out depending on his readiness. The mother, pleased with his improvement, said that he talked, acted and looked like other children, but appeared different from them in his "limited social ability, restricted interests and peculiar way and rate of learning." In general, he had become "a happy and pleasant child to live with," although he "obviously had a long way to go."

At seven, Edward entered a class for the retarded where he stayed for two years. The family felt that his stay in this class under a sympathetic and interested, although not too well trained, teacher was of incisive importance for Edward's growth. Although at first difficult to control, he made much progress there. When punished by being kept home a day, the child "got the point." The principal agreed to take Edward into the second grade. He had done so well at the end of the year that advancement to fourth grade was recommended. After that accomplishment he was able to keep up with the school work, although his social difficulties continued. An attempt at participation in a scout troop proved too difficult.

Edward had always been musical. At 12 years of age, he took music lessons and seemed to have great facility in composition. The parents were unhappy when he dropped the music at the end of the year, fearing that high school work would require too much. His obsessiveness was not as bad but he continued to show "fixed ideas."

When seen at the Clinic at 13 years, Edward was doing moderately well academically in the eighth grade of a public school. He still suffered from major disabilities in his interpersonal contacts, had an idiosyncratic way of expressing himself and great difficulty in comprehending social situations.

In 1970, the mother wrote that he had gotten along so much better than they had ever expected. Edward finished high school at 19 and wanted to go to college. She attributed this to the pressure he felt to do like the others in the family. Tests were arranged which showed him high on verbal ability and mediocre in performance. It was felt, however, that he could try. Edward went to a state university and took courses in horticulture. He could not master the chemistry, shifted to history and got his B.A. degree at the end of five years. He lived at the dormitory but made no lasting friends.

After graduation, Edward obtained a good horticultural position but he could not make the grade and was asked to leave. This event was very upsetting to him. For the last few years, he has been working at a government agricultural research station in a "blue collar capacity." Edward does not like this too well preferring to associate with "educated people." He has his own apartment and entertains himself with his Hi-fi set. He has bought a car with money that he has saved. He enjoys an active social life, belonging to hiking clubs and he has led hikes. His knowledge of plants and wild life brings him respect. He has begun to date girls. He comes home on weekends when he has time, and he is very welcome.

The mother adds: "We could, of course, write volumes on all the special things we had to do for Edward and with Edward at each stage of his life—but at this time he is completely independent and self-sufficient. I do believe that he enjoys life."

Case 4

Clarence B., born June 15, 1940, was first seen on May 31, 1945. The nursery school that he had attended for two years said of him:

Clarence is an awkward, tall, thin youngster who always seems glad to come to school. His tendency to be quite tense and to repeat certain behavior patterns has been very marked. He remains an individual resisting change and appearing oblivious to his surroundings. His responses have seemed more a matter of personality pattern than a lack of intelligence. He has shown increasing interest in letters and words, the clock and pictures. Clarence rarely comes directly into the school; he had varied from stopping in the hall to look at the clock to listening to the sound of the drinking fountain. Any of these things, once started, persists day after day and week after week. Though he takes no interest in other children, he has shown real excitement over their name tags. When he entered school, he talked little or none. The few things he said, as in naming pictures in a book, were incomprehensible to most of us. Now he speaks distinctly. He repeats questions asked him rather than making a reply.

Pregnancy, birth and motor development were normal. Verbal utterances began at about two years, but were poorly enunciated. There was marked echolalia. "As a baby," the mother recalled, "he did not care much for cuddling." He had "an excellent memory for places, names, happenings, and stories."

A thorough pediatric examination proved Clarence to be in good physical health. In the Binet test, at 6 years, and 4 months, he scored at 5 and 9. He passed the third grade clinical reading test.

Clarence remained at home and went to public school. He was followed regularly by a psychologist who often informed us about developments. The parents, who also kept in touch with us, by 1951 said that he was "making a fair adjustment," that "there are times when he exhibits normal behavior," that "he is relating to people much better." Clarence read a great deal, made some progress in oral work, but did not join in conversations with his classmates. He had gone through a stage of preoccupation with "volcanoes, fires, diseases, sudden death and destruction." At one time, the parents were concerned about strong sibling rivalry.

In July, 1954, after finishing the eighth grade with A's and B's, Clarence spent the summer at the Devereux Camp, where he did well. At the Devereux Schools where he was enrolled, it was noted that he began to show concern about being accepted by his peers. He "made many continuing efforts in social relationships."

Clarence graduated from high school in June, 1958, with excellent marks and superior achievement test scores. After spending the summer with his parents, he was admitted to a college in Illinois, where he received his B.A. degree in 1962. While there, he "socialized" with a girl for a while. Going then to a college in Massachusetts on a scholarship, he felt isolated, and went home to write his thesis. After obtaining his Master's Degree in economics, he studied accounting at his home state university. Clarence got a job with the state planning office and promptly decided to study planning; he did everything required for another Master's Degree except for the thesis.

He might have done well at the job he obtained if it had not been for the fact that he was given a supervisory position. This was too much for him and he was dismissed in October, 1970. For a year he remained idle, for a time having a newspaper route. Finally, he applied for a job more in keeping with his education and is now employed as an accountant, at $7,500 a year.

Clarence gets along well now and has his own apartment. He obsessively tries to make social contacts. "He is awkward socially but can make a superficial adjustment," states a recent report. He senses embarrassing situations to the point of asking: "What am I doing wrong"? Although he dated a girl, she "broke off" after about nine months. Clarence feels that he ought to get married but that he "can't waste money on a girl who isn't serious." He likes driving a car and, as a hobby, collects time tables to maintain his interest in trains.

One sister has a Master's degree in education, the other sister in the history of art. Both are married; one has four children whom Clarence likes to play with; "he gets on the floor and they crawl all over him," the sister says.

Case 5

Henry C., born December 13, 1943, was first seen on May 26, 1947.

> He could not carry on even a simple conversation, a matter of considerable concern to his parents, even though with some coaxing he managed to say a few words. At the same time, the boy could identify every letter of the alphabet and also the punctuation marks. The child had a sizeable repertoire of tunes and exhibited considerable skill with blocks. He handled the Seguin formboard at his age level.

Both parents were college graduates. The father returned from the armed services in April 1947, having been away since Henry was 6 months old. He spoke of himself as a perfectionist ("bugs on keeping things in order"). The mother, who in her earlier years had to struggle with adjustment to her epileptic condition and to her mother's obsessive domination, was extremely tense whenever she picked up the baby for fear of dropping him during convulsion. In fact, she did so on one occasion which, though not injuring the child, increased her anxiety. She left the child alone most of the time, feeling that this was what he liked best.

On the boy's sixth birthday, he was placed by his parents in a foster home where he improved remarkably: "He does beautifully with words now" (March 1949), using good syntax, though occasionally reversing pronouns. In 1950, he was "no problem" in regular kindergarten: "He seems to be happy within himself and is slow in making overtures toward other children." There was a good relationship between Henry's foster parents and his mother. Henry's parents were considering divorce: the father was referred to as "an isolated iceberg."

In 1952, Henry decided to change his name, at first to that of his foster parents; then, retaining his first name, he gave himself a middle name after his patron saint and a last name after a movie actor. Eventually he had his name duly legalized.

When seen at the Clinic in July 1954, Henry related personal interests and incidents in a dramatic fashion but became uncomfortable when others tried to have him elaborate. He was passing into the fifth grade even though his school work was of a marginal quality; "the school recognized his difficulties and has agreed on a policy of promotion." At home, he was preoccupied with death and killing, both in his remarks and in his drawings.

In August 1956, Henry's mother was found dead (the janitor had to break into the apartment) when he and his foster mother went to visit her. The coroner's autopsy reported "natural death" (?). Henry, when informed, "cried a little but it was not difficult to distract him."

While Henry did well in school, at home he was rude and insistent, especially after visiting his father. He spent much of his time writing "horror stories, murder, science fiction." After learning to use the typewriter, "the stories became longer, more vivid, bloodier, and very often did not make much sense."

In the fall of 1958, Henry was entered in a boarding school, which he liked. Spending his weekends with the foster parents, he declined his father's invitations to stay with him.

In our usual efforts to follow the destinies of our patients, we corresponded with the father, the foster parents, and a financial guardian who for a time looked after a small sum left by Henry's mother and who, having moved to India, wrote us from there on October 4, 1971:

> . . . I first saw Henry at 2 or 3 years when my wife and I visited his
> parents and played bridge in their apartment. He was somewhat like a

wild animal running back and forth across the living room until he became exhausted. The next time I saw him, he was 15 and we had a very interesting conversation. I felt at that particular time that he appeared to be quite normal. His letters also indicated to me that he was being fairly well adjusted. I thought that it was quite remarkable that he was pretty much on his own since then.

We wrote to Henry himself when we learned of his address. Early in January 1972, he sent us a lengthy autobiographic letter; regretfully, we cannot reproduce it word for word but the following is an abstract:

On June 29, 1962, at 19½ years of age, he entered the armed services. Upon completion of basic training, he was assigned to one of the intelligence services, received a top security clearance, took courses until December 6, 1962 (the nature of which he could not disclose because they were of a "highly confidential nature"), and received an honorable discharge on January 18, 1963. Then follows a list of various jobs held in California and later in Pennsylvania, (six altogether) mostly as a "general office worker"; at present he is "chief inventory controller in a Motion Picture Laboratory" where he has received "several healthy pay increases." After drifting around, he feels that "perhaps at last, I have found a place worthy of my talent for settling down in." All six jobs were described in great detail, giving dates, description of responsibilities, names and telephone numbers of supervisors, and reasons for leaving the jobs. Generally speaking, "I have never been dismissed from any place of employment because of any working habits or lack of working habits."

The letter addressed "To Whom It May Concern," starts as follows:

> I am writing this resume with the intention of giving any person who would wish it a lucid account of my life, educational and working background, and experiences. I am 6 feet tall, weigh 145 pounds, have medium brown hair and hazel blue eyes. I am in excellent health with no history of any severe illnesses or injuries. I have an automobile and a permanent residence. I am also draft exempt and have no criminal record of any kind.

Elsewhere he writes:

> As for my future, I have absolutely no worries whatsoever. I live each day as though it were my last, and let the devil take tomorrow .... I am 28 years old and single (though several girls I know had hoped to change that) with no desire to get tied down for a good

long time . . . . I neither smoke nor drink but I do have an uncontrollable urge to gamble. (We all have to have a few bad habits.)

The letter is concluded as follows:

For as long as I live, I shall always remember you, Dr. Kanner, and how you have opened many doors for me. I cannot thank you enough for the limitless kindness you have shown me while rekindling the spark of living within me that had nearly died so very long ago.

Case 6

George W., born February 27, 1944, was first seen on January 11, 1951. His mother complained:

Although he has talked clearly, using big words and sentences since he was 18 months old, he still had never spoken *with* us—that is, carry on a conversation or even answer simple yes and no questions. He lives completely in a world of his own. As an infant he had not smiled like other children. At 2 years, he knew the alphabet and numbers. He never used the first person in speaking.

George was born 5 weeks past term, weighing 8 pounds at birth. He was on a rigid schedule and was awakened for feedings. His first words were spoken at 13 months, he walked alone at 18 months, and bowel control was established at 18 months; bed wetting continued until the age of 6 years. Gross motor development was described as poor and fine motor coordination as good; he could open and close a safety pin and replace the top on a toothpaste tube.

The boy's father, of Spanish (Latin American) descent, was a civil engineer who went into the armed services when George was 6 months old; he was away for about 2 years. On his return, he "had difficulty relating to George" and "kept looking for a physical (glandular) cause of George's problems."

The boy's mother had 3 years of college. "Intellectual pursuits" were important to her and she started George very early with letters and numbers. The case history is full of her expressions of conflicts with her father—fear of his displeasure and resentment of his domination. She blamed herself for anything that went wrong with George, at the same time hoping for some quick, miraculous cure. When the child was about 4 years old, she resorted to drinking for several years until she joined Alcoholics Anonymous.

Because George was not able to get along in kindergarten, he was referred to the Clinic where he developed a tenuous relationship with his therapist. He echoed things he heard, repeated names that came over the hospital's loud speaker, and used many neologisms. Also, he was preoccupied with traffic lights and with elevators.

At the age of 9, George was admitted to a center for emotionally disturbed children where he remained for 6 years. While there, he had many consuming obsessions, mainly focused on mechanical devices (plumbing, lighting), travel, map making, and physical health (he washed many times a day because of his fear of germs). These preoccupations gradually subsided and he became more interested in group activities, regressing occasionally, usually in association with changes in personnel. However, he did fairly well with his school assignments.

At the age of 15, George returned home and entered in public school in a "slow" sixth grade where "with encouragement but not much pressure" he was able to do the work. His teacher reported:

> He conforms to rules and regulations as well as any immature sixth grade child. He plays the violin well, he appears to enjoy the company of his classmates, he is quite friendly and likes to joke. He is particularly fond of poems and plays on words.

George's mother took him out of school when he was in the eleventh grade so that he could concentrate on music. He had played violin in a number of youth orchestras and took courses at a prominent Conservatory. Concerned about not getting a high school diploma, George has, in recent years, spent much of his time subscribing to correspondence courses. He is especially interested in languages, having learned Spanish in school, teaching himself French, and having "a working knowledge" of Italian. At present George is employed as a page in a library and is also in charge of mailing books (mostly to foreign countries).

George lives with his parents. He is helpful with chores at home (to make things easier for his mother who describes him as "dependable") but has no friends and "girls are not interested in him." His major preoccupation now is an overconcern about pleasing people: "He is not relaxed and afraid of doing wrong."

Case 7

Walter P., born June 16, 1944, was first seen on July 8, 1952. He had seemed normal until he was about 3½ years old when his mother noted that his speech was not progressing, he had become unusually quiet (sitting for long periods looking aimlessly around), and finally had just about stopped talking altogether. The child became unduly interested in spinning tops and other toys, was upset when things were moved from their accustomed positions, paid little attention to the people in his environment, and was slow in responding to being called.

Walter's parents gave the impression of being sociable, well-adjusted people. The father had 2 years of college and worked as an ordinance engineer for the federal government. He was able to give more specific and accurate information about the child than his wife. The mother also had 2 years of college and worked in a bank to provide money for the child's care and treatment. Both parents emphasized the harmony of their relationship. A brother, 3 years older than Walter, was getting along well.

Walter was born at term. At 3 weeks, he developed pyloric stenosis which was relieved by an operation from which he recovered uneventfully. There were no feeding problems. The boy began to talk at 2½ years of age and was fully toilet trained by age 3 without any apparent difficulty or conflict.

When seen at the Clinic, Walter was an attractive child who cooperated in a stiff, automatic way. While he did not relate to the examiner, looking vaguely out of the window and responding only to the simplest questions, he immediately placed all the pieces in the Seguin formboard. The boy would respond to "What is your name?," "How old are you?," "Sit in the chair," but would not cooperate in any verbal tests. His behavior was repetitious, obsessive, and withdrawn.

At 9 years, Walter was still obsessive, used little speech but had progressed some in "play school," he had learned to copy and to spell some words, and was very destructive with anything chipped or broken.

At 10, the child's mother reported that he was "progressing well." Walter attended a school for retarded children, was learning to write and to do simple arithmetic, seeming to enjoy it, but reading was causing him some trouble. Also he was playing and talking better with other children and could give simple messages over the telephone (he was able to say what he wanted). The boy had a variety of rituals, first, tapping his chin until it was red, and later, rubbing his eyes. His mother found him a "lovable little boy" who behaved well when they took him out.

Arrangements were made with a psychiatric clinic near his home for follow-up consultations.

In 1971, the mother gave this follow-up report:

> Walter attended a boarding school for exceptional children from 1956 to 1962, coming home on weekends, and then lived with her (his father had died). For 2 years, he attended a day school and then worked for a short time in a sheltered workshop. "Since June 1968, he

has worked at a small restaurant as a dishwasher and bus boy, earning $1.25 an hour. He seems to enjoy his work, has pleased his employers, and has never missed a day. He is a handsome young man, takes complete care of himself and of his room, and is neat and clean at all times. There are no behavior problems. He helps with the housework and takes care of the yard, including complete care of the power mower. His main difficulty always is in communication. What he says, he says well and in a fairly clear manner, but there is no voluntary conversation. Walter talks enough to make his wishes known, will answer the phone and tell me who is calling, but when I am not home, unless I ask him, he will not tell me if someone called.

Case 8

Bernard S., born August 3, 1949, was first seen on June 7, 1952. He was referred by the nursery school which he attended. His teachers reported that he seemed "more alone than most children" and that he was "in the school but not a part of it." The child showed some bizarre behavior and echolalia. He referred to himself in the third person and often had a smile on his face which was unrelated to anything obvious to the onlooker.

Bernard's father was a pharmacist who spent long hours in his drug store. His mother had manic-depressive episodes and had been hospitalized for a few months 9 years before Bernard was born. She did not become pregnant until 14 years after her marriage, which came as a "delightful surprise."

Very soon after Bernard's birth, his mother became ill again and was hospitalized for over a year during which time Bernard was cared for by a nurse in her home. When the mother took him back, Bernard was 15 months old and was walking "but not feeding himself." The mother was a perfectionist, especially about his eating. She continued to have mood swings and was under the care of a psychiatrist.

The parents separated when Bernard was about 2½ years old. Six months later, the mother disappeared with the child to Florida. The father fetched him back, and placed Bernard with a paternal aunt. One of the nursery school teachers who visited at the time, described the boy as relaxed and happy with his aunt: "For the first time, I heard him speak quite volubly." The aunt did not return him to the nursery school as she wanted him to remain at her home "where he could get some much-needed love and attention, so that he could feel someone really cared for him." The parents came back to live together again and took Bernard home. He was reentered in the nursery school at 4 years of age. The boy had a good memory; he knew the names of all the children in the school and noted who was absent before the teacher did. However, he could be brought into group activities for only very brief times. In the neighborhood, he stayed in the house because the children would not play with him and called him "that crazy kid." Their attitude improved when he bribed them with cookies.

The father gave a follow-up report when Bernard was 20 years old:

> He had graduated from high school at 19 and was struggling with junior college in a general course. His marks had been mediocre. He is not the studying type, seeking a job and a simple uncomplicated life. He lost 2 years of school in shifting around. One year he spent in a "progressive" boarding school, but that proved to be "more of a hippie colony" and his work was poor. The mother died while he was there and then he did not want to go back. After the paternal aunt who had cared for him as a small child came to live with them following her husband's death. Bernard showed marked improvement.

The father remarried in 1968 and Bernard got along well with his stepmother. He had had "no real psychiatric treatment."

Bernard is "backward and shy but that is the way he is." He did approach a girl once for a date in a very negative manner. He hates clothes, drives a car, does best if not pressured and helped his father in the drug store (he did not wait on customers but would fill the shelves). His chief interest is the streetcar museum. He is a member of a club that goes there on Sundays, laying track, painting cars, etc. They take trips. He used to like history, is up on world politics, and reads the newspapers.

Case 9

Fred G., born December 11, 1948, was first seen on August 11, 1952. His parents gave a history of difficulties dating from colic for 6 weeks after birth. He was carried around constantly by members of the family; when the colic subsided, he continued to demand attention. A practical nurse handled this by letting him "cry it out." At 3 months, the child was taken to visit his grandmother and placed unceremoniously into her arms on arrival. He reacted with terror, screaming for the 3 weeks, and since then had a great fear of strangers.

> In spite of Fred's ability to go through some of the motions of the Binet test, it was not possible to get his full cooperation. He placed the small formboard figures. When asked to match forms, he named them

first. He ignored people in the room and repeated questions rather than answer them.

Fred was born by Ceasarean section, walked at 14 months, and began to talk at one year. His speech was good and he had a large vocabulary but would not use the first person and repeated a phrase rather than say "Yes." Weaning from the bottle was difficult and slow, and there was also conflict over bowel training.

At home, he was preoccupied with music, being able to recognize records just by looking at them when he was 3 years old. He could identify compositions after hearing them by saying: "That's the Moldau," "That's Beethoven's Fifth," etc. Six months before coming to the Clinic, he had been sent to a nursery school where he was fearful of the children. After his mother stayed with him several days, he calmed down but ignored everyone, refused to participate in any form of group activity, and "was just there." The mother said that "at home there could not be a better child." "He likes to be by himself," she added. He would go into rages over inanimate objects that would not do just as he wished.

The father, who wanted to be a physician, took up a related course of study because family finances did not allow him to go through medical school. After 3 years, he abandoned it for government work involving secret documents and assignments. The mother, a college graduate, had taught school several years and quit a year before Fred's birth. She came from "a family of pushers" and had great intellectual drive. The woman expressed a fear that she might be blamed for the child's difficulties. There seemed to be no particular domestic problems. The home atmosphere was one of emphasis on such cultural pursuits as music and intellectual discussion.

For approximately 2½ years, from 1952 to 1955, Fred regularly attended a day care center for emotionally disturbed children. He formed an attachment to the director and saw her often in the years that followed.

When tested at 16 years, he was found to have a full scale WISC IQ of 118 (verbal 126 and performance 104). His arithmetic score was at the ceiling with quick answers on the tests, and comprehension, similarities and rote memory were rated as being of high average. On the Rorschach, he showed "sharp alterations between impulsivity and repression" and "a struggle between feelings of relationship and isolation."

At 23 years of age, Fred is doing well at a university where he has a B plus average and is gifted in mathematics.

He has adjusted well in college life and his schoolmates respect his academic prowess. The young man has sloughed off his obsessive preoccupations. For instance, he dresses well but is not as compulsive about clothes as he used to be.

Though described as "awkward and intellectual," he tries, at least on the surface, to take part in the concerns which he knows should be those for his age, even "experimenting" once with a double date arrangement (not repeated). Fred drives a car skillfully, with full knowledge of all the parts, and in his spare time has done some composing and built a telescope.

Until his first year in College, Fred had always lived with his parents. After some hesitation, particularly by the father, they supported his decision to move to a dormitory.

DISCUSSION

Now that 29 years have elapsed since the identification of early infantile autism, the children so diagnosed in the first decade of its recognized existence have reached adulthood. Despite considerable mobility of some of the families, it has been possible to learn about the patients' present status. The first of an anticipated series of follow-ups appeared last year as a report of the destinies of the eleven children whose condition had suggested and crystallized the specific syndrome (Kanner, 1943, 1971). Altogether, 96 patients had been designated as autistic before 1953 at our Clinic, the "birthplace" of the syndrome. Of this number we have selected those now capable of functioning in society. Besides the two presented in 1971 (Donald T. and Frederick W.), we have sketched the biographies of nine such persons (one female and eight males), currently ranging in age between 22 and 35 years. The nosological criteria, set down in 1943, had been uniformly applied to all 96 children.

The value of catamnesis has been sensed for quite some time. As far back as the early 1940's, Cottington (1942) compared the results of shock treatment, psychotherapy and socialization of a few psychotic children, none older than 14 years. Lourie, Pacella, and Piotrowski (1943) in a review of 20 children "with schizophrenic-like psychoses," saw three types of "adjustment": (1) Apparently normal (4 cases); (2) fair to borderline (5 cases); and (3) low grade (11 cases). These reports were pioneering innovations at a time when interest was centered mainly on description and speculation about etiology. However, they dealt with categories rather than individuals, whose subsequent fate after childhood or at most the early teens has remained unknown.

Continuous curiosity about the patients' progress has always been one of the primary concerns of our Clinic (Kanner, 1937a, 1937b). Names, symptoms, diagnoses, and any other relevant items were cross-indexed for all. Since, except for our own communications, early infantile autism did not enter the public arena until about 1950, our Clinic saw itself as a quasi ex-officio archive for all that pertained to the syndrome, to be kept in flux and added to as time went on. This gave helpful information for a study (Kanner & Eisenberg, 1955) which comprised children with an average age of 14 years and yielded one finding of potential predictive value:

> The prognosis has shown to vary significantly with the presence of useful speech at the age of 5 years, taken as an index of the severity of autistic isolation.

Many are now in their 20's and 30's; all but two of them were available for "check-ups" in 1971. Their biographic profiles are—and will continue to be—a part of the "archive" and have aided us in picking out those who have gone farthest in terms of social adjustment.

Eleven autistic children (9 in this series plus Donald T. and Frederick W. reported in 1971) have emerged sufficiently to function as adults in varying degrees of nonpsychotic activity. Three have college degrees, three had a junior college education, one is now doing well in college, one graduated from high school, one passed the eleventh grade, one went to a private "boarding school for exceptional children," and one received vocational training in a sheltered workshop.

Their present occupations are bank teller, laboratory technician, duplicating machine operator, accountant, "blue collar job" at an agricalatural research station, general office worker, page in the foreign language section of a library, bus boy in a restaurant, truck loading supervisor, helper in a drug store, and college student. Two (Thomas G. and Henry C.) had enlisted and been accepted by the armed services but were "honorably discharged" within a year.

What distinguishes them from those who, remaining wholly isolated, did not make the linkage with society?

In comparing the two groups, no difference could be found with regard to ethnic origin, family characteristics, or specific intercurrent events. Nor is there anything in the features of physical health that stand out as a contrast, though Thomas G. began to experience convulsions after his twentieth year.

We did, however, find a number of items which were shared by the patients who form the nucleus of this study. They have to do with a variety of maturational and environmental issues and with the patients' type of reactions to the growing awareness of their peculiarities.

All of them used some speech before the age of 5 years. This in itself cannot be taken as an all-valid prognostic sign because many who had done likewise have failed to reach a similar degree of emergence. What characterizes our group is a steady succession of stages: No initiative or response—immediate parroting—delayed echolalia with pronominal reversals—utterances related to obsessive preoccupations—communicative dialogue with the proper use of personal pronouns and greater flexibility in the use of prepositions.

Not one of them had at any time been subjected to sojourn in a state hospital or institution for the feebleminded. This seems to be significant in view of our experience that such an eventuality has invariably cut short any prospect for improvement (Kanner, 1965). All of our eleven patients here considered have remained at home at least before school age and some quite a few years longer. Three still live with their families, the others—whether in foster homes or boarding schools—had regular contact with their relatives. However, many other autistic children who stayed at home did not advance as those eleven did.

One recurrent theme, though, could be noted as specific for our group in clear contrast with the non-emerging autistic children: a chronicle of gradual changes of self-concept and reactions to them along the road to social adaptation.

In the first few years of life, there was in this respect no difference between any of our 96 patients now over 20 years old. Their isolation with all its corollaries—neither chosen nor imposed from without—was a form of existence which was had, lived, experienced rather than contemplated or reacted to. It was part of an innate illness not perceived as such by the ill child who was contentedly (though pathologically) "adjusted" unless threatened by external interference with the status quo. There was a minimum of centrifugal reaching out and a minimal response to centripetal incursions. As time went on, some of the incursions began to be tolerated in varying degrees. Unless they became too overwhelming and the child was pushed back into self-incapsulation until his status was barely distinguishable from extreme mental retardation, he was making compromises to the extent of verbal interplay, demanding parental assistance with his rituals, falling in line with I-You identification, superficially going through the symbolic acts of shaking hands, hugging and kissing, and generally yielding to the rudiments of domestication. This carried over to nursery school and kindergarten, at least in terms of joining mechanically in routine activities, first on invitation and then more or less spontaneously.

Our eleven children went through the same stages. It was not until the early to middle teens when a remarkable change took place. Unlike most other autistic children, they became uneasily aware of their peculiarities and began to make a conscious effort to do something about them. This effort increased as they grew older. They "knew," for instance, that youngsters were expected to have friends. Realizing their inability to form a genuine buddy-buddy relationship, they—one is almost tempted to say, ingeniously—made use of the gains made by their obsessive preoccupations to open a door for contact.

> Thomas G. joined the Boy Scouts and found recognition by teaching astronomy and playing the piano; he also joined a swimming and athletic club. Sally S. utilized her good memory, of which she was fully aware, to merit acceptance in high school and college; when she failed as a student nurse because the maintenance of a genuine relationship with the patients was beyond her capacity, she became a laboratory technician and has made a reputation for "excelling in chemistry." Edward F. enjoys an active social life belonging to hiking clubs, and his knowledge of plants and wild life brings him respect. Clarence B. "obsessively tries to make social contacts; he is awkward socially but can make a superficial adjustment." Henry C. enlisted in the Army, had several well-paying jobs and "has an uncontrollable urge to gamble." George W. is "over-concerned about pleasing people." Walter P. satisfies his social needs as bus boy in a restaurant and "pleases his employers." Bernard S. is a member of a street car museum where he lays tracks, paints cars, and goes on trips. Fred G. is respected by his schoolmates because of his academic prowess.

Again and again we note a felt need to grope for ways to compensate for the lack of inherent sociability. Out of this developed a paradoxical use of the previously self-serving, isolating obsessions which instead come to serve positively as a connecting link with groups of people.

The contacts thus established led to the discovery that the boy-meets-girl issue was paramount in the talks of the companions. Again, there was a vaguely felt obligation to "conform." Those attempts were sporadic and short-lived. The "explanations" offered indicated that there was not too much displeasure with the absence of any real involvement.

> Henry C. reported that he was single, that several girls "had hoped to change that" but that he had "no desire to get tied down for a good long time." Thomas G. declared categorically that girls "cost too much money." Clarence B., who "socialized" with a girl for a short time in college, stated that he "ought to get married but can't waste money on a girl who is not serious." Bernard S. was said to have approached a girl once for a date "in a very negative way" (inviting rebuff). Fred G. "experimented" *once* with a double date arrangement (never repeated).

George W. made things easy for himself by deciding a priori that girls were not interested in him. Sally S., the only girl in our group, once asked seriously at 23 years of age what she ought to do if ever she fell in love with someone, an experience she had never had before. She said: "I have never had the interest in boys most girls my age have." At 30 years, she dated a man for a few months but gave this up because she was "frightened by any intimacy."

COMMENT

On the basis of the recorded and discussed observations, the question raised in the title of this paper can be answered with reasonable certainty. Not counting the gifted student of mathematics killed accidentally and the young man whom we have so far lost track after 1962 when he was in college, eleven of the 96 autistic children known to our Clinic since before 1953 are now in their twenties and thirties, mingling, working, and maintaining themselves in society. They have not completely shed the fundamental personality structure of early infantile autism but, with increasing self-assessment in their middle to late teens, they expended considerable effort to fit themselves—dutifully, as it were—to what they came to perceive as commonly expected obligations. They made the compromise of being, yet not appearing, alone and discovered means of interaction by joining groups in which they could make use of their preoccupations, previously immured in self-limited stereotypies, as shared "hobbies" in the company of others. In the club to which they "belonged," they received—and enjoyed—the recognition earned by the detailed knowledge they had stored up in years of obsessive rumination of specific topics (music, mathematics, history, chemistry, astronomy, wild life, foreign languages, etc.). Reward came to them also from their employers who (as confirmed in statements sent to us) remarked on their meticulousness and trustworthiness. Life among people thus lost its former menacing aspects. Nobody has shoved them forcibly through a gate which others had tried to unlock for them; it was *they* who, at first timidly and experimentally, then more resolutely, paved their way to it and walked through. Once inside, they adopted some of the values they found there. Material possession became an object of ambition. Those who are not with their families (eight of the eleven) live by themselves; one (Thomas G.) even owns a house which he bought several years ago. All drive automobiles and there is no record of accidents or traffic violations.

There have been equally duty-bound, though haphazardly pursued attempts to form personal friendships. These were far less successful. Failure apparently was not met with major frustration, self-reproach or accusation of others. There even was a sense of relief in matters of dating; ready rationalizations were: "a waste of money," "cost too much,"; Sally had a dread of "intimacy," Henry did not feel like being tied for a long time. No one in the group has seriously thought of, or is now contemplating, marriage.

This, then, is the profile of eleven autistic children, now adults, whose social adaptation does not run counter to the general run of the populace. It differs essentially from that of at least 83 of the 96 other autistic children in the series. Fascinating as it is, it does not offer a definite clue for the cause of the difference. The presence of speech before the age of 5 years and the fact of being kept out of state institutions are helpful hints but, being shared with some of the non-emerging children, they can only be viewed at best as straws in the wind pointing to prognostic probabilities.

Hence, at least for the time being, there is no alternative to the idea expressed at the close of our 1971 follow-up: "It is well known in medicine that any illness may appear in different degrees of severity, all the way from the so-called *formes frustes* to the most fulminant manifestation. Does this possibly apply also to early infantile autism"?

It must be kept in mind that our "emergers" grew up in the days before the introduction of therapeutic techniques especially intended to remedy the autistic illness, be they based on circumscribed psychotherapeutic, psycho-pharmacological, or behavioristic orientation. Would any of those have in any way altered the outlook for our 96 children? Will any of those increase the ratio of "emergers" in the future? What can we make of the fact, documented in this study, that almost 11 to 12 percent "got there" without any of those techniques? Now that a number of state hospitals have divisions for the personalized care and treatment of children, can we look upon admission of autistic patients to them with better expectations than before? Will the biochemical research now vigorously under way uncover early indications pointing to prognostically reliable assessments of the degree of severity of the autistic illness?

All these are justifiable curiosities with important practical implications. It will take time to satisfy them. Continual follow-up or even better follow-along, will—as we hope that this study does—prove in the long run to be of great importance. Our astute readers have undoubtedly noticed that this paper is being presented with a twofold purpose. One is, of course, patently announced in its title. The other, more implicit aim is an attempt to set up a sample for follow-along and follow-up studies hopefully to be conducted in clinical and research centers as the intervals between childhood and adulthood of autistic patients keep lengthening.

REFERENCES

Cottington, F. Treatment of schizophrenia in childhood. *Nervous Child,* 1942, **1,** 172-187.

Kanner, L. Problem children growing up. *American Journal of Psychiatry,* 1937, **94** 691-699. (a)

Kanner, L. Prognosis in child psychiatry. *Archives of Neurology and Psychiatry,* 1937, **37,** 922-928. (b)

Kanner, L. Autistic disturbances of affective contact. *Nervous Child,* 1943, **2,** 217-250.

Kanner, L. Children in state hospitals. *American Journal of Psychiatry,* 1965, **121,** 925-927.

Kanner, L. Follow-up study of eleven autistic children originally reported in 1943. *Journal of Autism and Childhood Schizophrenia,* 1971, **1,** 119-145.

Kanner, L., & Eisenberg, L. Notes on the follow-up studies of autistic children. In P. H. Hoch and J. Zubin (Eds.), *Psychopathology of childhood.* New York: Grune & Stratton, 1955.

Lourie, R. S., Pacella, B. L., & Piotrowski, Z. A. Studies on the prognosis in schizophrenic-like psychoses in children. *American Journal of Psychiatry,* 1943, **99,** 542-552.

15

APPROACHES:
RETROSPECT AND PROSPECT

A little more than 60 years ago, the foundation of the National Committee for Mental Hygiene evoked an unprecedented amount of enthusiasm which soon spread over the civilized portion of the globe. Its banner carried a lofty slogan: The prevention of insanity and delinquency. It had an exciting message: Give us people at the earliest age at which they have personal difficulties and we shall help them to stay out of mental hospitals and prisons. There is no earlier time for this task than the years of sprouting and budding. As predicted in 1900 by Ellen Key, the noted Swedish sociologist, we found ourselves moving in what she said would be the "century of the child."

For the first time in the history of mankind, the welfare of children was ushered in as an acknowledged and loudly acclaimed concern of scientists, social agencies, and governmental planners. In rapid succession, juvenile courts, special educational facilities, and child guidance clinics entered into the cultural texture as ingredients of communal responsibility. Child psychiatry came into its own as

215

Long ago, the moral and political philosophies started with exalted ideals for the benefit of humanity, with emphasis on eternal values which are the noblest aspirations of the species.

Have they, in the course of several millennia, brought about the abolition of fratricide, tyranny, greed, and prejudice? *They have not.*

This is because the basic goal has been split off into a variety of "approaches," each claiming the sole possession of the key to redemption. Ideals degenerated into ideologies, the golden rule into iron-fisted injunctions, religion into sectarianism. Inflexible sets of tenets and arrays of *sine qua non* procedures, each unique to a specific "approach," have done very little for the furtherance of the goal on whose behalf it has been inaugurated.

How does this apply to our own concern? A few examples may suffice:

(1) The mental hygiene movement resulted in the creation of communal clinics which wisely recognized the benefits to be derived from the collaboration of all those who had a hand in the guidance of troubled children and their families. There could have been no more promising start than such a multidisciplinary arrangement. But what happened? The breadth of vision was promptly narrowed down to the much vaunted "team approach" of psychiatrist, psychologist, and social worker. The pediatricians, the educators, the juvenile courts, and all other groups were kept away from active participation and viewed superciliously as hopefully obedient recipients of the wisdom emanating from the established trinity.

Were the portals of the clinics open to all children with developmental difficulties? The "approach" deemed it inconvenient to admit those in the first few years of life, the intellectually handicapped, the organically damaged, the psychotically non responsive, and the offspring of "uncooperative" parents. Thus the services were limited to an elite of patients considered worthy of being "approached."

(2) Since the dawn of civilization, many outstanding thinkers have said wise things about the soul, the mind, the morals, the destiny of man, as if "man" were a homogeneous category. In the past two centuries, anthropologists, physicians, teachers, and civic-spirited statesmen were increasingly impressed by the heterogeneity of the members of the species. The rights of the individual became the sacrosanct basis of the new democracies.

It was in the field of education that the first concretely measurable criteria for heterogeneity were worked out, at least so far as application to scholastic aptitude was concerned. Standardized developmental assessments accentuated the need for special facilities attuned to the difference and adapted to the requirements of individual children. When these were set up, the administrative a widely ramified discipline devoted to the study, treatment, and preclusion of developmental and behavioral distress. Hardly ever had so much been achieved in so short a time in terms of man's efforts to improve the lot of his fellow men.

Has all of this led even to an infinitesimal reduction of "insanity and delinquency"? *It has not.* Can we sit back with Pollyannish delight in contemplation of anticipated fulfillment? *We can not.* Should we, therefore, despairingly, sardonically, or with shoulder-shrugging abandon turn our backs to the festive glee with which all these innovations were brought into existence? *We should not.*

Dissatisfaction with things as they are is unquestionably an indispensable step toward progress without which there would be unimaginative stagnation. But it must be supplemented by curiosity about practical, attainable means of amelioration. This requires patient, self-critical inquiry and the setting of realistic goals without premature hosannas or excursions into pseudo-omniscience.

Goethe has tried ingeniously to deal with this issue in the famous confrontation between Faust and his famulus. Wagner represents the hosannas. Behold!, he declares, we have reached the acme of wisdom and we can forever bask in its resplendent glory. Faust cannot concur. Smarting from a conviction of ignorance, he succumbs to the ghostly phantom of omniscience.

The Wagnerians in our midst, like their prototype, marvel at the advances made after ages of inertia, point with pride to the mushrooming proliferation of professionals, paraprofessionals, buildings, and monetary appropriations, and look for more and more of these accoutrements for the mental hygiene brigade. Local and national policies are set down, statistics are paraded, functions are delineated, and all is well with the world.

The Faustians, like their prototype, are restive in the face of the slowness and imperfections of human endeavor. Impatient with its piecemeal and often zigzagging pace, they grope for an all-encompassing breakthrough that would enable them to find an answer, *the* answer, to every question. Some of them, imbued with impeccable idealism and creative urge, have startled their contemporaries with revelations proclaimed with evangelical fervor and generally known as tightly systematized "approaches."

This is a semantically fascinating term. You might think that it is the patient who approaches you with his problem and that you might take it up from there, depending on its nature, its varieties, implications, and complexities.

No, say the approachers, it is we who have a ready-made, universal set of premises and techniques applicable to all comers. All you have to do is learn the catechism and the rituals and you are safely on the way to salvation.

"approachers" lost no time imposing rigid regulations centered around the IQ and would-be diagnostic labeling. All of us know of children who were kept out of classes for the retarded because they were emotionally disturbed and were refused admission to classes for the emotionally disturbed because they were retarded. We know of the heated battles, which have not yet fully subsided, between the advocates of continuous and of contiguous grouping—battles in which the theories of the two sets of "approachers" took precedence over practical planning for each child in accordance with his personal needs.

(3) In no area of scientific search for the betterment of health has there been such a plethora of "approachers" as in contemporary psychiatry. It would be unfair to deny to any of them the acknowledgment of underlying earnestness and of a sincere desire to be of help. In fact, one often senses an overdose of goodwill and an impetuous straining to anticipate the ultimate triumph of etiologic omniscience and therapeutic omnipotence.

Out of the multiplicity of factors which, in a vast variety of fusions, make up the complexity of human existence, each one of different leaders picked out a special set for the top hierarchical role as the basis of a supposedly all-valid "approach."

The past few decades have witnessed a fascinating procession of approaches of varying longevity, some with few and others with many adherents.

Who still remembers the days when the apostles of the focal infection credo preached and practiced the removal of teeth, tonsils, appendices, gall bladders, and parts of the colon as a sure cure of schizophrenia (Cotton, 1921)?

Who remembers the excitement created by the breathtaking discovery of the functions of the innersecretory glands, promptly seized upon by some as the unrivaled source of all human behavior and the promise of a therapeutic elixir? The "glands of destiny" (Cobb, 1927) and the "glands regulating personality" (Berman, 1921) were declared to hold *the* answer to all psychiatric curiosity.

Who remembers the stir aroused by some of the new typologies, the reams of literature on anthropometric measurements claimed to be the infallible guides to characterologic predestination (Krasusky, 1927)?

These "approaches" have had their day, not too long ago, in the lifetime of some of us. Most of them have their "kernel of truth"; some have made a few factual contributions which can be incorporated as fragmentary addenda to our body of knowledge.

There are other approaches which still hold powerful sway. We are here concerned mainly with child psychiatry and more especially with the childhood psychoses. There are those who look on infantile sexuality alone, others on early mother-child relationship alone, others on faulty conditioning alone, still others on neuropathology or biochemistry alone as the open sesame to the gates of understanding and the passkey to therapeutic planning. What happens to a psychotic child and his family has often been "programmed" not so much in accord with the specific circumstances of each patient's illness as by the predictably uniform ritualism of the approacher's orientation.

*   *

Of course, this state of affairs could not go unnoticed. Adolf Meyer persistently spoke out against what he called "exclusive salvationism" of the splinter groups which, far from seeing themselves as such, paraded their credo as the infallible guardian of the truth, the whole truth, etc.

At long last, in 1956, the situation reached a point when the Committee on Public Health of the New York Academy of Medicine convoked a conference headlined: *Integrating the Approaches to Mental Disease*; the proceedings were superbly edited by Kruse (1957). The broad aim was "to afford an opportunity to a group of experts who hold different views on the causalities, pathogenesis, and therapy of mental disease to come together, to engage in cross-exposition, and to plan research in common." Prominent representatives of four "major categories" (1. organic, 2. experimental psychological, 3. psychodynamic, 4. psychosocial) took part in the discussions. "Each of these four groups," the editor said, "has its distinctive methodology, vocabulary, and doctrine; to the others the methods of each are unfamiliar, the language strange, and the concepts esoteric." Throughout the debates, the terms "approaches," "positions," "viewpoints," "doctrines," and "schools of thought" were used synonymously. There was quite a bit of airing of intradoctrinal acceptance and unacceptance, common ground, communication and concept barriers. All this was intended to find a way out of "provincialism," "insular grouping," "segmentation," "fragmentation," "narrow vista," resulting in "restricted objective and approach."

It cannot be said that those sessions have changed the situation perceptibly. At the meeting itself, augmented in its second portion by men who had no doctrinaire commitments, politeness prevailed. The spokesmen for the four groups gave expression to their loyalty oaths, with elaborations, explanations, "defense mechanisms," and ever so subtle bows in the direction of the infidels. Tepid handshakes took the place of distant nodding acquaintances. The summary stated: "It was manifest that on a theoretical level there was much tolerance (*sic!*) on all sides, but that differences developed rapidly in concrete situations. The transactions clearly reveal the basis of difficulties of mutual understanding and of planning a combined research project by the four approaches." One of the participants put it a little differently: "When we act in our role as scientists, we begin to see one another's problems; when we act the role of teachers of our pet theories, we tend to become more welded to our respective doctrines."

After this memorable meeting, which constitutes a milestone in the history of psychiatry, the participants went home and, apparently unimpressed by what had happened, took up where they had left off. They had brought with them their neatly tied packages, had done their best to market their ware and, finding no takers in the other three groups, lugged them to their respective lairs.

Since then, however, there have been signs of a greater desire of an approximation between the sundry sets of approachers. The heated battles for hegemony have simmered down to less passionate skirmishes. In fact, one occasionally catches followers of the various "schools" somnambulating in each other's camps.

*　　*
*

These reminiscences and reflections appear to be particularly appropriate at the conclusion of the first (1971) volume of the *Journal of Autism and Childhood Schizophrenia*. This journal was inaugurated with the determination to serve as a vehicle for those studies and observations which would lead to a better understanding and to more effective means of prevention and treatment of the childhood psychoses. It set out to invite and encourage the reporting, coordination, and eventual integration of data obtained from factual investigation of the problems which knock at our door, which *approach us*, instead of entering the arena equipped *a priori* with somebody's ready-made approaches for the readers' comparison or contrast, approval or disapproval. We have managed to steer clear of the kind of frustrations which resulted from the talkfest arranged by the New York Academy of Medicine.

We were, as the record shows, amply rewarded by receiving worthwhile contributions centered around the children, not around the claims, promises, sophisms, or pugilistically rolled-up sleeves of approachers. These efforts came from scientists representing, in accordance with the plans announced in the first issue of the journal (Brown, 1971), many areas of patient-centered, rather than approach-centered, curiosity. They were concerned with refinement of diagnostic criteria, epidemiology, phenomenology, neurology, biochemistry, ethological correlates, results of ameliorative endeavors (educational, psychotherapeutic, psychopharmacological, behavioristic) and follow-up studies. Abstracts of pertinent work published recently (1970-1971) in other-language periodicals (thus far—Russian, Japanese, and German) have been arranged to give the readers familiarity with important research not easily accessible to them in the original.

Under these circumstances, there is no room for doctrinal strife, for a contest of opinions. There is no call for the oratorical cleverness spent on proving or questioning the supremacy of a specific "approach." Nobody can argue about established, carefully documented facts presented so that, if there is any doubt, an experiment can be duplicated and an observation can be checked by anybody with a healthy Missourian "I-want-to-be-shown" attitude. The immediately following pages, which tabulate the contents of this journal's first volume, are an indication of the caliber of the contributions to come. The editor wishes to thank the authors for the high standards attained by the journal from its incipiency. Their work paves the way for the accumulation of pertinent, scientifically unchallenged knowledge.

REFERENCES

Berman, L. *The glands regulating personality*. New York: Macmillan, 1921.

Brown, B. S. A task force with a goal. *Journal of Autism and Childhood Schizophrenia*, 1971, **1**, 1-13.

Cobb, I. B. *The glands of destiny*. London: Heinemann, 1927.

Cotton, H. A. *The defective, delinquent, and insane: The relation of focal infection to their causation, treatment and prevention*. Princeton: University Press, 1921.

Key, E. *The century of the child*. (English rev.) New York: Putnam, 1909.

Krasusky, W. S. Kretschmer's konstitutionelle typen unter den kindern im schulalter. *Archiv für Kinderheilkunde*, 1927, **82**, 22-32.

Kruse, H. D. (Ed.) *Integrating the approaches to mental disease*. New York: Hoeber-Harper, 1957.

16

LINWOOD CHILDREN'S CENTER: EVALUATIONS AND FOLLOW-UP OF 34 PSYCHOTIC CHILDREN

The observations sketched in this report were made in conjunction with a research grant from the U.S. Department of Health, Education and Welfare to Dr. Charles B. Ferster, at present Professor and Chairman of the Department of Psychology at the American University of Washington, D.C. At Dr. Ferster's invitation, I accepted an assignment to evaluate the patients treated at the Linwood Children's Center in Ellicott City, Md. This was done in two series of all-day visits, one extending from September to December 1966 and the other from April to June 1968, with two intervening visits in October 1967.

The Linwood Children's Center was inaugurated in 1955 under the leadership of Miss Jeanne Simons, who has since organized, directed, supervised, and personally participated in its activities. I proudly take some credit for encouraging this dedicated woman to utilize her unusual abilities for the benefit of psychotic and near-psychotic children. Undaunted by the din of the markets with their loudly advertised "schools," "approaches," and "techniques," she has brought with her a combination of empathy, understanding, patience, and ever-expanding experience together with a uniquely integrated blend of realism and idealism.

In order to appreciate fully the status of the children presented in this report, it is necessary to give at least an outline of the therapeutic procedures which have been developed at Linwood. There is no more appropriate way of doing this than to quote a summary prepared by Miss Simons in collaboration with Dr. Kathryn Schultz, her consulting psychiatrist:

> The main considerations in our treatment procedures would seem to be as follows:
>
> (1) The child comes in with a fresh start. Staff members who deal directly with such a child have not read the records, know nothing of his background, and are in a position to perceive him and respond to the youngster on the basis of their immediate and personal experience. They are encouraged to look for and build on the rudiments of health which may be apparent in even the sickest boy or girl. Each child is dealt with from the beginning on the basis of his unique characteristics. It is felt that this will be an essential element in his developing later a self of which he is aware—someone with his own name, likes, aversions, privileges, limitations, and his own bodily and emotional feelings.
>
> (2) Staff members are prepared, through experience and training, to deal in some practical way with the compulsions and need for sameness that make it so difficult to live with most autistic and other psychotic children. Briefly, these include limiting the area of compulsive activity, ignoring the compulsion (in which case it may subside if the child develops other interests), broadening the compulsive activity into related more constructive pursuits, and using it as a reinforcer for an unrelated constructive activity. None of these measures depend on understanding the meaning which the compulsion has for the child, though presumably it has some. Cutting through a compulsion, which has finally become a weapon to exert control over people (rather than a self-protective device for maintaining an unchanging environment) constitutes a skilled therapeutic maneuver to be undertaken only *after* the given compulsion is used as a weapon.
>
> (3) Self-aggression, like compulsiveness, is a rather frequent problem which may require special handling during the initial as well as the subsequent stages of care.
>
> (4) Verbalizations, and the choice of experiences to which the child is exposed, are geared to the children's characteristically concrete way of thinking, especially in the case of autistic children.

(5) The child's treatment is generally individualized within the group, rather than viewed as taking place in individual sessions away from the group. Individual therapy, however, is indicated in some cases.

(6) There is a highly flexible use of periods of residence incorporated into the day treatment program in which all children start. Residence, however, is not prescribed for all children. It is rather indicated for the working through of special problems and as a component of the experience of the child who becomes ready to attend public school in the community.

(7) Communicative speech is viewed as a behavior that develops within the context of relationships with people. It is therefore not the object of special therapeutic endeavors until the child has developed a firm enough capacity for relatedness and an ability not to withdraw under the pressures and frustration created when speech is required of him.

(8) Once a basic capacity to relate to human beings has begun to develop, and more complex aspects of personality to emerge, the program is adjusted to meet a variety of individual needs. There is a pre-school and academic educational program, and provision for participation in the ordinary experiences of a school-aged child. At such more advanced stages, therapeutic help continues to be needed due to the limitations imposed by the child's concrete way of thinking and also lack of social experience.

This statement is an indispensable prolegomenon to the case reports, because all of the 34 children, when seen for the evaluation, had been treated at Linwood for varying lengths of time. The outlined procedure had thus been a significant part of their "biographic" background. At the same time, it was highly instructive to learn about the influence of the Linwood experience on each child since their arrival there. This was especially noteworthy with regard to the 22 children (17 boys and 5 girls) who were revisited after the lapse of about 18 months, though the impact of the experience also showed itself unmistakably in the other 12 patients (11 boys and 1 girl) who were seen only once for the purpose of our evaluation.

The arrangement was such that each child was at first discussed with all members of the staff who had any contact with him. The case history was gone over in every available detail, including the child's pre-Linwood existence, the family's situation and emotional constellation, the physical status (prenatal, paranatal, and postnatal), and the observations made at Linwood. Then the child himself was led into the conference room after an appropriate preparation and the examiner was introduced to him by Miss Simons. Wherever possible, the parents were interviewed in a manner which helped us to learn more from them about each child, and helped them to gain as much clarification as we could possibly offer. That which followed will become evident in every individual case.

Miss Simons has subsequently completed a follow-up investigation which together with her concluding note is incorporated in this report. In collaboration with Dr. Schultz, she has arranged for a presentation whereby the children are grouped into five diagnostic categories. Reflecting the frequently apparent perplexities of nosological nomenclature, the grouping was nevertheless deemed appropriate for an effort intended, in part, to add to our knowledge of diagnostic differentiation of psychotic disturbances in childhood.

EARLY INFANTILE AUTISM

Case 1

September, 1966. I saw Mark about a year ago when the parents applied for the child's admission to the Children's Guild. At that time, the boy had no difficulty separating from his parents. He immediately occupied himself with some toys, which he handled without any particularly evident purpose. There was no verbal response to my remarks or questions, and no eye contact. He seemed neither to accept nor reject me. Though he did not seem to object to my presence, so long as I did not interfere, Mark shrank from physical contact of any kind. He was as ready to leave the office as he had been to enter it. Pinprick reaction was typical.

In my interview with the parents (and it was really *my* interview) both waited for spontaneity or initiative to come from me. The mother did most of the talking, always in response to my questions. The father, who has a not too severe but noticeable speech difficulty, entered only sporadically and briefly into the conversation. When he did so it was when I addressed myself to him personally. I was impressed by the mother's vagueness in her responses and also by her inability to focus on me, on her husband or on anything else in the room. I felt that this child needed more than the Guild could offer at the time, and suggested the Linwood Children's Center. The parents accepted this, and it surprised me that neither of them asked for any specific information about Linwood.

When I saw Mark today, I could not help but feel that he has gained a great deal since I first saw him. There is still the typical pinprick reaction, and still a failure to communicate other than with my foot placed on top of an object in which he was interested. But, on the other hand, an occasional fleeting eye contact was in evidence. He tolerated or, to put it more strongly, seemed to accept my holding him on my lap for a few seconds and certainly seemed pleased when Miss Simons took him on her's. I understand that after some difficulty fecal control was established, and that Mark has some contact with other children. His fine motor coordination is adequate, while speech, even though not directly communicative, is mostly limited to preoccupations with letters and numbers. The boy was able to identify pictures and look for initial letters corresponding to names of items in such pictures. He seems to be able to accept gaps. In the letters of the first test series, "7" was somehow missing; I know some autistic children who would become panicky and not be satisfied until the letter was restored. But Mark just left a gap between "6" and "8" and went on failing to show any particular enthusiasm when the "7" was finally found.

When invited to shake hands with the people present, he conformed in a rather mechanical manner. Mark went up to the person, waited until a hand was held out to him, and then used either his right hand or his left. In this, as well as all of his other activities, definite handedness had not as yet been established.

While not uncomfortable in the presence of people, the boy walked between them without paying attention to anyone. I guess that our behavior did not suggest the threatening possibility of unwelcome interference. On one occasion, however, Mark came up to me and said repeatedly, with quite a bit of pleasure, "Thank you, thank you very much."

Diagnostically, I should not hesitate to speak of this youngster as an autistic child with some emergence from aloneness, a reduction in compulsive behavior and also in desire for the preservation of sameness. Thus far, it has been easier to reach the child than to reach his mother, and the father is still a puzzle with respect to his role in the child's life. Regretfully, I did not understand what Mark said when I asked him about his sisters and the whereabouts of his daddy and mommy. He did say something, which did not sound to me or to any other person in the room like an answer to my question. This is a child who will need protracted help from the Linwood Children's Center. With it, I think that his prognosis is better now than a year ago.

April, 1968. Mark, who is now 6 years and 8 months of age, has made tremendous progress since September, 1966. He is one of those autistic children who can associate themselves with reasonable comfort and demonstrate some eagerness for mechanical reading and number work. The boy has acquired a sufficient capacity for reading which might be at a level of high 1st or low 2nd grade. But while he does very well mechanically, he is not quite able to integrate this sufficiently to talk about what happens, answer questions, and consistently or even inconsistently correlate the concept with the happening reported in his reading matter.

As he came in, he did well at first in answering questions and performing on the blackboard. Very soon, however, it became obvious that such conformity was too much for Mark and be became quite noisy and slightly rambunctious. Some behavioral inconsistencies are in evidence. The boy did remember the pinprick I gave him in 1966. He came in reluctantly to get his new pinprick, and then said "*I* hurt myself," apparently identifying himself rather than me with the pain. Later on he refused to come close to the pin, though from a distance, he good-naturedly waved goodbye. While leaving, he was quite ambivalent, at first expressing a wish to stay and immediately thereafter a desire to depart. I am quite optimistic with regard to this child's progress. Contact with people is an area in which Mark has to advance quite a bit more, and he will do so in the course of time. It is fortunate that he has been here since an early age and that there is an opportunity to keep him at Linwood for several years. Prognostically, these are good signs.

January, 1973. Speech, which was not in evidence at the age of 3 years and 3 months when Mark came to Linwood, had developed rather rapidly within one year. Temper tantrums and frequent screaming, almost endless to those who had to endure, have subsided after 2 years. Discharge from Linwood in September, 1972 was possible after the boy had already adjusted himself to public school. This 10½-year-old child speaks fluently and shows very few signs of his psychotic behavior in childhood. Good at a variety of competitive sports, a diligent boy scout and excellent student, he has a number of friends of his own age.

Case 2

September, 1966. I had an opportunity to see Gary in 1964 while attending the Children's Guild for a period of time. When he entered the Guild it was not an exaggeration to say that outwardly Gary seemed to be merely vegetating. At that time he would tolerate no physical contact with people. There was no eye contact and the child was impervious to any kind of verbal approach. A nurse from the University of Maryland, who spent some time at the Guild, took on Gary as her special assignment. It took some time before she could win him over to the extent of letting her carry him around, even though, at times, he would slip out and run to the corner of the play yard trying to hide in the hedge. On such occasions Gary stood stock still and it was obvious that he sought comfort in his complete isolation. Awareness of other children went only so far as staying away from them. The nurse was able at least to give him the feeling of wanting to be with her, and at times he would adjust to her embrace in the manner of a few-months-old infant.

When I saw him today, he was both the same and a different Gary. The boy still ran out a few times, but this time his act was more of an invitation to be brought back than a mere escape to aloneness. There was "method in his madness." He still had a typical reaction to the pinprick; yet I felt that it was somehow not entirely depersonalized.

Gary has by now achieved definitely right-handed tendencies as well as adequate fecal control. He is still, with one or two brief one-word exceptions, not a speaking child though already a communicating child. Instead of being completely away from people, the boy invites and enjoys playful physical contact delighting in his own spontaneous physical romping.

From a diagnostic point of view, even though there is not too much of "a desire for the preservation of sameness," this child responds to the criteria of early infantile autism. He certainly has shown emergence from what I would not hesitate to call absolute isolation, and has reached a point when people are no longer as threatening as they must have been. The boy is even able to go through the motions of stroking cheeks with what seems to be an attitude not devoid of fondness. Since he is now showing a capability for sound imitation, I wonder whether this could not be used playfully for the introduction and repetition of syllables with varying consonants. In his motor development, Gary has taken an interest in cutting and scribbling. This, as well as general behavior, indicates good coordination, at least in the finer motor activities.

If one was to sort out the diagnostic categories at Linwood to come up with a nosological label, I would not hesitate to consider this child among the group of autistic children.

June, 1967. Gary's discharge from Linwood in June, 1967 at the age of 6 years and 2 months was prompted by his family's move to Pennsylvania. A day-care center for severely disturbed children which he began to attend did not provide us sufficient information to judge the child's progress.

Case 3

September, 1966. This child, who has been at the Linwood Children's Center for more than 18 months, has shed a great bit of his destructive behavior and joined in the erect posture of the species. While this marks a change from his previous existence, Frank still presents a picture of extreme aloneness with so much self-capsulation that, when absorbed, he is impervious to sound and sight that is not within the range of his absorption.

This morning was very remarkable in that I had an opportunity to see three youngsters who may be termed autistic. And yet, there is such a remarkable heterogeneity of the total picture that they impress one as children who are very different from each other. Frank, at least as he appeared today, offered an impression of the extreme. Within the period of undisturbed observation at Linwood and thereafter, he has reached a point of dispensing with his destructiveness and porcupine contortions. On his good days, the boy was able to establish some peripheral contact with children and follow one person around when in need of something.

It is my understanding that the parents, who are cooperative and (one should pardon my use of the cliche) well-motivated, have a sense of some progress in the child. We certainly cannot present a Pollyannish prediction, but at the same time it would be inhuman to play Cassandra toward them, and perhaps even toward ourselves. From a purely realistic standpoint, we are far from being entitled to shout "hosanna" when confronted with a child who, at 6-years of age, is so maximally away from the world in which he lives. But, even though knowing this as an empirical reality, we cannot allow ourselves to capitulate even if it were only for the sake of our peace of mind.

Since this child has responded so little in his ability to be reached, I wonder if it might be worthwhile to see what more intensive operant conditioning may achieve. This method of modifying behavior may possibly have something to offer that less mechanized therapy cannot do at the present time.

January, 1970. Upon discharge from Linwood in November 1968, Frank was reportedly making some progress at a special school for severely disturbed children in Virginia. After being exposed for about one year to operant conditioning, the principal focus of treatment in that setting, he left the area together with his family. His parents were reportedly pleased with the residential treatment center which provided the type of care that this child might require for quite some time.

Case 4

October, 1966. Having known Brad, now almost exactly 8 years old, since he was not quite 3 years of age, I see at this time a remarkable change in his behavior even though some basic features are still in evidence. During the course of the first 4 years of our acquaintance, the child had no contact with people and definitely no eye contact. In my office, he would run around without giving any kind of positive or negative cognizance of my presence, would immediately go after objects, open and close doors, not respond to any form of verbal communication and shrink from physical contact. Brad would spot a round ashtray and spin it with considerable skill.

When led in by Miss Simons today, he sat down in the chair opposite me across the table and, at first, spent quite some time looking intently at me. Even when trying to fit forms into the formboard or cylinders into the cylinder board, the boy still took time out either to look at me or to look into space, returning to his task at Miss Simons' gentle invitation. He used both hands indiscriminately, guided mostly by the proximity of the object to either hand. When the formboards were removed, I started playing with him in a manner that one would with a 2- or 3-year-old child. He responded to this promptly and with pleasure. Even in the formboard situation, Brad on one occasion seemed pleased with the performance to the point of saying "That's good." After some persuasion, more so on the part of Miss Simons, he played with me using one of the educational toys (a ring tower) and got the idea of taking turns. When I was remiss, he would guide my hand to the ring when it was my turn to play. On request, Brad picked up one of the rings that fell down on the floor. We continued playing putting our foreheads together, establishing contact which the child enjoyed very much, at times opening his eyes widely and expecting me to do likewise (which I did). He often held my hand, at times gently, and sometimes squeezing it with delight. A few times, he did wave some of the toys very closely to my face but never to the point of touching or hitting me. There was a mutuality in the relationship and it seemed as though he did some "operant conditioning" of his playmate, involving me as his "subject."

I understand that toilet training has been accomplished by this time with some infrequent and erratic "accidents." Brad still has some obsessive food habits but there has been a mild improvement; joining the other children in food intake is one of the few signs of entering into group activity. He has on occasions used one other child to satisfy his compulsive needs. Mrs. Nash's examination shows Brad to be a child whose performance would not transcend the level of a 2-year old. However, his handling of the formboard goes somewhat beyond that level. If one had not followed his development, it would be possible to conclude that we deal with a severely retarded child. But early history of complete self-isolation and compulsive behavior indicates that he shows signs of a slow emergence from both. There is no cause for being sangfroid. Further progress may be very slow and reach a level that would not quite prepare him for social living. Nevertheless, there has been some emergence and the child's behavior gives one the impression that he has stored up verbal and other means of communication, which are beginning to come to the fore. I was particularly impressed by the way in which Brad rewarded me for playing with him with "speech," which was essentially a pleasant and pleasing utterance of "badabadabada." I may add that on one occasion while working with the formboards, he hummed some tunes, and on another spontaneously started a song, in which a bit of "Old McDonald Had a Farm" could be recognized.

On the basis of the history and today's performance, I would not hesitate to consider Brad as an autistic child with some degree of at least partial emergence.

April, 1968. Brad, now 9½ years of age, would, if we depended entirely on psychometric measurement, not go beyond the 4-year level. Since the last evaluation (more than about a year and half ago) he has been doing quite a bit of echolalia and also indulged in very limited spontaneous speech, some of it in terms of gibberish. The main impression is that the boy has very little awareness of himself in relation to the world of people. He has tried, in an infantile teasing way, to acquire some concept of people that is only partially realistic. I should say, that while this child has shown additional signs of partial emergence, he is still basically very psychotic. Thus, the prognostic assessment formulated in 1966 still stands. I think now that no thought of living on his own can be entertained and this child will need a sheltered environment in the future. Meanwhile, I do not think that anything better can be done for him than continued residence at Linwood. We may hope for somewhat better formal relationships with people and also affective relationships which would, nevertheless, prove very difficult for him to develop.

January, 1973. Brad managed to develop communicative speech which he used spontaneously. Reasonably good relatedness was in evidence at the time when he left Linwood in July, 1972. Also, food habits were nearly normal. This child, initially extremely self-destructive, could not be reached at a level where some learning could be projected beyond random recognition of letters, numbers, colors, pictures or words. He lives at home and arrangements are being made for limited training at a day-care center.

Case 5

October, 1966. This child's arrival was preceded by a report from Georgetown University, very helpful in providing unusually good and detailed background information. I was further helped by Dr. Schultz who, having seen Kent with Miss Simons, was able to make very pertinent observations.

I saw the boy's parents again. Even though they sat facing me, next to each other, their closeness was merely geographic. The father was a bit more spontaneous and direct in answering questions. The mother seemed to weigh each question first before deciding on an answer. Some of such answers were either contradictory or modified a bit to suit the purpose. She tried to intellectualize but went about it not too intelligently on several occasions. Both parents described themselves as not too sociable. They are "friendly" with neighbors but there is very little real contact with them. They have, as Kent's father says, "acquaintances" but no friends. The mother reported feelings that there was something unusual about her child from the first week of life. His way of crying and persistent frequency of such crying prompted her to wonder.

I gave them an opportunity to be spontaneous by asking whether there was anything that they wished to tell me about matters not covered by the questions. Nothing of significance was forthcoming; I had to make it easy by asking another question. Not spontaneously but in answer to that question, they observed that Kent spanks himself on the bottom. The mother added that this was an imitation of what was done to him, making sure that it meant that the child is never punished severely. Between them, there was quite a bit of fast talking until one or the other changed or modified something stated by the partner. They said that both could be affectionate with the child but there was not much compensation, though the father gave an impression of somewhat greater warmth, mostly in terms of providing material needs and some physical contact. Both parents felt they would like to enroll their child at Linwood and faintly expressed a wish of wanting to know what was done here.

The child allowed himself to become engaged in play while waiting for the interview. When he came in, Kent showed no interest in contact with people and yet seemed a bit more aware of persons and what they did than some of the children I have seen here. While, as the mother said correctly, Kent "lives in a world of his own," he does so leaving the world not entirely outside of the range of his awareness. There is some eye contact, more as a matter of curiosity than of relationship. When given one of the eductional toys, he handled it fairly adequately but became easily frustrated when parts of it could not be maneuvered as he wanted. However, when our back was turned, Kent rearranged the whole thing. He was adept with cylinder blocks and I am not sure that he even got the concept. The boy allowed me to pick him up and started climbing up on me, and a while later also on Miss Simons. Physical contact did not seem obnoxious to him. He reacted to the pinprick in a manner which included me as a person rather than dealing with a depersonalized hand.

This child though autistically remote, shows signs of readiness to accept approaches from others; he wanders on occasions but allows you to resume negotiations. I anticipate noticeable growth at Linwood.

June, 1968. If one were to see Kent for the first time without the benefit of knowing his background, one could be easily misled into believing that this is basically a very retarded child who at the age of 6½ years is still not speaking. He appears to enjoy very infantile play. On the basis of my observations in 1966 and also impression of present condition, I would be inclined to feel that there has been a great deal of progress. A change of environment yielded a remarkable change in the child himself, who is emerging from a state of passivity to one of making approaches to people. Entirely different than in 1966, he has now the courage to tease and to find himself in a relationship with people. There is a great deal of babbling, repeating sounds, and putting some words into sounds that are connected with a tune. I understand that Kent has also begun to use some real words which he pronounces intelligibly. I think that the shift of his status from commuter to resident which served to limit exposure to two entirely different patterns of relationships proved to be most beneficial. I would say that this child's newly-gained naughtiness is a sign of great progress, and hope that he will have an opportunity to remain here for a good long while. I can foresee no miracles, but look forward to considerable advances.

January, 1973. Accidental death of the boy's mother necessitated a sudden departure from Linwood in early 1970 after a stay of more than 3 years. Although much better relatedness, reasonable self-care, and some verbal communication were in evidence at discharge, Kent's progress since the 1968 evaluation was rather disappointing. Our prognosis in this case was not really favorable, chiefly due to the increasingly unsuccessful attempts to advance his very meager intellectual development.

Case 6

October, 1966. Tammy is a well nourished, round-faced, dark-haired little girl who will be 8 years old in two months. When she entered the room, accompanied by Miss Simons, she took fleeting notice of the people, fleetingly acknowledged introductions, and disregarded my invitation to shake hands. At Miss Simons's invitation, Tammy sat down in a chair near the table, facing me, though she looked at me only when specifically asked to do so by Miss Simons. Then the eye contact was brief.

The child seems to be in good physical shape. She used the right hand most of the time, especially in drawing and handling the toys, even though she also occasionally used the left hand, especially so when shaking hands at the time of departing. Her coordination seems adequate.

Tammy showed spontaneity only when asking for objects that she wanted. On such occasions, the sentence formation was proper, the pronouns were used adequately and there was natural intonation. Things were quite different when questions were asked of her. There was quite a bit of echolalia if she chose to respond to the question at all.

When given a sheet for drawing, Tammy first produced a complete figure which had in it all of the things that usually go into the drawing of a human. There were eyes with glasses and a nose, a mouth, and a short trunk with arms and legs with attention to hands and feet. But at the lower end of the abdomen, the girl produced another figure which she called "rabbit." Ears were the only missing components. When asked what all of that was meant to be, she said "double" and proceeded to write some letters, starting with a small "b" (which she called "d") and inserting another not identifiable letter next to it. Then, at the other corner of the paper, she wrote a capital "J" with a double outline. It is possible that "double" may have indicated a combining of the human and rabbit figures, but I am not sure that this properly interprets what she meant by saying "double." At Miss Simons request, Tammy drew and colored a girl again, a well organized drawing. That girl had much hair on both temples and on both sides of the forehead. There were buttons on the dress and generally quite a bit of detail such as a large hat around the head down to the neck. She then drew a boy, producing a drawing quite different from that of the girl. Again, the ears were missing. The hair was appropriate for a boy's hairdo. But while her girl's hat and clothes were yellow, the boy's suit was black. Tammy then spontaneously drew another picture of a girl who was crying with tears coming down from both eyes. This being Halloween, she gave the new girl a pointed head. When asked why the girl was crying, she said something about going out in the street and then, when asked again, a word or two that sounded like "don't throw." One of the figures she identified as "Tom." There is no Tom at the Linwood Children's Center but she has a brother so named.

I asked Tammy if she had any brothers. There was no response but a bit of a mischievous smile. When I asked how many brothers she had, the child said "many." There was again no response when she was asked about sisters, where she lived, where her daddy lived and where her mother was. When Miss Simons asked who would call for her in the afternoon, there was no response and a pause followed by quite a bit of echolalia.

Tammy's school book shows that she had learned to write nicely. She copied adequately, except that at one time, one "2" was reversed in a row of several 2's. On one sheet she wrote October entirely backwards, beginning at the right upper corner of the page. All during this time Tammy was sitting in her chair, getting up only once or twice to point to the toys for which she asked.

An airtight diagnostic formulation is not easy. The girl's behavior certainly does not present the picture of the so-called brain-damaged or typically hebephrenic child. The pinprick reaction may be considered somewhat equivocal, though she did not respond to me in any pleading or angry fashion, saying however, "it's hot," thus acknowledging the experience. Tammy does not exhibit the general physical appearance of the typically autistic child. The difference between her spontaneous remarks, properly addressed to Miss Simons when she asked for toys, and her answers to questions is most remarkable.

It is reported that this child had manifested a bit of compulsive behavior at home, insisting on flushing the toilet after any member of the family has used it, and throwing temper tantrums when this was not allowed. There are other reports of similar compulsiveness. It is difficult to say what role her behavior may have played when she initiated some sex play with other children. Is this another stage in her compulsiveness? I do not think that we would be too far afield if in view of the compulsiveness, of her good contact with objects and poor, though graduated, relationship with people, the echolalia or lack of responsiveness (whenever questions are asked that come too close to matters pertaining to her family) to think of this child as autistic. We must keep in mind, however, her well organized reproduction of people in drawings and the remarkable difference between spontaneous communication and response to other people's requests.

On the whole, this child has certainly shown considerable improvement. Her latest IQ was shown to be 79, and the drawings disclose a capacity which is not below the girl's age level. She has "learned to learn" as her notebook shows. What the strephosymbolia will mean in terms of reading readiness remains to be seen.

April, 1968. Tammy has gained a great deal in ideational aspects. Physically, she has maintained her good nutritional status and appearance of well being. The girl has responded sufficiently to learn to read and write. She reads at the pre-primer level which is quite behind her general age expectations, but is beginning to show more interest, at least in reading material which she can manage. Tammy responded to the pinprick, this time with definite recognition of the culprit and ability to tell me off, in no uncertain terms. From the viewpoint of professional diagnosis I would say that we might see her as a child who is emerging from a more definite autistic condition. This child has reached a point where some more emergence can be expected, gaining so much at Linwood that one would recommend continuation in this setting for quite some time.

May, 1970. Tammy's capacity to conceptualize, which became more apparent during the last 2 years of her stay at Linwood, tends to suggest some reservations with respect to the diagnosis of autism. At the age of 12½, she left us for California to enter a day-care center focused on special education.

Case 7

November, 1966. David, 7½ years of age, has been at the Linwood Children's Center since October 1964. Referred by the Walter Reed Hospital, the boy has presented problems from the beginning of life. He was born after a pregnancy in which the mother was suffering from hypertension and labor was protracted. However, his weight was adequate and motor development presented no particular difficulties. It was reported that David shunned physical contact. As early as in the child's first year of life his father noticed that he did not like being picked up. There was some speech development, not specified in any prior reports though mention was made of limited speech. After some time, he used less speech until it stopped altogether for a period. There is no way of connecting this reduction of speech chronologically with the aseptic meningitis, which David had at the age of 3 years and 11 months. Prior to this illness, he was described as a loner, not an affectionate child and also a rocker and head banger. When seen at the Arlington Health Clinic at 4 years and 9 months of age, he tested 79 at a non-verbal IQ creating the impression of organic difficulty with possible autism. When the boy came to Linwood, he screamed compulsively and was, for all practical purposes, mute.

David is the older of two children; his sister is approximately 2 years younger. There have been no complaints about her development. The father has been hospitalized for ulcer and arthritis and is also said to have had a mental breakdown. At the time of this child's enrollment at Linwood, he expressed some guilt about beating his son. The mother has been described as "helpless, angry, frustrated, anxious." David has never been in residence here, and there was quite a bit of anxiety on at least two occasions when his continuation at Linwood was threatened by financial contingencies.

David was seen by Mrs. Nash, the psychologist, about 5 or 6 months ago. She felt that this was a bad day for him; he had temper tantrums and seemed to have tested at an approximately 4½-year level. It is quite possible that the boy performed not as well there because of the unaccustomed surroundings.

This morning when he was brought for the interview, David automatically shook hands when requested to do so; the first had the quality of a "dead fish handshake" (later handshakes had less of such quality). On request, he sat in the chair and remained there throughout the performance, except that from time to time he would get up and wander, leaving the room and returning when asked to come back. By now, David uses language with occasional echolalia. He brought his schoolwork, decidedly above the 4½-year level. There was evidence of quite a bit of organization and discrimination in that he could point correctly to numbers. David wrote his first name and proceeded to read the words on his work sheet; this was accompanied by rhythmic movements of body and arms. The boy read in a quiet voice which he would not raise when asked to do so. The pinprick reaction was somewhat equivocal though David returned promptly when I called him back. He did look at me when I pricked him and later on said, "No, no." Before he left the child said very distinctly, "I want to go downstairs."

I do not believe that the meningitis as such has had a decisive part in the etiology of this child's problem, which existed long before the illness. A certain degree of compulsiveness is reported; he would not leave the bus until a staff member in the group said "Goodbye." I understand that the child's capacity for learning has developed during the past few months. His performance is definitely on the first-grade learning level so that the low IQ can be discounted as a permanent indication of his endowment. In view of the inability to relate to people, compulsiveness, and better ability to relate to formboards and the usual educational toys, I would not hesitate to view David as an autistic child.

April, 1968. David presented himself today, about a year and a half after the first evaluation. It is obvious that in his contact with people there is very little, if any, show of affection in the relationships. At one time, he seemed to become angry at Miss Simons when a specific question was asked about his father who is now in Viet Nam. David seemed to have some contact with his father and it is said that he wrote an unexpectedly long letter to Viet Nam in which he reported some items of the household routine. However, no special feelings were expressed in that letter. The boy has made progress in learning and read a passage from his reader. As he read it, one became aware that this was not meant for anybody's hearing or participation of any kind. Also, there were quite a few peculiar movements with his hands during the course of the reading, almost like a ritual connected with such reading. The pinprick reaction was more typically autistic today than it was a year and half ago.

I do not think that there is any question about the diagnostic formulation. This is a typically autistic child in the sense of self-isolation, ritualism, and more interest in mechanical performance than in any affective meaning. The report from school about aggressiveness may be interpreted positively at the present time. It was apparently a response to attempts to stimulate some contact with children rather than a matter of particular hostility or animosity toward other children. On the whole, I should say that this (to me at least) unquestionably autistic child has improved and should remain in the Linwood setting. I anticipate further progress in the mechanics of reading, number concept acquisition and writing, with a slow and gradual attempt, to be brought a little closer into the world and feelings of people.

January, 1973. In 1964, this child did not use communicative speech, spending his time away from other children, rocking and twirling and also avoiding eye contact. Attempts to reach him were so unsuccessful that the initial suspicion of deafness was almost difficult to refute. Gradual progress, accelerated by transfer to a more advanced group in 1969, prepared the boy for the 4th grade of public school which he now attends while spending four nights in residence at Linwood. It is noteworthy that David managed to verbalize his wish to participate in the program of our advanced group and also readiness to go to school. He keeps up with his schoolwork, plays a musical instrument, participates in competitive sport games and develops plausible social contacts with his peers.

Case 8

November, 1966. I have known Drew when he was at the Children's Guild at the age of approximately 3½ years. He was then a markedly withdrawn child who had extremely little contact with the teachers and other children. In the course of his attendance there, the boy began to make slight and fleeting overtures toward one of the teachers. There was hardly any speech except for limited echolalia.

Drew came to the Linwood Children's Center in January, 1964. The boy is now 7 years and 5 months old, a rather small child for his age that can be described as physically attractive. He certainly does not have the dull expression of a child of his age who due to retardation tests as low as Drew does. When examined by Mrs. Nash, he did not exceed the age level of 3 years in any sphere.

When seen today, Drew upon entering took almost no notice of the people present and, at first, did not even immediately proceed, as many autistic children would, to examine some objects in the room. He responded to Miss Simons' invitation to draw. In order to secure some degree of responsiveness, Miss Simons made use of his preoccupation with vacuum cleaners, starting a primitive drawing of one. He got the concept but did not accept her invitation to add parts, finally agreeing to add a cord. Drew was asked to cut out the completed drawings. He used the scissors impatiently and, again while understanding the concept, cut through the drawing and eventually began to tear the paper. The boy did not spontaneously do any spinning, but did so with pleasure when, after a demonstration, he seized some round objects. While Drew has been ambidextrous for many years, he seems recently to have shown predominant left-handedness. He reacted to the pinprick in typically autistic fashion, relating himself only to the pin, rubbing the place which had been stuck, but not referring the act or injury to the person who pricked him.

There was quite a bit of speech, some of it clearly pronounced, and some so slurred that one could not understand it. Drew is capable of forming sentences and his understandable speech had quite a bit of self-admonition. When he got on a bed he said "off bed." At one time, the boy asked for lunch, and, when told that this was not lunch time, said, "make it . . . make it." He spontaneously said "not going home." During the process he ran around the room without any particular aim though some of these excursions took him to the door. Mere calling of Drew by name did not bring him back, though some activity had to be connected with this for he sometimes responded and at times did not.

In simple jigsaw puzzles, Drew placed things properly. In one involving parts of a man that have to be put together, he was definitely guided by space rather than content. He tried several times to find a space for the man's face in different parts of the puzzle, locating the proper opening only after all other pieces were in place and the face seemed to fit the remaining space.

Prognostically, one is entitled to considerable skepticism, especially since Mrs. Nash found no area in which Drew's responses went beyond the middle of the third year. This, however, is somewhat deceptive as it is very difficult to get the boy to respond to the demands and instructions necessary for the test. He performs somewhat better, but not very much, in his spontaneous activities.

When the child was about to leave, Miss Simons said to him "Say goodbye Dr. Kanner." He said "Say bye Dr. Kanner." That incident is reminiscent of the difficulties which autistic children have in separating parts from the whole. This, as well as the boy's compulsiveness, the difference in his relationship with objects from that with people, typical pinprick reaction, and self-admonitions distinguish him sufficiently from inherently retarded children with such low IQ. I should think of Drew as a child with the syndrome of early infantile autism whose outlook for the future is not too promising. It is difficult to say to what extent the Rh incompatibility and early history of diarrhea with high fever are of any etiological significance, though one might certainly think of psychological factors that may have played a part in view of the personality of his parents.

December, 1967. Drew's discharge from Linwood in August 1967 was followed by severe illness in his family that appears to have impeded the child's mild progress observed during the course of his 8½-year association with Linwood. We were informed towards the end of 1967 that he was attending a day-care center for the mentally retarded.

Case 9

December, 1966. Dan, a boy who has been at Linwood for about 2½ years and celebrated his 12th birthday yesterday, was a very severely withdrawn youngster. He was, as Miss Simons expressed it, "invisible when he first arrived." Dan had been examined from time to time in various settings and, with one or two exceptions, was thought to be very severely retarded. One or two diagnosticians tended to describe the child in terms of early infantile autism. In the course of residence at Linwood, the boy emerged from his extreme aloneness. He has remained compulsive to the extent of remembering license plates of cars that come here often enough, the name of every person who accompanied me to the center, telephone numbers and birthdays. Dan has learned to read fluently and even acquired some knowledge of French. At the same time, his writing is "sloppy," largely because it does not seem to be meant for other people's perusal.

Dan is paying a price for his emergence. It seems to be so terrifying to him that the boy's responses to conversation comprise a manic-like type of behavior, more than possibly a defense against coming closer to people. Conversation, which includes to the point answers to some questions (even recognizing and explaining two of the Rinet 10th year absurdities) is accompanied by various excursions and mergers. He can report some of the happenings at Linwood, chronicling the events pertaining to some of the children as a matter-of-fact occurrence without any kind of emotional participation, sympathy or anger.

April, 1968. Dan, whom I saw in December 1966, has gained a great deal in terms of further acquisition of factual knowledge. He has developed curiosities in certain areas, and has done some reading and inquiring in order to add to his knowledge. At the same time, his behavior during the course of the evaluation session does not differ too much from that which he manifested during the first meeting. Dan becomes very much upset by the requirement for closer contact and communication, and still tends to become manic-like in general demeanor. A feeling that Dan would not differ from a person in an acute manic state would have been engendered by one who did not know Dan and saw him for the first time. It is possible, however, to find reasons for some doubts in this respect. The boy managed to verbalize quite a few things during the interview which seemed spontaneous, and referred to matters which had no possible meaning to anyone but himself. It was evident, however, at least on a few occasions, that he referred to very specific incidents which one can understand only if one can share his frame of reference or have some ideas of what the boy is speaking about. Obviously, while he has good sixth grade knowledge and probably better than that, one cannot think at the present time in terms of an attempt to have Dan attend regular public school like some of the other children residing at Linwood. This would be too much of a challenge to him and make his behavior in the classroom in a regular school impossible. Eventually, his present experience might slowly and gradually lead to such an arrangement, but it is still at least a year or two off. Miss Simons plans occasional visits to a class in which no demands are made of Dan.

January, 1973. At a point where the staff had serious doubts of reaching this child to facilitate further progress, Dan responded to a temporary measure to allow him to play alone with a favorite toy (transistor radio). When given an opportunity to detach himself from the group, the boy turned away from the transistor and proceeded to indulge in stereotypic rocking and twirling which he had not done for some time. This was correctly interpreted as a clue that Dan wished to emerge from his aloneness, which after some prodding he finally verbalized. From that point on, after a brief period of fierce temper tantrums, progress was rather spectacular. This autistic child, who at the age of 10 (when he came to Linwood) did not use his limited speech to communicate, refused to relate to anyone and spent most of his time scribbling unintelligibly, became a happy adolescent capable of verbalizing his feelings, and relating to most adults and some of his peers. Presently a successful student at a public high school, he earned A's and B's in the 9th grade. Dan's hobbies include ice skating, track, piano, participation in spelling contests, and a variety of other age-appropriate activities. Awareness of his incapacity in childhood and pride in overcoming the handicaps is about the major characteristic of this remarkably successfully recovered young man.

Case 10

December, 1966. There are few children at Linwood who have not at one time or another been "diagnosed" as autistic. This child's disorder was correctly recognized as autistic, first by a psychiatrist in California and then by Dr. George Frankl at Winston-Salem. Jackie's history as well as present performance are very much in keeping with the criteria described in my first publication on the subject of autistic disturbances of affective contact (Kanner, 1943). There is the aloneness and the compulsive desire for preservation of sameness. Jackie is able and has been able for quite some time, to read fluently. While at first such reading was more mechanical with little comprehension of semantics, he is now much more aware of the contents. In one of his papers, where he was to designate opposites to a number of words, he wrote "parents" as an opposite of "peace." His parents are now divorced and Jackie and his brother are with their mother. The father is described as detached from people, somewhat on the passive side.

Jackie disliked the interview situation, declaring that he would not do certain things asked of him by saying "No" and, when he left, declaring just as openly that he did not enjoy the experience. However, he immediately sat down to do an intricate jigsaw puzzle being guided by the shape of the pieces rather than content of the picture.

This child has made progress at the Linwood Center even though his relationship to people is still tenuous. One looks forward to the time when it may be possible to arrange for public school attendance while he is still at Linwood. Jackie will relate himself well to books and to matters of memory, the teachers serving mainly as opportunities for leading him to this kind of activity.

April, 1968. Jackie is now 11-years of age, a boy who has made considerable progress during the time of his stay at Linwood. Even though, his general scholastic achievement is at the 3rd grade level, I think that one might say that this child offers promise of further growth and development in terms of scholastic achievement. The one thing that impresses me most is his coming much closer to being reasonably comfortable with people since the time I saw him in 1966. At the time, there was no question about his wanting to stay away and declaring definitely that he would not do things, and would not progress. The boy now answers questions quite readily, again a bit uneasily when the conversation relates to members of his family. This extremely serious-minded child whom I saw about a year and 4 months ago, is now amenable to some degree of amusement and responds to humor much more than in the past. I have no cause to change the diagnostic formulation. How soon and to what extent he will emerge to become a full fledged member of a group, I cannot predict, but I certainly think that Jackie can make progress in learning and also in terms of approaching a greater sense of reality and contact with people.

January, 1973. When admitted to Linwood in April, 1964, Jackie presented a variety of autistic symptoms that included near-mutism (rare use of few words at a very high pitch level) and extremely compulsive behavior with no tolerance whatsoever for any disruption of ritualisms and stereotypies. There was no eye contact, lack of social smile, and no signs of relatedness. After 8 years and 4 months at Linwood, Jackie lives at home and attends a public high school. An intelligent 8th grade student, he is still unable to fully overcome some of his compulsions which he can nevertheless frequently interrupt, with a smile, when admonished to do so. Increasingly uninhibited relatedness and ability to meaningfully communicate with peers and adults alike tend to justify much optimism with respect to Jackie's future.

Case 11

December, 1966. This 9½-year old boy has been at the Linwood Children's Center since June, 1962. He presented problems from a very early age, so much so that the parents became concerned and consulted someone when Ken was in his third year of life. He was satisfied to stay in his playpen, fearful of leaving the house, afraid of drinking glasses and also of strangers. There was a very small number of words which he pronounced but which, according to the anamnesis, seemed to have no communicative connotation. In his fourth year of life, Ken's mother committed suicide by hanging in the basement. After this, he had a great fear of basements and, when first introduced to Linwood, was panicky about going into the Center's basement. The boy had certain peculiarities such as entering a room only on one side of the door. There is a history of long food capriciousness, and living through a period of holding back his feces. Improvement began approximately a year ago, when Ken developed good sphincter control and when it became possible to change his status from a resident to a day patient. This was due to the fact that his father remarried, and the stepmother, a warm person, knew how to handle him as well as the six other children from the father's previous marriage in addition to her own child.

Ken, when seen today, appeared to be in good physical condition. He is sturdily built and has a somewhat large cranium and rather high forehead. He has gained speech to the extent that there is considerable echolalia. His voice is high pitched; for want of a better term, I would say that it resembles somewhat the voice of "Donald Duck." Much is not intelligible, but his echolalic expressions are pronounced more clearly than naming of things. Obviously most of Ken's speech is not intended for communication. Echolalia assumes the inflections of the way the sentence has been presented to him. In between, he interjects frequently something that sounds like "da-da-da-de-da," again in a high-pitched tone. All the while, the boy seems reasonably comfortable in the situation. There is no evidence of the self-destruction, often such as choking himself and others, which existed at the time when he came here.

Ken does simple jigsaw puzzles adequately, and erected a tower at least 12 blocks in height before it collapsed. He put the blocks down, making sure that the upper side matched the rest. The boy allowed changes to be made in the order but then rearranged all blocks in the same manner, returning two that I deliberately handed to him with the wrong side up.

His pinprick reaction is definitely in relation to the pin rather than to me. When I stepped on a block which he wanted to retrieve, the boy struggled with my foot not seeming to connect me with the process.

The anamnesis and his behavior today make me feel that this is a typical autistic child who is just beginning to show signs of emergence. He has learned to sing "Jingle Bells" with a reasonably good reproduction of the tune, and to draw a Christmas tree. Ken even made a primitive attempt to draw a person, named some of the elementary colors, and responded to Miss Simons' correction of some not too well pronounced words. The child is now ready for more intensive instruction and I strongly recommend that he remain at the Linwood Children's Center. There has been definite progress since his arrival at the Center and more can be anticipated.

April, 1968. There was much progress in many respects since I saw Ken in December, 1966, even though basically, he remains as autistic as in the past. A great deal of echolalia is in evidence. Hardly have I ever seen an echolalic child who could use his echolalia in a way as efficiently as this child. It serves the purpose of keeping away from any involvement. This is also true of singing and true of doing the kind of formboard work reminiscent of cos blocks. In fact, I do think that it might be a good idea to have him practice on the cos blocks for he might come up very high in comparison with many other functions. Ken has acquired some need for contact with people. It was remarkable how he managed to again and again point spontaneously to one of the teachers, seeming to rejoice in being able to refer to her as "Marsha." When the boy sat down next to me, he did not shrink from physical contact except when singing a song. While he did that, I could hold his hand and it was a good contact; as soon as the song was over he immediately withdrew his hand. Ken thus almost noticeably uses his activities such as singing, working with blocks, or his echolalia as a means of keeping away from the need to establish more intimate contact. At the same time, he occasionally answers a question sparing no more than one or two words for such purpose. He was able to give his address and at one time spoke of Washington, D.C. It was not possible to get Ken to use the word "Washington" without the word "D.C.," another bit of echolalia. There is evidence that echolalia or similar activities "designed" to keep a distance from people made him feel more secure. While indulging in such activities, he tolerated my hand on his and seemed to feel comfortable. I understand that Ken will receive speech therapy in the near future. This is a good idea, not only because of his ability or inability to speak (I think he has a good basic ability) but also because of the additional opportunity to establish a relationship. As time goes on, mechanical repetition of words becomes less mechanical, stimulating more intimate contacts with one and possibly more of his teachers.

January, 1973. After more than 7 years at Linwood, Ken was transferred to a day-care center where operant conditioning techniques are being used to facilitate further progress. His physical strength coupled with some aggression became increasingly difficult to manage in a setting where most of the younger children are easily frightened by such behavior. This seemed to be less of a problem in Ken's new environment. Also, life at home was reported to be increasingly enjoyable so that institutional care is no longer under consideration.

Case 12

December, 1966. Sandy is the third of four children. The second and fourth are said to be healthy and reasonably well adjusted. Allen, the oldest brother, is also a resident at Linwood who will be seen later in the day.

Unfortunately, at this time we do not have a history of Sandy's early development and know nothing of the early milestones. This will be obtained from the parents because I think it essential for his evaluation. I understand that Sandy, after an initial period of day care, is now a Linwood resident. A thorough physical examination has not been performed or reported by any of the agencies that have been interested in this child. I would suggest that this be done, with special emphasis on neurological status and metabolic studies. A PKU test was found to be negative. Mrs. Nash found this 10-year-old boy's functioning to be at an age level of approximately 2½ years.

Within the last 2 or 3 months, Sandy has been accessible to some degree of learning. The boy has learned to spell simple words and became preoccupied with spelling. He counts up to 6 correctly and then uses numbers indiscriminately. In the course of an educational test comprising rings of different sizes, he placed the rings back to make a pyramid; when a mistake was made, he was able to rectify it. All the while he seemed cheerful, exhibiting a facial expression which would not indicate a severe functional retardation. Sandy occasionally answered a question directly, but had to be urged by Miss Simons to pay attention to what was said to him.

The boy's college educated parents are people with many peculiarities. They are interested in their children to the extent of maintaining a very orderly household which seems to run within a framework of meticulousness. The children are not called by their names but referred to as brother and sister.

It has taken the major part of 5 years before Sandy could be induced to the limited degree of learning that he is now capable to follow. An adequate diagnosis would depend on a better developmental history and the results of an intensive physical workup. We do know that, at least functionally, Sandy is very severely retarded and that there is a possibility of metabolic involvement.

Now that he has been sufficiently responsive to formal instruction it will be interesting to see what the next few months will come up with. Personally, I do not share the optimism expressed at the Linwood Children's Center.

April, 1968. One has the right to be greatly encouraged by the progress made by Sandy since his first evaluation in December, 1966. Within this year he has emerged sufficiently to be able to start first-grade learning while a year ago he was rated as having a developmental level of 2½ years. This does not necessarily mean a gain of approximately four years in one. It just means that the child is more receptive to teaching than he was at that time. I regret that it has not been possible to obtain the additional information that a thorough physical examination and a more detailed report about early developmental milestones might have provided. However, his general demeanor and typical pinprick reaction make it more probable, if not certain, that we can now include Sandy in the roster of our autistic children at Linwood. He seems to be more or less repeating the history of his older brother Allen who is doing rather well. I think it quite possible to anticipate a similar development in this child who is making great strides in comparison with his performance in 1966.

January, 1973. Sandy, a mute 5-year-old autistic child in March 1962 when he entered Linwood, has managed to develop relatively normal though not age-appropriate speech, cope with 4th grade arithmetic and read at the 5th grade level. Discharged at 15½ years of age to enter a public school class for the educable, he was no longer as difficult to manage as in the past when severe temper tantrums and self-destructive behavior were limiting his progress. Somewhat anxious, and still not ready to function in a competitive environment, Sandy is nevertheless able to verbalize his feelings and adjust to living at home. One might reasonably anticipate further growth, even though a period in a sheltered workshop is in sight.

Case 13

December, 1966. Allen, a 15-year-old boy, has been at the Linwood Children's Center for approximately 6½ years. He was very withdrawn at first and had very little communication. In the course of his stay, he has improved to the extent that makes it possible for him to attend the local junior high school.

The boy has a large repository of factual knowledge. At the mention of Vietnam, for instance, he was able to draw a map of North and South Vietnam, Laos and Cambodia. He knew the capitals of many states and could name the European countries through which the Danube River flows. Allen knew the dates of the Civil War and seemed comfortable in answering all those questions. He seemed really to enjoy the questions connected with the so-called absurdity test and promptly recognized all absurdities. Able to define abstract terms, such as pity, revenge, and jealousy, the boy was even telling us that he had been jealous, though refusing to disclose the details.

Things were different when it came to issues involving his personal feelings. When dropped on a desert island and allowed to take along only one person with him, he would select a person whom he likes but could not come up with a particular name, neither someone from home nor from school. When asked whom he liked best, he referred to himself but could not name a person liked next to best.

Allen was able to say that he did some day-dreaming which at times was pleasant and at times unpleasant but would not disclose any contents. He said that he had some ideas about what he wishes to do in the future but again refused to specify. When asked how he would feel about going into military service after reaching appropriate age, he doubted the possibility of being accepted, referring to his thinness and saying that this was the only reason.

The boy is emerging to some extent from a more severe autistic condition. He is still very self-contained and leads a private life from which other people are excluded. However, he is able to function sufficiently to attend school. Contact with people is tenuous but still, with definite reservations that he makes, Allen can carry on a conversation about things that are not emotionally loaded. His world is still static, in that he is unable to make concessions. It is a world filled with facts which are not integrated into interpersonal relationships. He knows, of course, that his younger brother is also at Linwood and seems to have strong feelings about it. Allen has no real contact with Sandy, having spoken to him "rarely." While he thinks that he "may" go home next year, he does not think that Sandy will be ready to do so and, it seems, would not cherish the idea anyway. But he is making scholastic progress which may be a wedge to further his reaching out to live with people.

April, 1968. Allen has done well in school. His last report card has B's and C's, and also good marks concerning general behavior, courtesy, and respect for property. With quite a storehouse of knowledge, he has his preoccupations with certain data. Allen is impressed by power and has no friends. He has formed a peculiar relationship with a male staff member whom he teases, orders around, and treats as though Allen were the teacher and the other person the pupil. It is a rather ambivalent relationship with which he is quite preoccupied and does not know what to do with. The boy feels that he is ready to enter a regular public school class in Montgomery County; the head of the school's personnel department, a man who can be of help, is aware of this. Allen is receiving individual psychotherapy from a local psychiatrist who may help by prompting him to discuss personal matters more intimately than he has been able to up to this time. He shrinks from any kind of commitment about anything like covering a subject in school or a preference for food. I was pleased to note, however, that this serious minded person has developed a sense of humor in appreciating some answers to riddles which he did not provide. I think that Allen will need continued therapy over a long period of time, but it is good to know that this is a boy with a history of a very severe disturbance in childhood, who has been able to respond to the kind of help that made it possible for him to become a good student at a regular school. It would be interesting to see Allen after a year or two and assess his progress.

January, 1973. At 22 years of age, Allen graduated from public high school, and began to work as a filing clerk on a part-time basis. He lives at home, has hobbies, reads a lot, draws exceptionally well, is interested in computers and enjoys history. Some older friends, chiefly people who can gratify his quest for facts and information, have broadened his social horizon. Interest in the opposite sex is thus far not in evidence.

Case 14

October, 1967. We are seriously handicapped by the paucity of essential information about Gerald's development prior to his admission to Linwood during the summer of 1967, at the age of approximately 3 years and 10 months. We know roughly that the boy's mother had vaginal bleeding during the last trimester of pregnancy, that some measures were taken "to prevent prematurity," and that he weighed about 6 lbs. at birth though thought one month premature. At 13 months of age, he had a febrile convulsion, and in the course of the first 3 years of his life which commenced in Washington, journeyed to Hawaii, Korea and then came back to the city of his birth. We know little about the circumstances, living conditions and the family's emotional constellation during that time. Seen at the Walter Reed Hospital prior to arrival at Linwood, the boy was unresponsive, had no demonstrable vocal communication and was not toilet trained. A persistent habit of bumping his head, to a point of requiring occasional stitches, was in evidence at intake; it is still in evidence at this time.

As seen today, Gerald has only a limited and fleeting contact with people, relating to objects in a rather specific way. He is a skillful spinner of objects that can be spun, can—but does not always—place the cylinders in the proper holes of the Montessori arrangements, and has a limited concept of how to handle a ball. There are some grunt-like sounds that appear when he is pleased and especially when displeased. At one time, though, Gerald did (for the first time, I am told) indulge in some gibberish in which vowels and consonants could be distinguished. At times he was able to smile, but it was difficult to correlate such smiles with any particular situation. His response to pin prick was one which he related much more definitely to the pin than to the person who pricked him. There were several types of bizarre behavior which seemed ritualistic. These included tapping objects (cylinders) against his mouth, beating the backs of his hands against each other, and performing something like a dance, a ritual manifested when leaving our room. At the age of 4½ years, Gerald acquired the ability to whistle better than most children of his age can, and at one time whistled to a tune which was sung to him. On the whole, his contact with people is extremely limited and there was hardly any interest in the people around him or in anything that happened in the room.

I would not hesitate to say that the child presents the basic features of the autistic syndrome. There is the aloneness and there are some ritual features like spinning with fine coordination that is better than gross coordination. Nevertheless, I feel that we cannot disregard the history of prenatal bleeding, the possible gynecological or pre-obstetric manipulation, and the record of one convulsion.

I would also say that during his 3 months at Linwood, the child has shown some signs, though minimal as yet, of progress. There is some smiling, there was a first instance of gibberish, and there is a whistling to a tune. I thought that on a few occasions it was possible to deflect him a bit from the spinning to which, however, he returned again and again.

June, 1968. Casual observation might initially lead one to believe that this child presents almost exactly the same pattern that was in evidence last October. On the other hand, closer observation brings out that while there is still no verbal communication of any kind, his vocalization shows quite a bit more modulation than before. Gerald is still interested in the ritualism of spinning. When confronted with any spinning which stimulates a great deal of excitement (almost ecstasy), he jumps up and down, simultaneously bringing his arms together and very frequently combining this with other ritualisms of tapping against his cheek or mouth. One thing that came out of this observation: while the boy was interested in the spinning top at a time when he did not know how to handle it, he learned to manipulate it, and gradually developed a special technique that required skill. Once he managed, it was very difficult to divert him from it. I am sure that this could have gone on for a long, long time with repeated ecstasy and repetitious jumping up and down and tapping his mouth and cheeks. I feel that this child is now getting ready for some form of behavior modification with tokens, or operant conditioning that might be of some help in getting him away from the extreme preoccupation. This might also facilitate some learning to develop patterns that go beyond his present limited repertoire.

January, 1973. Three years at Linwood can be summed up as follows: no progress in speech development, adequate participation in group activities, good sphincter control, reasonably adequate relatedness and some advances in imitative play. Indiscriminate temper tantrums and self-destructive behaviors were on the whole no longer in evidence. Gerald is now in a day-care center where operant conditioning techniques are used to modify his behavior.

Case 15

October, 1967. While this is the first time I saw Tina for any length of time, I had seen her previously, once in my office, once at the Children's Guild, and also from time to time fleetingly after the girl's enrollment at Linwood. I remember her as a child who did a great deal of crying which sounded almost inconsolable. I also remember the beautiful work done by Miss Simons in trying to bring about a separation between mother and child. Tina's mother gave me the impression as though she were concerned with the child in utero, meaning interested in and concerned without having anything to do about the infant—you carry the child, do everything to avoid danger to the embryo, but you do not have to have a person-to-person contact with it. This seemed to me to be a continued type of relationship with Tina after the girl was born.

When I saw Tina today there was no crying whatever. She was much more of an acting and interacting person than I had known her to be. The girl exhibited quite a bit of spontaneity in carrying out some of the tasks given her, showing reasonable understanding of things said to her and demonstrating good coordination. Handedness (right) is now definitely established. There was also spontaneity in a different area: when frustrated, she would stop, turn to something else, or just turn her head away. Tina gave evidence of some of the negativism which one encounters as a developmental milestone in many 2 to 4 year old children. When she succeeded in some tasks, she quickly looked up seeming pleasurably to expect a word or glance of approval. It is significant that this 4½-year-old child knows colors, identifies numbers up to 10, and places some of them in correct order. She identified words like "pig" or "chair," and enjoyed, *really* enjoyed, playing with and catching a ball which was almost one third of her size.

On the whole, this youngster has made remarkable progress and offers a far better prognosis than I would have thought possible a year ago. I think much of the future progress will depend on her diabetic condition rather than on psychological development, provided that the child can continue in her present setting for quite some time.

June, 1968. I first saw Tina when the parents questioned me whether the Linwood Children's Center was the best place for her. Linwood, which she entered in October, 1966, had been recommended by a social worker whose comprehensive notes provided a very good general background for the evaluation. From all appearances, anamnesis and the girl's behavior left few doubts that this was a child manifesting all the peculiarities and nosological particulars of early infantile autism.

Today, I can see considerable emergence from the autistic pattern. Tina eventually established a good relationship with me, but only after many compromises which I had to make. It was very interesting to observe how she made her first approach to me when she proceeded to the blackboard and wrote the abbreviation "Dr." Since no one paid any particular attention to her, or knew what she was saying, she made sure to change it to "doctor." Later on, Tina came closer and closer, but only after a time of not even turning around to look at me. I understand that she has made one "friend" at Linwood. In conversation, there was always the need for an attempt at some compromise. At first she gave no answer when I asked her about a sister. Eventually, I learned that Tina has a sister whose name is Dora, and eventually that Dora is now 3 years of age. There was always some negotiation necessary to get a response, and she appeared to enjoy her negotiations and the eventual coming around.

I would say that this child is very much in the process of emerging from a profound autistic condition. Her mother, I think, will need more counseling or guidance in the course of time. Of course, the child also has a diabetic condition for which she is being treated, and as a result of which she once experienced a coma. There is also the evidence of Rh incompatibility of her parents and the story of difficult delivery. How all these things fit together and contribute to the picture is difficult to say. However, we can conclude that this girl is making progress demonstrating considerable emergence from the originally typical autistic picture.

January, 1973. Remarkably well adjusted at the age of 8½, Tina left Linwood to attend the 1st grade of a public school. She is not only a good student, girl scout and an outgoing classmate, but also a responsible child who manages to properly regulate the intake of drugs prescribed for her diabetes.

CHILDHOOD SCHIZOPHRENIA

Case 16

October, 1966. Here is a child who came to the Linwood Children's Center 4 years ago when he was inaccessible, severely disturbed, hyperkinetic, and destructive. Not relating to people, and only moderately to objects, this boy was wetting and soiling indiscriminately. This condition persisted for quite some time, regardless of whether Phil was at Linwood as a day student or resident. He came accompanied by notes detailing a neurological examination and summarizing 2 years of weekly therapeutic sessions at a child guidance clinic. From these sources, we have a history which describes the child's behavior, reports inconclusive or altogether negative EEG and pneumoencephalographic findings and also sketches a family background that was not too helpful to the child. We know that a second child was born to the parents when Phil was about a year old, and that the family moved when he was 2 years of age.

At Linwood, the hardly manageable behavior went on for better than 3 years, whereupon a noticeable change occurred during the summer of 1966.

When Phil was seen today, he immediately manifested his awareness of all people in the room, accepted introductions, and repeated names identifying Miss Simons, Mrs. Mitchell and Dr. Ferster, whose name he did not quite remember until Miss Simons provided the first letter. Phil sat down on invitation and agreed to play with the toys, handling the cylinder blocks adroitly, though ambidextrously, and generally showing good coordination. He has learned to count and to identify the letters of the alphabet. When asked to draw a boy, he first printed the word *BOY* and then produced a Humpty-Dumpty-like creature, into which he spontaneously invested a mouth and, on special request, also eyes and ears. There was much repetition of questions asked of him, but not quite in the form of real echolalia. It seemed that Phil actually enjoyed the sound, and there was quite a bit of inflection in all of his repetitions. I could not help but feel that he derived some pleasure from the novelty of the situation and his own participation in it, almost as though the child was making discoveries. He was able to repeat 5 digits forward, could not do it with 6 digits, but did not get the concept of repeating 3 digits backwards. When asked what a chair is, he replied "green," properly identifying the color of the chair in which he was sitting. By the same token, a pencil was "yellow". When asked what a horse was, he said "h-o-r-s-e." It seems that this child is groping for communication, yielding that which occurs to him immediately. On request, though after some hesitation, he even drew a horse which had four legs, a head, and a tail. Phil was friendly throughout and definitely *with* the people who spoke to him.

When I tried the pinprick reaction, the boy most certainly connected the act with me, looking up frightened and pleading. Later on, at Miss Simons' suggestion, he told me on the toy telephone not to do it again. However, this act was not fully completed by then. When he left, Phil properly addressed the three other people as "Doctor," and emphatically called me *"Mister* Kanner."

This child presents a diagnostic dilemma. We cannot say that his anamnesis or demeanor indicate that there are no ascertainable traces of CNS or metabolic dysfunction. While early history of supposedly normal progress for 2 years that was followed by regression may prompt one to think for a moment of Heller's Disease, the boy has certainly emerged to a point where this can be excluded. He may have appeared as a severely retarded child, but the last few months indicate an increased ability and desire to learn. Phil's hand printing is neat and he promptly spells out certain simple words. The pinprick reaction and his capacity for being with people keeps one from accepting the diagnosis of autism, unless emergence of such impressive quality had unexpectedly materialized. One may, because of the history and some of the described performance, think of a "schizophrenic" development in the broadest sense of this word.

Suffice it to say that, in light of the history and early observations at Linwood, this child has made phenomenal progress in a situation which provided an opportunity to discover his identity and establish contact with other people, less threatening to him than those in the child's past. At the present time, Phil is a friendly child, who developed adequate sphincter control, is learning to read and write and, to quote Miss Simons, has discovered the enjoyment of life.

April, 1968. When I saw Phil today, I was truly amazed that having seen me for the first time in October, 1966, he remembered me as the Doctor who took care of him and also used a pinprick. This demonstrated a phenomenal memory for certain specific events. Coming to Linwood in a dilapidated state, this child has socialized to an appreciable extent, to a point of behaving and achieving at a level of an approximately 6-year-old youngster. Having been rescued from a state of near vegetation, he is a likeable retarded boy who, if one were to think in terms of IQ's, rates about 50 to 55. This much had to be said in order to keep myself from indulging in new optimism.

January, 1973. After nearly 9½ years at Linwood, Phil was finally ready to move on to a more permanent setting provided by a local day-care center. At the present time, this 16½-year-old adolescent lives at home and functions in a sheltered workshop. There is no evidence that dramatic progress in any area is in sight.

Case 17

October, 1966. The major part of the 10½ years of this child's life has gone into intensive effort in several quarters to establish a diagnostic basis for his handicap as a framework for remedial activities. Purely an impression of schizophrenia has remained on the books so far. At the same time, we have the information that Greer did not walk until the age of 22 months and that sphincter control has not been fully established to this day. No objective physiometric evaluation has ever been able to find any area of performance which goes beyond that accomplished by an average 2½ to 3-year-old child. There is no question about the boy's ability to hear, and he comprehends the spoken word if it is within the limits of his intellectual level. Greer promptly sat down on request, handed me an object (in this case he understood the name of the object), blew a match, and even fetched for me an educational toy (indicated as "that thing") from the mantle. He had, on the whole, good eye contact when he felt like looking at somebody. On one occasion, he took me by the hand and led me to a bed where he lay down, inviting play of the order of tickling which he enjoyed thoroughly.

In the pinprick test situation, the boy definitely reacted to me as a person. At 10½ years of age he still has not developed handedness preference. When an object is at his left, he reaches for it with the left hand and vice versa.

It would be stretching the concept of schizophrenia extremely far if we were to consider this boy a schizophrenic. There is no basis, no performance that goes beyond, at best, a 3-year level. There is also no indication of any kind of catatonic, hebephrenic, delusional or hallucinatory content.

I understand that he has shown some limited positive response in operant conditioning experiments, but would not a retarded child show an equally limited response? Unless anything to the contrary could be demonstrated, I am convinced that these responses do not transcend the 2- to 3-year level of behavior. I have no doubt that continued effort of this kind may result in further additions of fragments within the same level, but would this warrant a general overall prognostic optimism? Would, in view of the excellent facilities at Linwood, the efforts expended be more warranted for children with a different outlook? After a considerable period of individual therapy, after efforts at Hillcrest and at Linwood, we find, through little fault of theirs or his, a picture which in no way has changed this child's status. We ought to have the courage of reality and gently, sympathetically, lead the family to the recognition of things as they are and suggest an extended residential placement.

January, 1971. After a period of care at Linwood lasting 4 years and 3 months, Greer left us in January, 1967. He now spends most of his time at a training center for the mentally retarded, an institution which may be of some benefit within the framework of his dim prognosis.

Case 18

November, 1966. Grant is a thin, physically healthy 5½-year-old boy who has been at Linwood for approximately 4½ months. Pregnancy and birth were reportedly normal. He did not walk alone until about 16 to 17 months of age, but then immediately began to run. The child seemed to have hearing difficulties which began to improve after a tonsillectomy at 2½ years of age. Since that time, his hearing improved. The hospitalization, however, was a highly traumatic affair; the mother was not allowed to see him and the child was force fed. Eating became even more of a problem than before that experience, and he was readmitted to the hospital due to dehydration. Grant was seen at the Children's Hospital in Washington where Dr. Reginald Lourie saw a combination of psychosis, retardation and possible minimal brain injury.

The parents report that since the hospitalization, this child has been running away from home without any particular aim. While at Linwood, he ran away several times; on three occasions the authorities had to be notified and he was picked up by the police. Grant would have run away more frequently save for the close supervision which became necessary. He has at times used almost ingenious devices to get away from the building.

When seen today, this child spent much of his time striving to get away from anybody who attempted to hold him, trying every exit, and saying several times "Goodbye." While not at it, some not too gentle persuasion prompted him to do some very simple jigsaw puzzles, singing or humming happily in the process, thumb through the pages of a telephone book, and occasionally utter a few words. Grant definitely saw me as the perpetrator when I pricked him with the pin, and said, "Don't you hurt me." I am told that he recognizes the names of states, though in this particular situation he made no effort to demonstrate such ability.

Diagnostically, one is very much impressed by this child's persistent and active desire to get away from people and from structured situations. He seems to be bent on this more than on anything else.

This child has had difficulties in relating from an early age but it is quite possible that the traumata of hospitalization may have accentuated the desire for withdrawal which, one may say, he keeps practicing constantly as a matter of perpetual urge. For the purpose of nosological classification, I would feel that this child fits best into the general diagnostic category of schizophrenia, without any particular sub-division or sub-specification.

April, 1968. In quite many respects Grant has shown progress largely in the area of vocabulary, reading, writing, and spelling. In these areas, he performed as much work as any 6-year-old child. The boy has also shown progress in the sense that he now tolerates the presence of people, unlike at the time of my first acquaintance with the child in November 1966, when he used to run away from people in similar situations. This progress is one of challenge, a certain attitude, a certain desire to want to get this child to grow much more in other areas. Diagnostically, I think this child fits in best with the conditions described in this country most aptly by Louise Despert (1968) as schizophrenia with insidious onsets. I don't believe that he fits into any of the more specified categories such as symbiosis or autism. So I think that we can reiterate that this child's behavior resembles most closely that of a schizophrenic child without any particular sub-categorization. The fact that he has learned more than mechanically the art of reading and writing at his age level would make one feel that remaining at the Linwood Children's Center is indicated. At this rate of progress, with emphasis on closer contact with people, one might reasonably look forward to further gains.

January, 1973. One might be tempted to reconsider Grant's diagnosis of childhood schizophrenia, admittedly in light of recent studies (Rutter, 1972) that are in favor of discarding this nosological label. There is an impression of an innate impairment that is beyond the diagnostician's ability to pinpoint. Persistent stereotypies and preoccupations, observed in the course of the past 4 years at Linwood, tend to suggest a pattern that is more typical of autism. Grant's ability to conceptualize is just beginning to emerge. Hyperactivity, mediated by small doses of Ritalin, has subsided rather considerably. Names, numbers and pictures are now increasingly meaningful to this child, whose capacity for purely "mechanical" recognition and rote memory was at times quite deceitful. Grant can imitate and utilize his visual memory in a manner that enables him to keep up with our educational program. While still not ready for public school, chiefly due to hyperactivity, the boy is nevertheless progressing most satisfactorily, reading and writing (printing) at the 5th grade level, socializing easily and displaying a good sense of humor. One might conclude that guarded optimism is not unwarranted.

Case 19

November, 1966. Before discussing my experience with Jerry, I should like to present a few introductory notes prepared by Miss Simons on the basis of her observation of the boy's parents; these seem very important in the evaluation of this child's development:

> The mother is an extremely rigid woman and looks it, always seeming close to tears; she has a high-pitched voice. Jerry's father seems easy-going on the surface. However, he cannot let anything interfere with his own rather narrow world comprising his job and his car. The man has no friends as he feels that people are dangerous species who can do harm. The sister, 9 years older than Jerry, is a miniature version of the mother. Just looking at her and talking, one is confronted with the same high-pitched voice, the same rigid face, although she has been able to express anger toward the father. The girl's reason for going to college at some distance from home was connected with her wish to be away from home and desire to avoid facing the father. In order to live comfortably, the father has sought complete obedience from the children. He does not quite know why, except that "children should be obedient," and his requests are to merit immediate compliance. He gives an order to perform and anticipates prompt obedience. The man has been known to spank or hit his children; the older girl was exposed to this even when she reached her teens. He has used a belt. While explaining, his face has a vague, friendly smile; he does not seem to feel bad or guilty about it all, for this is the way he wants things to be. With the same methods and attitude towards Jerry, he noticed, after the first few years, that hitting did not yield obedience. Thus, after being in counseling here for about a year, the man announced that he had given up hitting the child and also resigned himself to expectations that Jerry would never improve. The mother has been able to express some dissatisfaction or anger toward her husband. This came about in group sessions, when support was forthcoming from other group members. Her voice was never more natural or face more relaxed than she did this. But before she expressed herself freely, she proceeded to ask her husband if he would be angry at her thereafter.

I feel it is essential to be aware of this background as one tries to evaluate the child's present condition and the development which has taken place during the past 3 years since Jerry has entered Linwood at the age of 5 years and 5 months. Jerry's history discloses that he was born normally at term after a normal pregnancy. There was a slight delay in motor development and he did not walk until 17 months of age. Toilet training was not accomplished at the time when he came to Linwood, though at the present time he has adequate sphincter control. The parents report that this child was quite ritualistic. When taken out for walks, he had to proceed in the same direction. While there was little, if any, language, the boy is reported to have said to the parents: "Do you want to eat the baby?" I am not sure that this was what he really said, but it is what the parents seemed to hear.

When brought in by Miss Simons, Jerry responded to my request to shake hands, offering the left hand. A little later, when playing with toys, he used the right hand predominantly. When invited, he sat down on my lap, at first a bit uncomfortable in the chair when I tried to place him in an embracive position. It did not take a long while for Jerry to adjust, whereupon he was not only quite comfortable but even seemed to enjoy the contact. During the interview, he accepted some cuddling from me and, of course, from Miss Simons. This he did in a passive way but willingly, never showing any signs of fear or shrinking. The boy could be induced to play at a primitive level, such as running after him. This he enjoyed considerably, exhibiting rather good skill. Jerry performed the cylinder block test and the pyramid consisting of rings of different sizes. Again, he skillfully put the blocks in accordance with size, immediately noticing one mistake and correcting it. After some hesitation, he handed several objects to other people. On one occasion, when I placed a book of matches on the table and asked him to hand me a match, he literally took a match out of the book and handed one to me. There was no verbalization or vocalization or any noise during the entire performance, except that sometimes, when chased, there was audible laughter. At this time, I could find no evidence of any kind of compulsiveness.

As I see him now, Jerry does not present even one of the principal elements of autism; there is no ritualism, no repetitiousness, no insistence of the preservation of sameness. Also, he accepted closeness to people much more readily than an autistic child. There is quite a bit of passivity in his behavior, a facile acceptance of an approach that he enjoys, but with no reciprocity during the period of our interview. Any contribution on his part had to be guided manually. To this, he also conformed in the past.

From time to time, he looked away in a manner which would impress an observer of an adult with possible hallucinations. As he is now, I cannot possibly view this child as either inherently mentally defective or as atypically autistic. If I were pushed into a corner to make a diagnostic pronouncement, I would consider this boy as rather globally schizophrenic, without any kind of specific categorization.

I feel that if this child had an opportunity to have someone commence a one-to-one-person relationship over a long period of time, without the interference of his parents, he could be helped to form better relationships and even to initiate verbal interchanges. I do not know how this can be accomplished for I do not feel that the parents would have sufficient understanding to see the necessity of such therapy. It may sound superficial, but I might almost say that this child must have been terrified into schizophrenic withdrawal. He was certainly brought up in an emotionally morbid environment, and has now reached the stage, with the help received at Linwood, when he can start out on an infantile level of far greater comfort than he must have experienced. Jerry responds to warmth and seems to be beginning to learn to give back in kind. He has had many physical investigations, including electroencephalography which do not yield any diagnostic guidelines.

April, 1968. Since I saw Jerry about a year and a half ago, there has been a stationary picture, with minor exceptions. This concerns me in my own impression of a schizophrenic withdrawal, the child having remained in that state since a very early age. There is still no speech, though he does understand other people's speech at an early level of development. I can see no answer to this child's future needs other than eventual placement in a residential hospital. It is, fortunately, possible to retain him at Linwood during the period when the mother is being helped to accept life without Jerry. If and when this is accomplished, I think that hospital placement for the duration of his existence must be anticipated.

January, 1973. There was no progress during the 1½-year period from the last evaluation in 1968 and the date of discharge from Linwood. Jerry went to a day-care center for the mentally retarded where he remains at the present time. His mother finds it less difficult to keep the child at home having accepted the dim prognosis for the future.

Case 20

December, 1966. This 18-year-old girl has been "affiliated" with the Linwood Children's Center for the past 12 years. She is extremely withdrawn and there is very limited content in her communication or any other relations with people. Betty has not responded to any encouragement to formal learning. When asked questions, most of them very simple, she would repeat a question several times, not as a manifestation of echolalia, but rather as an act of avoidance of the necessity to answer. The girl is physically healthy, rather plump, and walks with a peculiar gait, supposedly caused by flat feet. She does not participate in any of the activities at the Center and is very much withdrawn, spending time in the classroom in the flesh but not in the spirit and often mumbling to herself.

Diagnostically, Betty fits better into the picture of simple deteriorating schizophrenia than any other classification. I do not believe that her continuation at the Linwood Children's Center is warranted. In a state hospital setting with therapeutic orientation, it might be possible to help her to become a member of the hospital community by being helped to learn how to do simple tasks of some usefulness, such as washing dishes, dusting furniture, or, hopefully, setting tables.

January, 1970. No apparent change in behavior was in evidence nor serious hope warranted that institutionalization can be avoided when Betty left Linwood in September, 1967. The girl proceeded to a day-care center integrated into a hospital community where she appears to live at this time.

Case 21

December, 1966. Drake, approximately 8½ years old, has been at Linwood for about 1½ years. He had been seen by various people from an early age, at first because of what seemed to be inadequate speech development. A neurologist who saw him in New York thought of him as intellectually retarded. This impression was soon discarded and when the family moved to Chicago he was seen for several years at a child development clinic where the boy was studied thoroughly and many contacts were made with him and his parents.

Mrs. Nash concluded that Drake is an intellectually normal child, with an IQ of at least 100. He is physically healthy, left-handed and left-eyed. The boy's school-work indicates reading and writing abilities reasonably commensurate with his age and requirements. While there is mention of ear trouble in early life and a "speech defect," he can communicate verbally except that sometimes at the end of a sentence there is some slurring. This also shows itself on occasions in his writing when after several words there is a slurring toward the end.

When seen at Linwood today Drake was at first somewhat reticent. He answered questions to the point, reporting his age, birth date, address, details about his brother whose age and grade in school he knew and volunteered quite a bit of information. The boy names two children with whom he sometimes played in the neighborhood, spoke of one child who has moved away to Philadelphia and told me that one of the boys at Linwood wanted to be his friend. He readily counted backwards from 20 to 1, copied a circle, square and a diamond, and then volunteered to recite a number of songs, telling me that he had learned one of them at the Ethical Culture Sunday School. He also told me about trips that he had made with his father and other people who seemed to be friends of the family.

All during this time, he made peculiar motions, waving his hands, whirling around on his axis, or hitting himself not too vigorously with a rhythmic motion. He reacted to the pinprick by seeing *me* definitely as a perpetrator, deciding on questioning that I had pricked him to see if it hurts.

In spite of an elaborate history from the Chicago clinic it is difficult to ascertain what role the child played in the home, or what the departure from New York, where the family lived with his grandparents, for Chicago meant to him. Drake spoke of being teased a great deal by his brother and said somewhat sadly that he does not know how to tease back, an art that he would like to learn and might master when he grows up.

He is now certainly much more reality oriented than in the past, and intelligently communicative, even though communication may at times constitute a strain. Seeming ready to leave, he asked me point blank whether there was anything more I wanted to say to him. But when I asked him whether there was anything he wanted to say to me, Drake remained and continued the interview.

I agree with prior diagnostic formulations that this child is not intellectually retarded, not brain-damaged, and not autistic. Nevertheless, his behavior, especially the peculiar motions and whirling, is at times bizarre, less so than it has been when he first came to Linwood. The best I can do diagnostically is to suggest that we deal with a schizoid child who has regained and is gaining more contact with people, has given up fantasies about an imaginary family of 3 (father, mother, and child) about which he talked previously and is seeking a relationship with adults and some of the children at Linwood. He offers a prognosis which is not too gloomy. In fact, I feel that after further reaching out at Linwood, it will be possible for Drake to enter a small school where he can make satisfactory progress in learning as well as in social conduct. This seems to be an attainable goal.

June, 1969. Drake's psychiatrist reported that upon discharge from Linwood in July, 1967 the boy went to a private school where he managed to function quite well.

Case 22

December, 1966. The door was opened to let in an 8½-year-old child in apparently good physical condition, with reasonably good motor coordination and handedness not as yet fully established. There was no verbal response either spontaneously or in answer to questions during the entire period of examination. There was, however, quite a bit of squealing, which seemed pleasurable to this boy. In the formal tests, Glenn rates at a level of about 2 to 3 years. Not entirely unresponsive, he was able to hand objects to people and also to retrieve such objects. He did the cylinder blocks and the simple formboards demonstrating concern when a form did not fit exactly into the hole and needing some reassurance that this was to have been anticipated. There was some repetitiousness in the performance, which one might designate as perseverance.

It is difficult to fit this child into a definite diagnostic category. He is obviously retarded in terms of general function. While there is no doubt about this functional retardation, the question of etiology is not as easily answered. I had some information having had an opportunity to see the father. It seems that there was a definite withdrawal and regression at the age of about 3 when the family moved back from France to this country. Still, in view of this child's emerging relationships with people, however limited, retention of sphincter control though with occasional exceptions, and the imitative quality of some behavior (he was said to have made consumable muffins at home), his development does not fit into the picture of Heller's Disease, of which one might think at first. In looking over all the possible and available diagnostic formulations, the picture comes more closely to schizophrenic withdrawal than to any other delineation that one can think of.

If one considers the progress that Glenn has made at the Linwood Children's Center, small progress to be sure, it is still very questionable whether this child can reach a level of independent social functioning within the foreseeable future. However, it is possible to think that, with another year or two at Linwood, he may reach a stage when one could help him to fit into a school group geared to the so-called trainable retarded child. The father seems to be quite aware of his son's limitations. I think that he is now well prepared for proper cooperation with Linwood and will be more of assistance than in the past when this was not the case. The child's younger brother, now 6 years of age, has also some difficulties of a nature which is not easy to determine, and a report from the University of Maryland, which follows his development might help us to round out the family picture.

January, 1968. Glenn would have soon commenced his fourth year at Linwood, had we not concluded that time has come for his departure. The boy is ready to enter the Search Light School, a facility for trainable retarded chilren which might advance to a degree his development.

Disorders With Evidence of Organicity

Case 23

September, 1966. Tod's chronological age is 6 years and 9 months. General longitudinal growth, however, is certainly not in keeping with the calendar for he gives the impression of a child between 4 and, at the utmost, 5 years of age. The history indicates that he is the fourth of 6 children, with no major developmental or behavioral difficulty in the other 5. History also reveals a lack of maturation in many areas, including motor development. This is not what one finds in children with difficulties that are primarily emotional. Nevertheless, in the approximately one year that he has been at the Linwood Children's Center this child, though still considerably retarded, has gained a great deal in the sense of parting with many of his compulsions and preoccupations. He certainly does not exhibit the kind of door-oriented obsession or fear of people described on earlier examinations. Mrs. Nash, who managed to elicit a good response, could not obtain performances that were above the level of 2½ years. Tod has still not developed definite handedness. In a formboard test involving 12 pieces of different shapes and colors, he approached the tasks rather promptly and carried them out satisfactorily.

While at Linwood, he has developed adequate fecal control, which may have been carried over to the home situation. Tod still exhibits a small area, approximately the size of a quarter, of alopecia which may be a residue of a small meningocele, as suggested by Dr. Schultz.

I certainly cannot see this boy as a basically schizophrenic, autistic or symbiotic child. There is no question about retardation, which is evident in his motor, linguistic, adaptive and social development. Tod's experience at Linwood shows that he is trainable in the motor and adaptive areas that represent his major gains. The relatively good adjustment of 5 other children in the family prompts one to feel that his parents have been reasonably competent five times. Thus, their difficulties in handling this child seem to have arisen more from bewilderment and anxiety than from rejection, coldness or lack of acceptance. I would help the parents to dismiss any false blame, which they seem to have attached to the child's fall, and encourage them in their acceptance of this child's handicap as something not attributable to human fault.

April, 1968. Tod, on the whole a somewhat more comfortable child, is nevertheless very markedly retarded. I doubt whether we can say that this boy, now almost 8½ years old, performs at a level that is beyond that of a 3½-year-old child. But even this is a rather overly optimistic impression. I understand that he may move on next September to a special public school class for markedly retarded children in Prince George's County. Tod has had the advantage of spending 3 years at Linwood where he received individual attention. It is hoped that parents' acceptance of this child, will enable him to live in his family's surroundings. I wish that the present-day public residential placement centers for the markedly retarded were able to give the child, any child, the facilities and care provided by the Linwood Children's Center. But even Linwood, with its ideal facilities and attitudes, has not been able to transform Tod into somebody less markedly retarded.

January, 1973. Tod's discharge in September 1968 was followed by a stay in a day-care center for the retarded. This gentle and easily manageable boy lives at home and continues to advance within the limits imposed by his neurologically determined handicaps.

Case 24

October, 1966. As we see Karen now, she presents a somewhat ambiguous picture of a child who *can* be induced to be playful in a motor way, once the initiative has come from someone else. I have an idea that on occasions she may even be spontaneous and initiate in her own way this form of play. When she entered the room where several people were present, Karen walked right straight between them without looking at any one person. In this interesting situation, I could not detect any eye contact except for some fleeting look in the direction of, rather than at the person. She is obviously more at home with objects than with people and has adequate motor coordination in putting things into holes. The girl handles educational toys with reasonable skill, except when it comes to screwing and unscrewing, the only occasion when she invokes somebody's help, leading her helper's hand toward the object. She has a good perception of color and an ability to arrange things by placing objects in appropriate compartments of a box with separate compartments for various colors. Karen can distinguish green from turquoise. In handling objects, she still has not developed a full handedness preference, using in most instances her left hand.

While the girl was occupied with educational toys she adhered to strict notions of what she wanted to do and became upset when the procedure that she felt was appropriate had been subjected to interference. Karen was most upset by the interference rather than angry at the person who interfered. When I picked her up, she struggled and was not reassured by pulling. More tolerant when a staff member picked her up at the time of leaving, there was even then more tolerance than pleasure at the experience.

I am impressed by the fact that, when tested by Mrs. Nash, she performed items at the level of up to 2 to 2½ years adequately, but not beyond such age level. Her whole demeanor in effect, impressed me as that of a disturbed 2½-year-old rather than that of a child nearly 5 years of age.

Nevertheless, Karen does show preference for objects rather than people, and is intensely interested in what happens to objects that she handles, at times making use of people's hands to receive help with objects that she cannot manipulate by herself. She does show displeasure, which is somewhat vigorous, when people interfere with her designs. When the cylinder blocks were taken out for her not exactly in the right order she became quite upset, but went on quietly when the order was restored.

The pinprick reaction was quite ambiguous. Karen did connect the pinprick with me and not completely with my hand.

Whatever the basic nature of the performance might be, the girl now functions at a markedly retarded level as shown by Mrs. Nash's experience and also by the child's general demeanor; yet features of autism are undeniable. It is difficult to say whether the unquestionable progress which has been made at Linwood is one of better than emotional adjustment or whether it is something which one might find in a markedly retarded child who has had the benefit of personal attention received at Linwood.

One wishes it were possible to obtain a more detailed and meaningful background to account for the first few years of the child's life. By the time this girl arrived, unclad, there were three small children around—the oldest yet at the beginning of school age. One wonders how much and what kind of attention the mother was able to give her at the time. It would also be interesting to know how these other children had progressed.

Nonetheless, I cannot get away from the conviction that this child shows an inherent, innate problem. The mother was unhappy from the beginning because of her feeling that neither she nor her husband could reach this girl. While the prognosis is guarded, the child is undoubtedly benefiting from her experience at Linwood, and she had best continue. Karen has developed a fairly adequate sphincter control, she has become physically nimble, feeds herself with some compulsive behavior connected with such feeding, and responds to an invitation for rough play with some evidence of pleasure.

April, 1968. Karen is now almost 6½ years old. As she appeared today, it seems that it will be necessary for me to revise the impressions which I had of the child about a year and a half ago. The outstanding feature now is that the child is beginning to imitate sounds, seems to derive pleasure from her apparently recently gained ability, works hard at it, and repeats words heard, at the same time in a very labored manner with some rather obvious suffering. I do believe that before we can come to any clear understanding of this child's problems it will be imperative to have a good speech and hearing evaluation and also a good neurological examination. The kind of speech that this child produces has, even though there are no signs of visible neurological impairment, very much of the quality that suggests a cerebral-palsy-type of athetoid speech. I would recommend that a detailed examination be made as soon as humanly possible and do not believe we can come to any clear understanding of what ails this child before we have the results.

January, 1973. Subsequent neurological examinations have not enlightened us as to the cause of the hearing and speech disorders that are not typical of the majority of our children who are autistic. After 8 years at Linwood, Karen has full sphincter control, self-care, reasonably good relatedness and an increasing ability to supplement her limited speech by pantomime. While self-aggressive behavior has virtually disappeared, the girl began to manifest infrequent but severe temper tantrums that can not be attributed to environmental stimuli. This problem, not as yet fully alleviated by medication (Ritalin) might yet provide a better clue to the possible brain injury and the child's inability to make better progress.

Case 25

October, 1966. If one were so inclined, one could build a whole textbook of child psychiatry around the experiences and behavior of this child. Organically, there is the history of a premature rupture of the membrane, of protracted labor, and of at least one or possibly two seizures of a convulsive nature. At the age of 8 years, Brent has still not established definite handedness preference and uses either hand with equal skill.

From the psychogenic viewpoint, there is a history of marital difficulties between the parents; after four months of this child's life, the father stepped out of the picture. The mother is said to be, to say the least, ambivalent about Brent, and both she and her adopted mother have visited many physicians and a chiropractor.

When the boy came to the Linwood Children's Center, he was extremely overactive, destructive and without visible direction. When seen today, a number of important features emerged. It was possible for him to sit through for about a one half of an hour, remaining practically all the time in his chair, and sustain interest in a number of activities. Such interest could be stimulated only by way of using visual means. Brent failed to respond to any verbal address, even to calling of his name, but promptly and correctly responded to gestures. This enabled him to handle simple, and even more complicated jigsaw puzzles and exhibit good space orientation, performing with some deliberation and not compulsively. Loud clapping of hands behind him produced no blinking of the eyes. He did blink when the clapping was close to his ear, prompting one to wonder about the nature of his responses. Was it a hearing response or a response to vibration? There is no question about the fact that this child has a marked hearing deficiency which extends not only to verbal communication but also to all kinds of noises. In other words, this is a deaf child and not one who suffers from receptive failure alone.

The Linwood atmosphere has been very good for this boy. He has calmed down, and is apparently less threatened by people than he must have been. Remaining here would help him to continue developing a greater sense of comfort, even though his educational needs call for a different highly specialized setting. Brent's progress has indicated that he is a trainable child. Moreover, it has helped to indicate that he is also educable if expert attention can be given to his hearing problem. I also feel that, in view of the peculiar home situation, a residential arrangement would be highly desirable. The Central Institute for the Deaf in St. Louis would be an excellent constructive possibility.

December, 1968. After 2 years and 4 months at Linwood, this severely handicapped youngster went to a private residential school that specializes in speech and hearing disorders.

Case 26

November, 1966. This well-nourished, somewhat pasty-looking almost 9-year-old boy has been in residential care at the Linwood Children's Center since June, 1962. Gene, the oldest in his family, was variously diagnosed as having hearing loss and receptive aphasia. His parents preferred residential care at Linwood so that they could give sufficient attention to subsequent children. However, they are sufficiently interested to look for further possibilities for this boy.

During the course of the interview, it is very obvious that Gene does not respond to the spoken word, but obediently, at times almost with automatic obedience, responds to gestural invitations to sit up, walk to the door, or hand me certain things. When invited verbally, there was no reaction and no facial sign of comprehension. Demonstrating fair space perception, he managed a rather complex jigsaw puzzle, being guided chiefly by space and less so by content. When frustrated, Gene resorts to peculiar finger motions. Persistent in his performances, he exhibits some facial anger when interfered with.

This child is at Linwood only because there is no other place that provides a combination capable of satisfying his emotional needs, while offering at the same time the specialized help which his aphasic condition appears to require. I still like the old term "congenital word deafness" better than aphasia, which in the course of time has been given so many different meanings. Gene must have given up a long time ago. I know such children who, no matter how frustrated otherwise, would eagerly look at other people for gestural communications. This child no longer does that and, in fact, must be touched bodily to communicate an invitation by gestures to do something. In his work, the boy is quite methodical. When leafing through a telephone book, he would not leave it until the book is properly closed. I wonder if something can be done to help this child through the Spencer Tracy Foundation. He must be helped quickly, for I think that the prognosis is otherwise bleak. One hopes that it is not too late to obtain such help.

June, 1971. This aphasic boy left Linwood in September, 1967 to enter a state hospital where he remained for a few months. He presently lives at home, attending a day-care center for the mentally retarded.

Case 27

November, 1966. If not properly informed, one can hardly believe that this little homunculus is 10 years and 4 months old. In size and appearance he is closer to a 5-year-old, in general demeanor he would hardly be rated as having reached the 3-year level. When Erik came to Linwood about 7 years ago, he was a little something rather than somebody and it is easy to agree with Miss Simons who thought of him at the time as a new born, covered with meconium. During his stay here as a day student, he has acquired adequate sphincter control, still does not use speech except for a kind of sing-song utterance of "Allan," occasionally whines in the manner of an infant and allows himself to be cuddled in a similar manner. The boy has good space perception and is able to match a considerable number of geometrical figures. He is consistently right handed, understands very simple commands, and reacted to the pinprick without any defensive or offensive movement.

This child is very markedly retarded in his general development and definitely not autistic or schizophrenic. One cannot possibly expect that he could ever be fitted in a setting that provides other than, I hope, good custodial care. I agree fully with the efforts planned at Linwood to assist Erik's parents in locating a good residential placement.

December, 1971. Erik's transfer to the Vineland School in January, 1967 marked the end of our efforts which, in the course of 7 years and 4 months, yielded no hope and no basis for reassurance sought by his parents. Residential care appears to be in sight for the remainder of this child's life.

Case 28

November, 1966. I am afraid that the report comprising my evaluation of this almost 10-year-old boy will have to be quite inconclusive. I saw him once before in February, 1964 at the Diagnostic and Evaluation Center, at which time Garth impressed us as a child lacking directions and quite undecided about his situation vis–a–vis other people. While he was unable to perform in a structured test situation and could not relate to me or to Dr. Robertson, who was also present, during the short interview, he made no move to leave the room, waiting for some kind of approach from one of us prior to deciding whether to respond.

When seen by the psychologist, Mrs. Nash, he did a great deal of verbalizing in a manner which she described as "reversed" speech. Occasionally however, Garth gave some factual answers to the point.

When seen today, the boy had to be literally dragged in by Miss Simons. At first, he sat on the floor, then allowed himself to be deposited in the chair, holding hands tightly before his eyes. At times, he permitted Miss Simons to remove his hands from the eyes and to hold them; at other times he would do that by himself. Even when Garth closed his eyes, he did occasionally peek through. When I lighted a cigar with some flames shooting up, the child was quite observant and later on seemed really to enjoy a repeat.

Garth's physical condition seems to be adequate. Unlike most of the children at Linwood, he developed definite handedness preference (the boy is right-handed), responded to the pinprick in a manner which indicated that he connected it with me rather than with a depersonalized hand, showed good coordination with cylinder blocks, and good space perception when handling the jigsaw puzzle (milk man). When he chose to answer a question, the answers were to the point. Garth wrote for me his brother's name, his own name, and knew the exact date, indicating this by writing "November 28". But at all times he played the game of doing things on his own terms, so that one could never tell when the boy would or would not perform at request. There was little spontaneity throughout except when he was ready to leave. Then he could be engaged in showing his muscles, accepted an empty cigar box, and upon leaving while trying a bit to delay the departure, said "Goodbye, Dr. Kanner," with a wave to me from the hall. Apparently, he could be more spontaneous when knowing that no further relationship would be asked for. I have a feeling that, while tested by Mrs. Nash, he used his incessant speech as a defense similar to that of holding hands before his eyes while here.

I have pitifully little knowledge of the interaction of the family members at home at any time during this child's life, or of the role that his older brother may have played. Diagnostically, I can only tell of the categories that Garth does not seem to fall into. The boy is, as his schoolwork here shows, not markedly retarded. He is *not* autistic. Garth's behavior today would not give any indication of the typical or even atypical constitutionally hebephrenic child.

If possible, I should have an opportunity to see both parents and the brother so that we can come closer to an evaluation of how this child fits into the emotional constellation of his family. If there is any kind of organic impairment, there is no demonstrable evidence of it neurologically, electroencephalographically, or otherwise pediatrically. I feel that because of his responses at Linwood, a form of therapy which includes reinforcement by rewarding (some may call it "token economy") might be intensified.

April, 1968. When I examined Garth about a year and a half ago at the Linwood Children's Center, I was again impressed by the behavior seen a while before when I met him at the Diagnostic Evaluation Center. At that time, I was especially impressed by a lack of direction and general behavioral inconsistencies. I made it a point, after seeing Garth at Linwood, to consult the parents and learned a few things which may be significantly important in this child's development. At the age of 9 months, he had measles associated with a very high fever, stiffening out in his mother's arms and, at one time, a mild convulsion. I cannot explain this child's subsequent development on a basis other than speaking in terms of "a postencephalitic condition." He certainly does not fit any of these other categories. It is not a matter of just plain simple retardation *nor* of autism. The mention of "symbiotic," as made by one examining psychologist, can be explained by the fact that this basically over-protective and anxious mother has so much more cause for clinging to this child and establishing a hope which, I see, is prevalent even among the professionals who have dealt with him. The Linwood Children's Center has done much for this child, enabling him, at least, to develop learning at the first-grade level. I cannot detect in any phase of his behavior a type of cognition that would make one feel that Garth has transcended the 6-year level. I agree with the management of the Linwood Center that his presence here has reached a point beyond which the Center cannot feel it can go. I also agree with the plan to think in terms of a hopefully good residential placement center, a goal that would seem more logical and effective.

January, 1973. After 4½ years at Linwood, Garth was transferred to a residential treatment center in November, 1968. He now lives at home and attends a special public school class for slow learners. There is more clinical evidence, though still inconclusive, that this a brain-damaged youngster.

Disorders With Evidence of Psychogenicity

Case 29

September, 1966. Dorothy is at 4 years of age a physically well developed, well organized, and rather agile child, who at the present time seems to feel reasonably comfortable with other people. This was apparent, at least so during the procedures of this afternoon when, in addition to Miss Simons, there were four other people around. It took the girl only a very short while to warm up to the situation; she responded to and sometimes invited playfulness. Dorothy took to the toys and handled them on the whole adroitly. Definitely right-handed, she scribbled, imitated a vertical line, was not quite able to reproduce a cross or a circle, and held the pencil somewhat awkwardly. Her pinprick reaction was decidedly not of the autistic variety. The girl reacted to the person who pricked at her rather than exclusively to the pin or hand. Eye contact was satisfactory and she enjoyed physical contact. At first, when I asked Dorothy to give me one of the toys, there was no response. But shortly thereafter she offered a toy and it was even possible to initiate a sort of give-and-take game, although this was not too consistent. The girl responded with a physionomic sign of pleasure when she was praised for putting two educational toys together. I understand that she swims beautifully.

There was some echolalia in her speech, but there were also spontaneous phrases, such as "Oh, boy," and "Look at." On one occasion she used the word "no" with emphasis but not inappropriately. After leaving, Miss Simons heard her say, "Room fun."

It seems to me that Dorothy must have been a very frightened, panicked child at the time when she came to Linwood. Most certainly, the story of the mother's horror when she found herself lying near the child and having her hands around Dorothy's throat, would lend substance to a great deal of anxiety in the relationship between mother and child, mostly emanating from the former. It is not evident from the history when the mother had her period of psychiatric hospitalization. Was this before or after the birth of the twins? If after, who took care of the twins while the mother was away? What was the major psychiatric problem that brought the mother to the hospital? The answers to these questions may throw quite a bit of light on the nature of the child's early emotional problems. Dorothy's mother has sought psychiatric help continued reluctantly because of fear of disclosing her therapeutic sessions to her husband. She seems to be crying out for help, and I feel that this cry should be heeded.

I should feel very uncomfortable if I were pushed into the corner and asked to make a specific diagnostic pronouncement. I can say that Dorothy is *not*, under any circumstances, a typical or even atypical autistic child. She does *not* impress me as schizophrenic. Even though she did not—at the last examination—test at a level higher than 2½ years, I am *not* convinced that the girl is seriously retarded. All I can say is that this is a child with major emotional difficulties during the first 3½ years of life, who has come closer to people and gained confidence and even pleasure in dealing with people during her stay at Linwood. A more telling history of interaction in her family may give more definite meaning to some of the things which now can only be surmised. At any rate, I feel that prognostically this child presents a better outlook than she did several months ago. I also feel that the mother should, and could be helped to verbalize her anxieties, which I am sure she has in relation not only to her daughter but also husband and one of her sons, presently on juvenile court probation.

April, 1968. Dorothy is now approximately 5½ years old. When I first saw her in September, 1966, I felt that this was not a markedly retarded child. She fulfills, I am sure, the requirements of a 4-year old child and a little better. Her speech has improved considerably, even though an appreciable amount of echolalia is still present. On one or two occasions, Dorothy gave evidence of echolalia with pronominal reversals. Today, she came without difficulty to the examining room, shook hands when requested to do so, and was amenable to physical contact which she occasionally seemed to enjoy, not shrinking from it at any time. There is not much physiognomics to evidence her feelings; she only smiled once or twice when I put my arm around her. This child, a member of a very disturbed family, has made considerable progress at Linwood. Because she does go home for three days during the weekend, it must be very difficult for her to be in two so discrepant environments. I am convinced that the girl would have made much more progress and come much closer to people if it were not for the need to divide her time between Linwood and home. Due to her mother's intermittent psychotic and always disturbed condition, it would be difficult, I am afraid, to change the arrangement. At any rate, I feel that this child should continue at Linwood for quite some time. She has made more and more friends, asking for them, in her echolalic fashion which she was able to substitute for proper requests with appropriate pronouns when prompted to do so. I do not believe that Dorothy's problem is innate. There is ample cause for the assumption that much of it is coming from a very disturbed and distressing home situation. The girl is certainly not as panicky as she was when first admitted to Linwood. She accepts people and their efforts on her behalf much better than in the past. If it were possible to make arrangements for a more consistent life involving one situation, namely Linwood, I would feel much more optimistic than under the present circumstances.

January, 1973. Dorothy left Linwood in early 1969 following the death of her father. During her 3-year residence, she became a reasonably happy though still hyperactive child. Echolalia was no longer present in her speech and sphincter control was fully established. Also, self-destructive behavior involving severe hitting of her head was no longer in evidence. The mother's inability to manage without her husband appears to have been chiefly responsible for the girl's placement in an institution.

Case 30

October, 1966. Ellen is a physically healthy, well-nourished, at least normally intelligent girl who, when she first came to Linwood, was self-destructive, and a manipulative, extremely negativistic girl. Lacking the experience of being accepted (and because of her reactions that made acceptance by parents difficult), she transferred her lack of self-regulation to a persistent effort to regulate the environment. As I saw Ellen today, she still showed signs of negativism and a more or less playful attempt to dominate the situation. However, the girl was able to yield to counter-manipulation which made use of her resistive tendencies. In this way, it was possible to deflect her from some of the shenanigans when they no longer seemed to serve a purpose.

In the examining room, Ellen had her hands before her eyes on arrival. She did not say anything in response to a greeting, but very soon, when challenged about her ability to do certain things, could not resist the temptation to prove that she was capable of performing. Thus, Ellen vacillated between resistance and compliance. This, I understand, represents one of her gains during the course of stay at Linwood. I certainly would not presently regard this girl as psychotic or even near-psychotic. If pushed into a corner in order to make a diagnostic statement, I would say that Ellen, who needed her remonstrations in order to maintain some strength, is learning slowly but noticeably that no one is threatened or angered by her resistance, which therefore does not serve the purpose needed by her in the home situation. I would say then that this is a 5½-year-old child who has not quite emerged from a protracted reliance on the oppositional syndrome, but with a gradual reduction of its virulence.

She is becoming more and more accessible to the kind of gentle firmness which, without making her feel guilty, can deflect intentions to more constructive and more comfortable activities. As the best next step, I foresee continuation at Linwood as a resident, as long as this can be maintained, with the hope that next year, when she is of school age, Ellen can be tried, and if necessary retried, in the nearby public school while she is still residing at Linwood.

April, 1968. Ellen who is now almost 7 years old has made remarkable progress since she came to Linwood. There is hardly any of the negativism observed when I first saw her in October, 1966. She is cooperative, highly intelligent, and easily handles the few sample test questions, performing at the 7-year level. She has been attending a public school kindergarten in Ellicott City and made a reasonably good adjustment in that setting. I think this is one of the Exhibit A's of the Linwood Children's Center. I should also say that this child offers an excellent prognosis, especially if allowed to remain in the Linwood situation for quite some time. It is remarkable that this child who has a very difficult family background has been able to function at the level which she has now managed to reach. A friendly girl, she even invited me on one occasion to come back and see her on a day which turned out to be her birthday. The best sign of Ellen's present condition is Dr. Hyatt's concurring statement to the effect that if he had not known of her background, he would have wondered why this child has to be at the Linwood Children's Center.

January, 1973. When admitted to Linwood in July, 1965, Ellen was not only self-destructive but also severely withdrawn. Scratching her face, tearing her clothes to shreds and lashing out at any adult who attempted to approach her, she used to spend hours in a catatonic-like state "rolled up like an embryo." Her behavior at that time was manifestly psychotic, except for visible signs of keen awareness of people and also of various objects which she could quickly seize and destroy. Now in the 5th grade of public school, Ellen functions normally, without any sign of deviant behavior that might have been anticipated on the basis of her clinical profile in the not so distant past.

Case 31

November, 1966. This is a boy, 7 years and 2 months of age, who originally was admitted to the Linwood Children's Center in June, 1964, withdrawn after about 4 or 5 months, and returned to Linwood less than a year and half ago. Ed and his younger brother, now 6 years of age, were abandoned by their mother when both were below the age of 2 years. The mother, herself the offspring of an alcoholic father and promiscuous mother with personality difficulties, has had no contact with the children since then. Though we have no specific details available, it is to be assumed with good reason that this child had little if any maternal affection, especially since his birth was followed in less than one year by that of another child. We thus know very little about the early development, even though the father assured us that early developmental functions progressed adequately. Suffice it to say that, when examined at the Children's Division of the Catholic University, Ed's speech was minimal and the general development estimated at about the level of a 2½-year-old child. Re-examination by Mrs. Nash in June, 1966, showed about the same results, indicating that hardly anything had been added during the intervening 2 to 2½ years.

When the child was seen here today, brought in with some initial resistance by Miss Simons, he was able to sit at the table opposite me. Ed did get up occasionally without any noticeable purpose but could be returned to the chair. He emitted noises which seemed to express discomfort but it was not the usual crying of a small child. Surprisingly, the boy showed good space orientation with the cylinder blocks and simple jigsaw puzzles or formboards. He exhibited definite right-hand preference and only on rare occasions used the left hand when the objects were within easy reach from the left. When two sets of cylinder blocks were mixed up, Ed showed good discrimination, guided by a very small difference in color. Given a somewhat more difficult jigsaw puzzle, usually workable at the 4-year level, he persisted with some help from Miss Simons until the whole thing was accomplished, not seeming frustrated with some of the difficulties which have presented themselves during the course.

At times Ed was able to smile, rather a bit mischievously, and evidence good eye contact. He reacted to the pinprick by connecting the source with a person rather than with a depersonalized hand.

Speech is still very limited. However, on one occasion when Ed wanted to leave, he uttered the word "door." I am told that he could be induced to form an occasional sentence, which he does with a somewhat peculiar intonation. On the whole, it is difficult to see any area in which the boy transcends a developmental level of 2½ or, at best, 3 years. Ed accepts fondling by Miss Simons but there is no sign of reciprocity or cuddling. He initiated some infantile games with her, at which time she had to soothe him. The child seemed to respond to her continued reminder to be gentle. She told us, however, that last week he broke her glasses.

It is amazing that it was possible here to teach him to identify the letters of the alphabet and to match identical letters. The most reasonable thing that we can say diagnostically is that Ed is a severely retarded child with an IQ that is below 35 at the present time. He has never had a thorough, or even cursory, physical examination. For the sake of completeness and with a possible idea of finding some organic diagnostic clue, I should recommend strongly a neurological work-up and, if possible, a determination of metabolic functioning.

Regardless of the findings, we cannot prognostically anticipate social participation in a non-residential setting. In view of the limited choices available, I think that plans might be made for admission to the Rosewood State Hospital. It would be kinder to this child to allow him to settle down in such a facility than to continue working for fractional attainments. Whether or not there are any organic causes, we do know that this is a child who has been psychologically deprived from the beginning, that he was abandoned by his mother at an early age, that there was a succession of housekeepers, and that he has had no opportunity to relate himself to any accepting adult until he came to Linwood. Such background made it difficult for him to benefit from the attention or advance beyond few fragmentary attainments.

April, 1967. At the age of 7 years and 7 months, Ed left Linwood for Rosewood State Hospital to remain there for an indefinite period.

Case 32

December, 1966. This 11-year-old boy, adopted by a high-ranking military officer and his wife, was taken out of a large German orphanage at the age of 10 months. The father is described as a person who seems to be incapable of forming warm relationships; the mother is said to be a tense woman. In his early days the child was reportedly intolerant of changes in his environment and had "strange fears." When Billy started in school, he did not associate with the other children. Little is known of the whereabouts and other vital details prior to his coming to Linwood at the age of 7 years. At one time, he was to have been given a Rorschach that supposedly characterized him as a psychotic child.

When seen today, Billy wanted to know where he was going to sit as soon as he came in. He sat down in the assigned chair, told me that he had inquired of another boy what was going to be said here and was told that he would be asked to state his age. When he noticed the number 11 behind his name on my sheet, he wondered why age was a matter of special interest.

While Billy answered every question, he was extremely guarded, avoiding specific answers with remarks such as, "various things" or "I'm not sure." He considered himself to be "fairly healthy," reminding that he had asthma due to being "allergic to my own sinuses." The boy was not sure whether he was bright, having mentioned something about problems with reading and writing. He said that he had friends but could not name even one friend, let alone a best friend. Not fully satisfied with either his father or mother, Billy would not go beyond this general statement. Sometimes he got mad at his mother and used his fists. He was not sure what he wished to do when he grew up, and after some urging decided that he wanted to be a scientist to explore things.

When asked to come up with three wishes, he had only one, namely when things were too hard he wanted them to be easier. Again this was as far as he would go. There is a statement in the anamnesis that his mother felt that Billy was clinging to her and that for some time, probably while abroad, he was sleeping with his parents; it is pretty hard to tell who suggested this.

The chief impression is that of a child who is utterly not sure of himself. He has asked questions about his origin, pointing out to me that he sought such information from his mother. However, neither she nor he remembered the names of his biological parents. Billy asked me once why I was writing down things and on the surface seemed satisfied when I told him that I did so in order to remember.

All the way through, you could not obtain a positive answer one way or the other about his feelings. He seemed guarded and a bit suspicious. One wonders about his earliest experience in the orphange. His relationship to people is reminiscent of the *hospitalism* cases described by Goldfarb (1943), Spitz (1945), Bowlby (1951), and other investigators. I do not think that this child is capable of forming real, genuine attachments. About himself, he is neither positive nor negative in any particular direction. I did not detect any tics or compulsiveness during the interview. Diagnostially, I see his general personality as related more to the hospitalism syndrome than to any other category.

April, 1968. Billy has in many ways made progress of which the Linwood Children's Center as well as the public school, which he attends since September, can be really proud. During his interview today, he exhibited very good formal behavior, talked about things almost philosophically and carried on a sustained continuous conversation without any sign of ideational scattering. I saw his school report card which details good progress in all subjects. This means so much more when we realize that this is the boy's first formal school experience. The report says that Billy gets along well with the other school children. I do not believe that he has close contact with any of them, but the boy has formed tenuous relationships with two children at Linwood. He has become philosophically tolerant of people and the world at large, and was able to say that he did not know of any one who was perfect. When I suggested the diety, he wondered whether even the diety is perfect because there is so much poverty, misery, and illness in the world. Billy will remain at Linwood for at least another year and I do not think that anything better could have happened to this child than being here for a few years. During the course of our conversation, he was rather tense; this came out in the form of labial and generally oral tics as well as facial tics which, I am told, occur from time to time. Of course, to this curious child, the interview was a very special occurrence. I learned from him that he remembered quite a few special items pertaining to our meeting about a year and a half ago, and that he reported some to his mother. It is thus possible that the tics were a little more than usually exaggerated because of the serious nature of this special occasion to the boy.

January, 1973. At 17½ years of age, Billy is attending high school, which he entered in 1969. At this time, plans are being formulated for continued education. The boy is reasonably well adjusted socially and has friends of his own age. He formed many relationships and has a variety of interests that are primarily scientifically oriented.

DEMENTIA INFANTILIS

Case 33

October, 1966. At approximately 10½ years of age, this physically small and immature boy does not transcend socially, communicatively, or in play and handling of objects, a level below that of a 3-year-old child. If the history given by the family is correct, Hal got along well until the age of about 19 months. He developed speech at about one year of age and was toilet trained at an early time. Then there was said to have been a regression and a "reversion" to simpler language. At 18 to 19 months of age, the boy was said to have had a low grade infection, after which there was a global deterioration except for sphincter control that has remained intact. At the present time, he has no intelligible speech save for a few words having to do with the naming of a limited number of objects. Hal seems to be generally at peace with the world, laughs heartily at times with little noticeable reason other than a general feeling of satisfaction. There are occasional noises, all associated with pleasure rather than anxiety or any kind of distress. He is by no means autistically withdrawn or resistive and does not seem to be threatened by requests or demands. At least in the interview situation, Hal generally tends to resemble the disposition of Elsie (Borden's Contented Cow) rather than that of a child in dread, anger, or pleasure derived from being with people. In the 10½ years of his life, he has learned to handle simple (very simple) formboards to replace the cylinder blocks in their proper holes without trial and error. Hal is able, with some prompting, to dress and undress himself, and also feed himself properly. When in the mood, he is capable of some degree of automatic obedience.

If one assumes that the early history, as given by the family, can be relied upon, one cannot help but think in terms of something akin to Heller's Disease, where a smooth development during the first 1½ to 2½ years of life is followed by complete regression, which may reach to a low plateau—so low that there is little prospect of trainability for social functioning. A brain biopsy has shown in many instances a ganglion cell dilapidation in the lower strata of the cortex. Whether or not this would be found in this case, we cannot get away from the fact that this child is now markedly defective in overall development. I have not even been able to elicit any of the usual play responses of an average 2 to 3-year-old child, such as "Peek-a-boo." Hal can come to fetch a piece of candy but, it seemed to me, only if he can see the candy itself. He also can explore pocketbooks when he knows that there is some candy in them. On one occasion, the child managed to utter the word "pocketbook."

None of this adds up to any justification for thinking in terms of psychotic development. This is basically a very severely retarded child. If one were to come up with an IQ figure it would be certainly below 35. Unless miracles happen, this child will need life-long care and supervision. A period of residence at the Linwood Children's Center may help the parents to prepare themselves for permanent residential placement of this child.

April, 1968. Hal will be 12 years old within about one month. His performance remains at a level that is certainly not above 2 to 2½ years of age. Since I saw him about a year and a half ago, he is the same happy, contented child with neither anger nor resentment towards anybody or anything. There is now even less of a question than initially that we are confronted with a problem along the lines of Heller's Disease or *dementia infantilis* (Heller, 1930). I think though that his residence at Linwood was beneficial for a child with so many difficulties was in a situation where he could feel comfortable. Also, his parents had had an opportunity to adjust themselves and accept the fact that Hal is a markedly defective child in all areas.

January, 1973. Discharged in August, 1968, Hal went to a day-care center for retarded children. Roughly 5 years of residence at Linwood did not result in major gains, except for some success in such areas as relatedness, sphincter control, and self-care. Occasional whispering did not develop into communicative speech, which might have been at best one of those miracles that wishful thinking had prompted some of us to hope for.

Case 34

December, 1966. Carl, a 12½-year-old physically well built boy with a handsome physiognomy, has been at Linwood Children's Center for approximately 3 years. His anamnesis, as documented by a pediatrician, tells us that he sat up at 7 months, walked at 11, and according to the parents said his first few words at about 10 months of age. There is a mention of premature rupture of the membrane, of severe colics after birth and of a convulsion, presumably febrile, at 10 months. The history of early toilet-training is not ascertainable. When Carl was 4 years of age, he witnessed a horrifying scene in which the father pushed the mother into the bathtub where she sustained multiple fractures that made it necessary for her to be immobilized in a cast.

As seen today, Carl does not exceed the 2-year level of development in any sphere of living. The best he could do was to copy a straight line with some help, to shake hands at request, to replace the cylinder blocks and, again with considerable help, to do simple jigsaw puzzles. At the same time, looking generally pleased and accepting caressing motions he babbled on, repeating syllables many times and jabbering away in a manner which impressed the parents as "Spanish baby-talk." There is the same type of behavior in his motor performances, accompanied by repetitious movements of hands.

It is true that the deterioration set in chronologically at about the same time when he witnessed the father's assault on his mother. However, we cannot get away from the fact that this happened to a 4-year-old child whose development was stopped and regressed along the lines of what is observed in Heller's Disease. Clinically, this child's behavior is an almost photographic replica of what I have seen in other children with this condition. Only recently has he reduced the frequency of encopresis.

I see no reason for retaining this child at Linwood. Placement at Rosewood State Hospital would be the logical arrangement. In view of the paranoid attitude, I shall refrain from a brain biopsy which, in the instances seen by me and by others, shows a ganglion cell dilapidation and shrinkage of the dendrites in the lower layers of the cortex. Also in view of the father's belligerence, one might present to him the alternatives of Rosewood or keeping the child at home, at least until such a time when the parents will be unable to cope with the situation. Even with the rosiest optimism, I cannot foresee anything but complete social dependence. For all practical purposes, this child functions in the range of idiocy.

February, 1967. Discharged on recommendations to commence residential care, after 3½ years of treatment at Linwood, Carl was still at home when last heard of in 1967.

CONCLUDING NOTE

The evaluations of 28 boys and 6 girls grouped into five nosological categories, all with histories of psychotic manifestations in childhood, have been greatly enhanced by the recent follow-up notes prepared by Miss Simons. In the first group of 13 autistic boys and 2 girls, whose age at follow-up ranged from 6 years and 2 months to 23 years (and treatment at Linwood, from 2 years and 4 months to 10 years and 5 months), at least six can be said to have attained a state of near-full or full recovery. This includes one boy who, while still at Linwood, is making encouraging progress in a public school where he successfully keeps up with normal peers. The outcome for all but one of the other autistic children was sufficiently satisfactory to permit them to go on to special day-care centers.

Among the 7 schizophrenic children, whose treatment at Linwood ranged from 1 year and 10 months to 12 years and 9 months, one managed to adjust to a normal school curriculum, and one, still at Linwood, is doing equally well. The remaining five in this group, however, proceeded from Linwood to a variety of sheltered environments.

The third group of six children whose behavioral manifestations could be more or less destinctly traced to organicity, appears to have moved in the same direction as the second. After a stay at Linwood that ranged from 2 years and 4 months to 8 years, four went to day-care centers for the mentally retarded, one child to a residential center, while one still remains at Linwood.

The four children whose psychotic behavior in childhood was more easily traced to psychogenicity than to organic causes, have gone on from Linwood (after a stay ranging from 2 years and 10 months to 6 years and 8 months) into two different worlds. Two children have been institutionalized, quite probably for the remainder of their lives, while two have adjusted themselves to normal lives in the community, attending school and functioning quite satisfactorily.

The two children with Heller's Disease went on, as might have been expected, to day-care centers for the retarded.

It would seem that the present state of the art does not allow us to meaningfully relate the outcome of any case to either the diagnosis or to duration of treatment at Linwood. Suffice it to say that of the 34 children whose stay at Linwood ranged from 1 year and 10 months to 12 years and 9 months, only a few have failed to demonstrate visible progress. If one were to attempt to think of the reasons why 9 youngsters have managed to emerge from their psychotic state in childhood and come up to levels which permitted them to function at home and attend schools for normal children, the *degree of severity* of their affliction comes to mind. With this as a point of departure, it is not unreasonable to think of the inner resources of each child, and to believe that the attention and care at Linwood Children's Center may have mobilized such resources to facilitate development and growth.

REFERENCES

Bowlby, J. *Maternal care and mental health.* Geneva: World Health Organization, 1951.

Despert, J. L. *Schizophrenia in children.* New York: Brunner/Mazel, 1968.

Goldfarb, H. The effects of early institutional care on adolescent personality. *Child Development,* 1943, **14**, 213–223.

Heller, T. Über dementia infantilis. *Zeitschrift fur Kinderforshung,* 1930, **37**, 661–667.

Kanner, L. Autistic disturbances of affective contact. *Nervous Child,* 1943, **2**, 217–250.

Rutter, M. Childhood schizophrenia reconsidered. *Journal of Autism and Childhood Schizophrenia,* 1972, **2**, 315–337.

Spitz, R. A. Hospitalism. In O. Fenichel (Ed.), *The psychoanalytic study of the child.* New York: International Universities Press, 1945.